MAGNETIC RESONANCE IMAGING

PHYSICAL AND BIOLOGICAL PRINCIPLES

Third Edition

MAGNETIC
RESONANCE
IMAGING

PHYSICAL AND BIOLOGICAL PRINCIPLES

Stewart C. Bushong, ScD

Professor, Department of Radiology
Baylor College of Medicine
Houston, Texas

with 475 illustrations

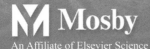
Mosby

An Affiliate of Elsevier Science

An Affiliate of Elsevier Science

11830 Westline Industrial Drive
St. Louis, Missouri 63146

NOTICE

Medical imaging is an ever-changing field. Standard safety precautions must be followed, but as new research and clinical experience broaden our knowledge, changes in treatment and drug therapy may become necessary or appropriate. Readers are advised to check the most current product information provided by the manufacturer of each drug to be administered to verify the recommended dose, the method and duration of administration, and contraindications. It is the responsibility of the licensed prescriber, relying on experience and knowledge of the patient, to determine dosages and the best treatment for each individual patient. Neither the publisher nor the author assumes any liability for any injury and/or damage to persons or property arising from this publication.

Previous editions copyrighted 1996, 1998

Library of Congress Cataloging-in-Publication Data

Bushong, Stewart C.
 Magnetic resonance imaging: physical and biological principles/Stewart C. Bushong—3rd ed.
  p. cm.
 Includes bibliographical references and index.
 ISBN 0-323-01485-2
 1. Magnetic resonance imaging, 2. Nuclear magnetic resonance, I. Title.

 RC78.7.N83B87 2003
 616.07'548—dc21

               2002045459

Acquisitions Editor: Jeanne Wilke
Developmental Editor: Jennifer Moorhead
Publishing Services Manager: Deborah L. Vogel
Project Manager: Claire Kramer
Design Manager: Bill Drone

Printed in the United States of America

Last digit is the print number: 9   8   7   6   5   4   3   2   1

This book is dedicated to the 309 Baylor College of Medicine radiology resident TOOLS who endured my medical physics classes, my easy exams, and my lousy jokes since I began doing this in 1967. They gave me much grief but much more pleasure, and most have become lasting close friends.

Achal Sarna **(MP)** '04 - Achilles Chatziioannou '96 - Akom Vutpakdi '71 - Angel Gunn '05 - Anjali Agrawal **(MP)** '02 - Anuja Jhingran^ '93 - Arnold Nitishian• '74 - Artie Schwartz '95 - Arturo Castro^ '82 - Augusto Merello• '82, '85 - B. Michael Driver^ '85 - B.A. King '72 - Barry M. Uhl^ '00 - Beatriz Lopez-Miranda '99 - Benjamin Wendel '80 - Berta Kvamme '94 - Bill Ketcham '02 - Bill Prominski '87 - Bill Reid '88 - Bin S. Teh^ **(NP)** '98 - Blake Hocott **(MP)** '91 - Bob Francis '84 - Bob Osborne '85 - Bob Stallworth '92 - Brandon Stroh '05 - Bruce Cheatham '79 - Bruce Morris '97 - Burton Spangler '71 - C.T. Morris, Jr. '80 - Candy Roberts '88 - Carl E. Nuesch^ '89 - Carl Harrell '81 - Carol Simmons '68 - Chad J. Goodman **(NP)** '99 - Chad M. Amosson^ '01 - Chad Mills '02 - Charles C. Trinh **(MP)** '99 - Charles L. Moffet^ '80 - Charlie Williams '73 - Charlotte Hayes '93 - Chitra Viswanathan '05 - Chris Canitz '97 - Chris Govea '04 - Cindy Woo '93 - Colin Bray '05 - Colin Dodds **(MP)** '03 - Craig Polson '89 - Craig Thiessen '89 - Daniel Miller '81 - Daniel Reimer '78 - Daniel W. Fang **(MP)** '01 - David A. Hughes• '76 - David Boals† '69 - David Diment '89 - David E. Goller '98 - David Feldman '93 - David King '87 - David L. Janssen^ '86 - David Walker^ '72 - Derek Bergeson Douglas Woo '77 - Doyle DePucy• '77 - Ebrahim S. Martinez '80 - Edward Knudson '74 - Elan Omessi '94 - Rhea '76 - Ellis Deville^ '77 - Candy '89 - Eugene Brown '88 - Arraiza '02 - Frank Hadlock '75 - '72 - Fred Johnson '77 - Fred Bourque '68 - Garrett Anderson '73 - Gene Smigocki '87 -

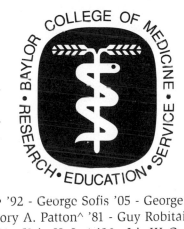

S. Conrow **(MP)** '00 - David '06 - Donald Holmquest• '74 - Simmons '68 - E. Gordon Delpassand• '90 - Eduardo Callaway '91 - Edward Elizabeth Koch '85 - Elizabeth Errol Anderson '85 - Errol Ezequiel Silva '01 - Francisco Frank Scalfano '89 - Fred Dean Quenzer '72 - Gardiner **(MP)** '02 - Gene Cunningham GeorgeBoutros '74 - George

Campbell† '72 - George Chacko• '92 - George Sofis '05 - George Soltes **(MP)** '94 - George Yama '71 - Greg Boys **(MP)** '04 - Gregory A. Patton^ '81 - Guy Robitaille '70 - Hal Jayson '83 - Harry Butters '78 - Hollis Halford III '81 - Hsin H. Lu^ '86 - Iris W. Gayed• '97 - Isabel Menendez '85 - J.P. Badami II '83 - J.P. Harris '03 - James Courtney **(MP)** '98 - James D. Green '70 - James E. Lefler '98 - James Fuchs '80 - James Lloyd '83 - James P. Caplan• '81 - James P. Willis '98 - James Teague† '78 - James Van Dolah '76 - James W. Cole '95 - James Wolf '91 - Jandra Kalus '73 - Janine Mele '03 - Jason Salber **(MP)** '02 - Jeff Sheneman '06 - Jeff Smith '91 - Jeffery Kass '75 - Jennifer R. Cranny '01 - Jesus Castro-Sandoval^ '83 - Jett Brady '97 - Jimmy Hammond '05 - Joel Dunlap '92 - John Barkley '04 - John Baxt '74 - John Brooks '69 - John Clement **(MP)** '04 - John Gundzik '91 - John H. Liem^ '77 - John J. Nisbet **(MP)** '00 - John K. Miller '95 - John L. Howard '90 - John Labis '03 - John Melvin '83 - John R. Bodenhamer '96 - John Romero '76 - John Thomas '93 - John W. Wright '90 - John Wilbanks^ '77 - Jon Edwards '78 - Jorges Gonzales '74 - Jose Guerra-Paz '77 - Jose V. Watson **(MP)** '01 - Joseph Chan '99 - Juliet Wendt• '92 - Karen Simmons '88 - Karl Chiang '91 - Kathryn M. Lewis^ '89 - Keith Light• '02 - Kirsten Warhoe^ '94 - Kuri Farid '78 - Larry Gaines^ '72 - Larry S. Carpenter^ '88 - Larry Yeager '79 - Lawrence D. Hochman^ '96 - Lawrence J. Scharf^ '88 - Lee Shukla '87 - Leroy Halouska '75 - Lillian Orson '89 - Linda Ann Hayman '76 - Lori Young '70 - M. Amir Ibrahim• '97 -

Marc Siegel '88 - Marcus Calderon• '73 - Maria Patino '05 - Marianne Greenbaum '99 - Mariano Nasser '76 - Marina Soosaipillai '80 - Mark E. Augspurger^ '00 - Mark Matthews '92 - Mark Miller '77 - Mark Pfleger (MP) '91 - Mark Sokolay '75 - Mark Stallworth '93 - Martin Cain '89 - Mary Round '92 - Mehmet Gurgun (MP) '93 - Mel Thompson '96 - Mian A. Ibrahim '97 - Michael A. Marks (MP) '90 - Michael Cagan '74 - Michael D. Bastasch^ '03 - Michael Driver^ '82 - Michael G. Gunlock '99 - Michael H. Hayman^ '77 - Michael Kerley^ '92 - Michael T. Sinopoli^ '03 - Mike Silberman '91 - Mike Sloan (MP) '91 - Mike Smith '91 - Milton Gray '69 - Modesto Sanchez-Torres (NP) '97 - Monica L. Huang '99 - Monte F. Zarlingo (MP) '00 - Munish Chawla '97 - Nan Garrett '03 - Nancy Anderson '84 - Nathan S. Floyd^ '02 - Nathan W. Uy^ '01 - Naveen Bikkasani '03 - Neil Cooper '86 - Nicholas Kutka• '71 - Nora A. Janjan^ '84 - Norman Harris '74 - Paul B. Horwitz (MP) '01 - Paul Weatherall '87 - Pedro Diaz '06 - Pekka Ahoniemi '73 - Peter Feola '95 - Peter Kvamme• '95 - Phil Mihm (MP) '97 - Philip Trover '77 - Philip Weaver '74 - Pieretta Ferro '71 - Rafael Aponte '88 - Raj Cheruvu '00 - Ralph Norton '75 - Ralph Sharman '74 - Ramesh Dhekne• '75 - Raphiel Benjamin '69 - Raul Meoz^ '76 - Ravi J. Amin (NP) '00 - Ray Ziegler '69 - Reed A.

'81 - Richard A. McGahan^ '90 - H. Oria '90 - Richard Parvey '80 - Robert A. Gilbert^ '94 - Robert Davidson• '91 - Robert Denman J. Feiwell (MP) '95 - Robert Jr.^ '84 - Robert Sims '85 - Robert Tien '88 - Rogue Ron Dillee '73 - Ronald Roy Longuet '79 - Russell D. Salmann Ahmed '06 - Sami Hatch^ '91 - Sanjiv Gala '06 -

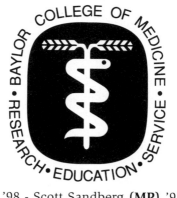

Shankwiler '90 - Reese James Richard Fremaux '81 - Richard Richard Wilson (MP) '94 - B. Poliner '90 - Robert '79 - Robert Francis '82 - Robert Malone '88 - Robert McLaurin, Robert Sonnemaker• '76 - Ferreyro '78 - Ron Brociner '85 - Eikenhorst '79 - Ross Zeanah '85 - Putnam '00 - Sager Naik '04 - Juma '84 - Sandra Sarina W. Fordice '98 - Scott

Dorfman '93 - Scott Meshberger '98 - Scott Sandberg (MP) '92 - Sidney Roberts^ '91 - Sima C. Artinian '98 - Simon Trubek '05 - Sophia Chatziioannou• '96 - Srini Malini '77 - Stanley D. Clarke^ '91 - Stanley Lim '04 - Stephen C. Greco^ '97 - Stephen Long• '81 - Stephen Parven '86 - Steve Hong (MP) '02 - Steve Sax '86 - Steven J. DiLeo '98 - Steven R. Rinehouse '95 - Susan Fan '89 - Susan Pinero '85 - Susan Weathers '81 - Tara Sagebiel '06 - Terry O'Connor '96 - Terry Reed '72 - Tex Clifford† '68 - Thanh John Van^ '02 - Thomas Dumler '79 - Thomas Hedrick '75 - Thomas L. Atlas (MP) '96 - Tim Dziuk^ '94 - Tim Tsai (NP) '96 - Todd Lanier '92 - Todd Minken '94 - Todd Samuels '79 - Todd Tibbetts '06 - Tom Kaminski '87 - Tom Lepsch '87 - Vasu Rao '94 - Vera Selinko '85 - Vivek C. Yagnik (MP) '01 - W. Sam Dennis^ '80 - Warren H. Moore• '82 - Wassel H. Beal• '74 - Wendy S. Carpenter (MP) '99 - William Cunningham '83 - William D. Permenter, Jr.^ '89 - William Jordan '70 - William Kent '80 - William Rogers '74 - Wilmer Moran '78 - Zachary Martin '86 - Zeke Silva (NP) '01

(MP) Highest Honors in Medical Physics
(NP) Naresh Prasad Scholar
• Nuclear Medicine
^ Radiotherapy
† R.I.P.

Preface

When I began teaching/research at Baylor College of Medicine (BCM) in 1967 and a few years later when the Houston Community College (HCC) was established, the subject matter *medical physics* was a piece of cake. All I had to teach were radiography and fluoroscopy. Today, all such students must know everything known in 1967 plus everything since . . . in the same length of time! Now, the required fund of knowledge is ENORMOUS, and the demands on students are exceptional.

In the early 1980s, magnetic resonance imaging (MRI) burst onto the scene as a diagnostic imaging tool with even more intensity than computed tomography (CT) had in the 1970s. Its similarities to CT are somewhat obvious, but the underlying physical principles are new and challenging to imaging physicians and technologists. Whereas CT is an extension of x-ray imaging and the basic physics has been well integrated into radiology training programs, the physical basis for MRI has not been well integrated because it is different. Formal courses are only now being developed. The person using an MRI system or interpreting the end result must fully understand the basic principles of how this modality works to obtain the highest quality image possible.

This third edition presents the fundamentals of conventional MRI and of the fast imaging techniques currently available. As in the first two editions, concepts continue to be presented in a way that is easily understood by students, technologists, and physicians who have little or no background in mathematics and physics. Interested readers will find a more complex mathematical development in Appendix A: "The Bloch Equations."

Since the first edition of this book, published in 1988, a wealth of advancements and changes has occurred in this fast-moving field. This accounts for the extensive revision throughout the book, four new chapters, and hundreds of new illustrations.

The text begins with an overview and an introduction of the fundamentals of electricity and magnetism (Part I). This is followed by an in-depth explanation of how MRI works (Parts II and III). Parts IV and V of the text discuss the latest imaging methods. The final section covers personnel and patient safety and administration issues (Part VI).

The American Board of Radiology (ABR) is developing a certificate of Additional Qualifications in MRI. The American Registry of Radiologic Technologists (ARRT) currently offers an advanced exam to qualify technologists in MRI. Both organizations will find that this text presents all the essential information needed for those advanced programs.

In preparing the third edition, I have incorporated the ideas and suggestions of many users and educators who were kind enough to communicate with me directly. The following people were especially helpful: Errol Candy, Dallas, TX; Luann Culbreth, Dallas, TX; William Faulkner, Chattanooga, TN; Roger Freimarch, Eugene, OR; Ed Jackson, Houston, TX; Jon Nussbaum, Boston, MA; Helen Schumpert, New Orleans, LA; Euclid Scerain, Burnaby, British Columbia; Wlad Sobol, Birmingham, AL; and Rees Stuteville, Kalamth Falls, OR.

Several of my colleagues have been especially helpful with this third edition: Scott Flamm, Houston, TX; Geoffrey Clarke, San Antonio, TX; and Erroll Candy, Dallas, TX.

I am also deeply indebted to Yvonne Young for her patient help in the assembly and processing of this manuscript. Kraig Emmert created the illustrations for this edition. His talents and clever ideas added humor and sense where concepts were sometimes difficult to express.

To test your skills, I have hidden an "error" in this third edition. Find this error and report it to me, and you will be appropriately honored and memorialized.

This volume continues efforts to make medical imaging understandable and medical physics fun.

Stewart C. Bushong

Contents

Part I

Fundamentals, 1

Part V

Applications, 317

Part VI

Safety, 363

MAGNETIC RESONANCE IMAGING

PHYSICAL AND BIOLOGICAL PRINCIPLES

Part I

Fundamentals

Chapter 1

An Overview of Magnetic Resonance Imaging

OBJECTIVES

At the completion of this chapter, the student should be able to do the following:

1. Define nuclear magnetic resonance and magnetic resonance imaging.
2. Identify the three imaging windows of the electromagnetic spectrum.
3. Distinguish between spatial resolution and contrast resolution.
4. Discuss the symbols M, B_0, B_x, FID, and T.
5. State the Larmor equation and discuss its significance.

OUTLINE

HISTORICAL TRAIL

If someone wanted to make an image of a patient 150 years ago, what could have been done? Actually, not much. At that time, only photography or hand-drawn images were available. Both types of such images use the narrow band of the electromagnetic spectrum called the *visible light region* (Figure 1-1).

Electromagnetic radiation can be characterized by any one of three parameters: energy, frequency, and wavelength. Although the only electromagnetic radiation that we can sense directly is visible light, we know that the range of electromagnetic radiation extends over many orders of magnitude and different types of radiation.

How does photography work? Visible light reflects off an object, and the reflected light is detected by a medium that is sensitive to that kind of radiation—a photographic emulsion or the retina. Therefore a photograph is made

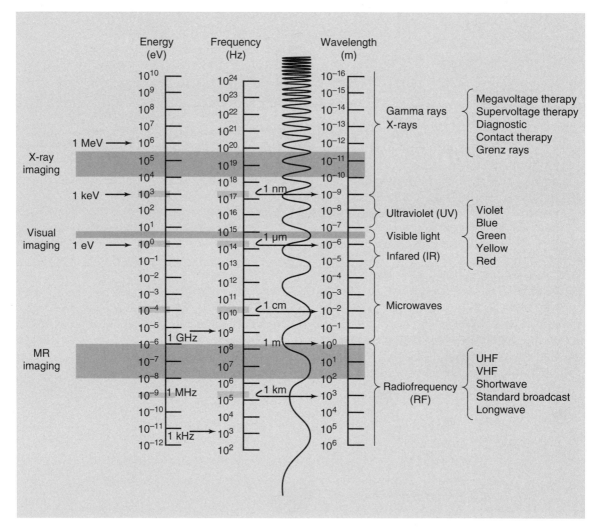

Figure 1-1   The electromagnetic spectrum showing values of energy, frequency, and wavelength for the imaging windows of visible light, x-rays, and radio waves.

with reflected electromagnetic radiation and a suitable receptor.

Nineteenth-century physicists studying visible light detailed its wavelike properties according to how it interacted with matter (i.e., reflection, diffraction, and refraction). Consequently, visible light has always been characterized by its **wavelength.**

 Visible light extends from approximately 400 nm (blue) to 700 nm (red).

When Wilhelm Conrad Roentgen discovered x-rays in 1895, there was suddenly another narrow region of the electromagnetic spectrum from which medical images could be made. In 1901 Roentgen received the first Nobel Prize in physics for his discovery. One reason Roentgen received this award was that within 6 months, he had conducted a number of cleverly designed experiments and described x-rays much as they are known today.

Some of his experiments indicated that this "x-light" interacted as a particle, not as a wave. As a result, x-ray emissions are identified according to their **energy.** Although we commonly refer to kilovolt peak (kVp), it is more accurate to use kiloelectron volt (keV) to identify x-radiation.

 Diagnostic x-rays range from approximately 20 keV to 150 keV.

How is an x-ray image made? Electromagnetic radiation (i.e., an x-ray beam) shines on a patient. Some of the radiation is absorbed; some of it is transmitted through the patient to an image receptor. This results in a shadowgram-like image from the transmission of electromagnetic radiation.

A Penguin Tale

By Benjamin Archer

In the vast and beautiful expanse of the Arctic region, there was once a great, isolated iceberg floating in the serene sea. Because of its location and accessibility, the great iceberg became a mecca for penguins from the entire area. As more and more penguins flocked to their new home and began to cover the slopes of the ice field, the iceberg began to sink deeper and deeper into the ocean. Penguins kept climbing on, forcing others that once were securely ensconced, off the island and back into the ocean. Soon the entire iceberg became submerged because of the sheer number of penguins that attempted to take up residence there.

Moral:

The PENGUIN represents an important fact or bit of information that we must learn to understand a subject. The brain, like the iceberg, can retain only so much information before it becomes overloaded. When this happens, concepts begin to become dislodged like penguins from the sinking iceberg. So, the key to learning is to reserve space for true "penguins" to fill the valuable and limited confines of our brains. Thus key points in this book are highlighted and referred to as "PENGUINS."

During the latter part of the nineteenth century, after Thomas Edison's early work, engineers and physicists worked to develop radio communications. Electrons need to oscillate in a conductor to create a radio emission. This requires the construction of an electronic circuit called an *oscillator*. The oscillator is the basis for radioelectronics.

The electromagnetic radiation produced by the oscillator is called a *radiofrequency* (RF) *emission*. Physicists identify this radiation according to the **frequency** of oscillation.

 RFs extend over a range from 3 kHz to 3 GHz.

Commercial broadcasts such as AM radio, FM radio, and television (TV) are similarly identified. The AM RF band ranges from 540 to 1640 kHz, and the FM RF band ranges from 88 to 108 MHz. TV broadcast ranges from 54 to 806 MHz, which includes both VHF and UHF.

 Magnetic resonance images are made with RF in the range from approximately 10 to 200 MHz.

Use of the RF region of the electromagnetic spectrum to produce an image is especially spectacular. It is based on an analytical procedure called *nuclear magnetic resonance* (NMR) and was first called *nuclear magnetic resonance imaging* (NMRI). Some of the leaders in radiology were concerned about using the word *nuclear* around patients. As a result, that word was dropped early in the development of this imaging process, and we are left with magnetic resonance imaging (MRI).

How is a magnetic resonance (MR) image made? For a visible image, radiation is reflected from the body. For an x-ray image, radiation is transmitted through the body. For an MR image, the patient is stimulated so that electromagnetic radiation is **emitted** from the body. Through the use of some clever methods, the emitted signal is then detected, interpreted, and used to produce an image (Figure 1-2).

Felix Bloch

Magnetic fields associated with atoms and nuclei were first described in the 1930s. Otto Stern and Isador Rabi each received a Nobel Prize in physics for their work on atomic and nuclear magnetism. Rabi coined the term **nuclear magnetic resonance.**

In 1946 Felix Bloch at Stanford and Edward Purcell at Harvard independently described NMR in a solid. They shared the 1952 Nobel Prize in physics for this work. Bloch continued

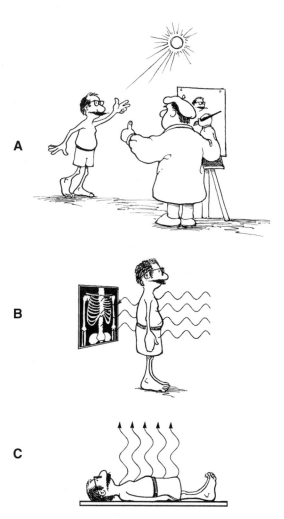

Figure 1-2 How images are made using the three regions of the electromagnetic spectrum. **A,** Reflected visible light. **B,** Transmitted x-rays. **C,** Emitted radiofrequency.

extensive studies with the NMR of water, thereby laying the groundwork for later developments that led to MRI.

Bloch is to MRI what Roentgen is to x-ray imaging, and Bloch is known as the father of MRI. As a theoretical physicist, Bloch proposed some novel properties for the atomic nucleus, including that the nucleus behaves like a small magnet. He described this nuclear magnetism by what are now called the *Bloch equations* (see Appendix A).

Bloch's equations explain that a nucleus, because it spins on an imaginary axis, has an associated magnetic field. This field is called a **magnetic moment.** Nucleons that have charge (e.g., protons) and that spin have even stronger magnetic fields.

Experimental verification for the Bloch equations did not come until the early 1950s. By 1960 several companies were producing analytical instruments called *NMR spectrometers.* During the 1960s and 1970s, NMR spectroscopy (see Chapter 9) became widely used in academic and industrial research. Such use of NMR enabled investigators to determine the molecular configuration of a material from the analysis of its NMR spectrum.

Damadian and Lauterbur

In the late 1960s engineer-physician Raymond Damadian, while working with NMR spectroscopy, showed that malignant tissue has a different NMR spectrum from normal tissue. Furthermore, he showed that the parameters associated with NMR (i.e., proton density, spin-lattice relaxation time, and spin-spin relaxation time) differ between normal and malignant tissue. Damadian produced a crude NMR image of a rat tumor in 1974 and the first body image in 1976. That image took almost 4 hours to produce.

At this same time Paul Lauterbur, an NMR chemist, was engaged in similar research. There is considerable discussion as to whether Damadian or Lauterbur should receive recognition, such as the Nobel Prize, for developing MRI. Both should probably share this recognition.

WHY MAGNETIC RESONANCE IMAGING?

When a plain radiograph of the abdomen is placed on a view box for interpretation, what can be seen? Not much. The image is gray and flat and shows little detail. A conventional tomogram or an angiogram may be done to improve image contrast.

Contrast Resolution

If such an image is unsatisfactory, what else can be done? A computed tomography (CT) image can be requested. The principal advantage of CT imaging over radiographic imaging is superior contrast resolution, the ability to image differences among low-contrast tissues. Contrast resolution allows visualization of soft tissue with similar characteristics, such as liver-spleen or white matter–gray matter.

The spatial resolution of a CT image is worse than that of radiographic imaging because it is digital and limited by pixel size. Likewise, the spatial resolution of MRI is worse than that of radiography. However, the contrast resolution is even better with MRI than with CT.

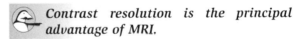 *Contrast resolution is the principal advantage of MRI.*

Spatial Resolution

Spatial resolution refers to the ability to identify an object, usually a small, dense object like a metal fragment or microcalcification, as separate and distinct from another object. Table 1-1 shows representative values of spatial resolution and contrast resolution for various medical imaging devices.

In x-ray imaging, spatial resolution is principally a function of the geometry of the system. Two important geometric considerations include focal spot size and source-to-image receptor distance (SID). In x-ray imaging, scatter radiation limits the contrast resolution. X-ray beam collimation and the use of radiographic grids reduce scatter radiation and therefore improve contrast resolution.

TABLE 1-1	Approximate Spatial and Contrast Resolution Characteristics of Several Medical Imaging Systems				
	Nuclear Medicine	Ultrasound	Radiography	Computed Tomography	Magnetic Resonance Imaging
Spatial resolution (mm)	5	2	0.05	0.25	0.25
Spatial resolution (lp/mm)	0.1	0.25	10	2	2
Contrast resolution (mm at 0.5% difference)	20	10	10	4	1

 CT has superior contrast resolution because it uses a finely collimated x-ray beam, which results in reduced scatter radiation.

In x-ray imaging, the x-ray attenuation coefficient (μ) determines the differential x-ray absorption in body tissues. In turn, the x-ray attenuation coefficient depends on the energy of the x-ray beam (E) and the atomic number (Z) of the tissue being imaged.

The basis for the MR image is different. It is a function of several intrinsic NMR characteristics of the tissue being imaged. The three most important tissue characteristics are proton density (PD), spin-lattice relaxation time (T1), and spin-spin relaxation time (T2). Secondary characteristics include flow, magnetic susceptibility, paramagnetism, and chemical shift.

There are two principal parameters to select in the production of a radiographic image: kilovolt peak (kVp) and milliampere-second (mAs). By carefully selecting kVp and mAs, radiographers can optimize the contrast resolution of an image without compromising the spatial resolution.

There are many parameters to select in the production of an MR image. The time sequence of energizing RF emissions (RF pulses) and gradient magnetic fields determines the contrast resolution. The principal pulse sequences are partial saturation, inversion recovery, spin echo, gradient echo, and echo planar. Each sequence has a large selection of timing patterns for the RF pulses and gradient magnetic fields to optimize contrast resolution for visualization of various anatomic and disease states.

Multiplanar Imaging

An additional advantage to MRI is the ability to obtain direct transverse, sagittal, coronal, and oblique plane images. Conventional radiographs show superimposed anatomy regardless of the plane of the image. In CT imaging, sagittal and coronal images are reconstructed either from a set of contiguous images or directly from the volumetric data of spiral CT. With MRI, a large data set is acquired during a single imaging sequence from which any anatomic plane can be reconstructed.

Viewing images obtained from various anatomic planes requires a different kind of knowledge on the part of physicians and technologists. Except for CT images, most x-ray images are parallel to the long axis of the body. The MRI interpreter may view anatomic planes that have not been imaged before. The required interpretive skills come with experience.

When students enroll in a radiologic technology program, the curriculum focuses on technique selection and positioning. Patient positioning in radiography is important to ensure that the structure being imaged is parallel and close to the image receptor. MR images are directly available as projections in any plane, when the patient is properly positioned at the magnet isocenter and with intended anatomy at the sensitive region of the RF coil.

Magnetic Resonance Spectroscopy

Another advantage to MRI is the possibility of doing in vivo spectroscopy. It is possible to make an MR image, see a suspicious lesion, put the cursor on that lesion, and encompass it within a region of interest (ROI). Then the radiologist could retrieve the NMR spectrum from that lesion for analysis.

An interpretation of the NMR spectrum could then tell whether the tissue is normal or abnormal. If the tissue appears abnormal, the NMR spectrum could reveal the molecular nature of the abnormality.

 Sensitivity *describes how well an imaging system can detect subtle differences in anatomy.* **Specificity** *refers to the ability to precisely identify the nature of such differences.*

MRI has excellent sensitivity. MR spectroscopy could provide increased specificity.

No Ionizing Radiation

Another advantage of MRI over x-ray imaging is that MRI does not require ionizing radiation. This lack of ionizing radiation has been effectively used to promote the safety of MRI to the medical community and public.

 MRI does not require ionizing radiation.

MRI uses RF electromagnetic radiation and magnetic fields, which do not cause ionization, and therefore do not have the associated potentially harmful effects of ionizing radiation. Some known bioeffects of RF and magnetic fields do exist, but they do not occur at the low intensities of MRI and are not associated with the induction of malignant disease.

MAGNETIC RESONANCE IMAGING HARDWARE

Just as a radiographic imaging system can be identified by its main components (i.e., x-ray tube, high-voltage generator, and operating console) so can an MRI system be identified by its main components (i.e., magnet, computer, and operating console).

The magnet is typically a large cylindrical device that accommodates the patient during imaging. Unlike a CT gantry, the MRI magnet does not have moving parts. The only things that move are electrons in a conductor. The patient aperture is usually approximately 60 cm in diameter. RF coils surround the patient in this aperture. Gradient coils, shim coils, and, in the case of an electromagnet, primary coils all surround the RF coils to produce the required magnetic fields.

The computer required for MRI is similar to that used for CT: very fast and with high capacity. During an MRI examination, more data are collected, and the computations required are longer and more difficult than those for CT.

The MRI operating console is also similar to that used for CT in that it has the same controls for postprocessing and annotation of an image. CT uses mechanical incrementation for patient localization and so does MRI. The patient undergoing MRI is moved to the isocenter of the magnet to ensure that the body part to be imaged is at that position. An MRI operating console has controls for the timing of RF pulses and gradient magnetic fields rather than kilovolt peak, milliampere, and exposure time.

AN OVERVIEW OF MAGNETIC RESONANCE IMAGING

The hydrogen nuclei in the patient, protons, behave like tiny magnets. Hydrogen makes up 80% of all atoms found in the human body, making hydrogen extremely useful for MRI. Because hydrogen is a single-charged spinning nucleon, the hydrogen nucleus exhibits magnetism called a *magnetic moment* (Figure 1-3).

The small arrows in Figure 1-3 represent these individual proton magnetic moments, which are also referred to as *magnetic dipoles*. Under normal circumstances, these magnetic dipoles (each has a north and south magnetic pole) are randomly distributed in space. Consequently, if the net magnetic field of a patient were measured, it would be zero because all of the individual magnetic dipole moments cancel.

Net Magnetization

When the patient is placed in the presence of a strong external magnetic field, some of the individual nuclear magnetic moments align with the external magnetic field (Figure 1-4). The Cartesian coordinate axis, X, Y, and Z, is always rendered with the Z-axis as the vertical axis as shown. Vector diagrams that show this coordinate system will be used to develop the physics of MRI.

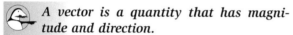 *A vector is a quantity that has magnitude and direction.*

The Z-axis in Figure 1-4 is drawn along the long axis of the patient. By convention, in MRI,

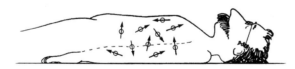

Figure 1-3   Under normal conditions, nuclear magnetic dipoles in the body are randomly distributed, which results in zero net magnetization.

the Z-axis coincides with the axis of the static magnetic field (B_0). In superconducting MR imaging systems, the static magnetic field (B_0) is usually horizontal, making the Z-axis horizontal, too. In a permanent magnet imaging system, the Z-axis is usually vertical, as in the vector diagrams that follow.

The intensity of B_0 is expressed in tesla (T). A frequent MRI question is, "How many rad equal 1 tesla?" The answer is none. A relationship does not exist between ionizing radiation and magnetic field strength. Nothing about MRI can be measured in rad because MRI does not use ionizing radiation.

With a patient positioned in a static magnetic field, proton dipoles align with the (B_0) field (see Figure 1-4). This statement is an oversimplification and is not entirely true. Only one of approximately every million dipoles becomes so aligned. However, once aligned, the patient is polarized and has net magnetization. The patient now has a north and a south magnetic pole.

Precession

In addition to polarization, another phenomenon occurs when a patient is placed in a static magnetic field. This phenomenon can be understood by considering the gyroscope. A gyroscope has an annulus of heavy metal attached by spokes to an axis (Figure 1-5). If the gyroscope is taken into space and spins, it only spins. However, if the gyroscope spins on Earth in the presence of a gravitational field,

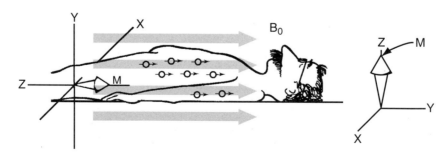

Figure 1-4   When a strong external magnetic field (B_0) is applied, the patient becomes polarized and has net magnetization *(M)*.

not only will the gyroscope spin, but it will wobble. Physicists call this wobble **precession**.

Precession is the interaction between the spinning mass of the gyroscope and the mass of the Earth that is manifest through the gravitational field. By spinning, the gyroscope creates angular momentum, which interacts with the angular momentum of the spinning Earth and causes the precessional motion.

Early space station designs were gyroscope-like saucers, spinning to produce an artificial gravity. Currently, hand and foot clips provide moorings for inhabitants of the International Space Station (Figure 1-6).

 The gyroscope precesses in the presence of gravity; the proton precesses in the presence of B_0.

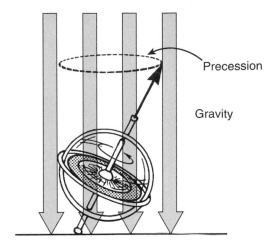

Figure 1-5 When spinning in outer space, a gyroscope just spins. On the Earth, however, it precesses as it spins.

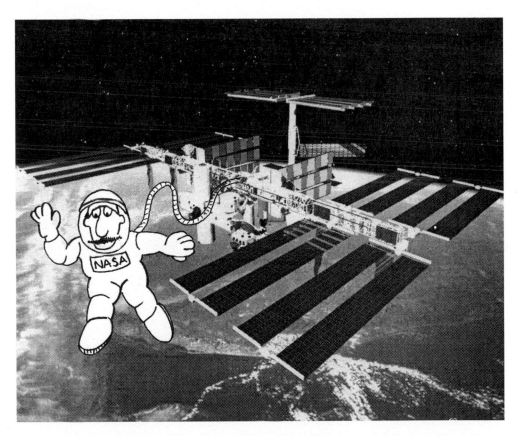

Figure 1-6 The International Space Station. (Courtesy National Aeronautics and Space Administration.)

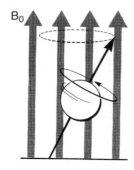

Figure 1-7 In the presence of an external magnetic field (B_0), a spinning proton precesses.

Similarly, if a spinning magnetic field, such as the magnetic moment of the proton (Figure 1-7), is in the presence of a static magnetic field, it will not only spin but will also precess.

The Larmor Equation

The following is the fundamental equation for MRI, the Larmor equation. This equation identifies the frequency of precession.

Larmor Frequency

$f = \gamma B_0$

where f is the frequency of precession and γ is the gyromagnetic ratio.

The Larmor equation relates B_0, the strength of the static magnetic field, to the precessional frequency (f) through the gyromagnetic ratio (γ), which has a precise value characteristic of each nuclear species.

Gyromagnetic ratio is to MRI what the disintegration constant is to radioactive decay. Each radionuclide has its own characteristic disintegration constant; each nuclear species has its own characteristic gyromagnetic ratio.

The units of the gyromagnetic ratio are megahertz per tesla. For example, hydrogen has a gyromagnetic ratio of 42 MHz/T. If B_0 is 1 T then the precessional frequency is 42 MHz. Likewise, at 1.5 T the precessional frequency is 63 MHz. The precessional frequency is also called the Larmor frequency.

TABLE 1-2	Nuclei of Medical Interest and Their Gyromagnetic Ratios
Nucleus	**Gyromagnetic Ratio (MHz/T)**
^1H	42.6
^{19}F	40.1
^{31}P	17.2
^{23}Na	11.3
^{13}C	10.7
^2H	6.5
^{17}O	5.8
^{39}K	2.0

Table 1-2 shows the principal nuclei of biologic interest in MRI. Medical applications of MRI concentrate on hydrogen because of its relative abundance and high gyromagnetic ratio. Compared with other nuclei in the body, hydrogen is the best for producing an MR signal.

Free Induction Decay

When a patient is placed in the B_0 magnetic field, the patient becomes polarized (see Figure 1-4). The proton magnetic dipoles have aligned with B_0, and the alignment is symbolized with one large arrow, M_z (Figure 1-8). This arrow represents a vector quantity called *net magnetization*. The symbol M_z represents net magnetization that lies along the Z-axis.

The MRI experiment begins with the emission of a pulse of RF at the Larmor frequency from a radio antenna, called a *coil*, into the patient (see Figure 1-8). For hydrogen imaging with a magnetic field of 1 T, the RF is tuned to 42 MHz.

If one plucks a string of a guitar and a harp is standing nearby, one of the strings on the harp will begin to vibrate (Figure 1-9); the other strings will remain still. The harp string vibrates because that string has the same fundamental resonance as the plucked guitar string. The "R" in MRI stands for **resonance.** The RF pulse transmitted into the body must

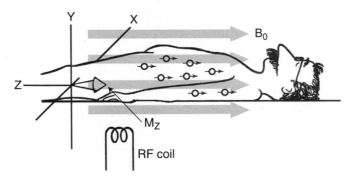

Figure 1-8 Net magnetization along the Z-axis is represented by M_Z and the large arrow.

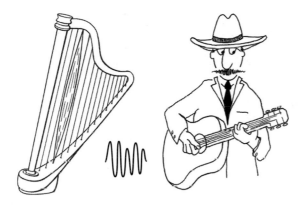

Figure 1-9 Plucking one guitar string causes only one string of a nearby harp, which has the same fundamental resonance, to vibrate.

be at the resonant frequency of the precessing hydrogen nuclei for energy to be transferred and imaging to occur.

Most objects in nature have a fundamental resonance. Energy transfer is always most efficient at resonance. For example, at a large hotel in Kansas City a few years ago, people were dancing on a suspended bridgelike walkway. They hit a resonance that was fundamental to the walkway. The walkway collapsed, killing several people. For this reason, marching military personnel are instructed to break cadence when crossing a bridge. A third example is the collapse of the Tacoma Narrows suspension bridge when it was subjected to harmonic buffeting winds (Figure 1-10).

With net magnetization in the Z direction, not only are the proton magnetic dipoles aligned, but each individual proton is precessing at the Larmor frequency (Figure 1-11). When the RF signal is pulsed at resonance into the patient, the energy state of each proton may be changed. This causes enough protons to flip into the negative Z direction, while still precessing about the Z-axis (Figure 1-12). This precession is always perpendicular to Z, in the XY plane, and is due to the phase coherence of the spins. This is the condition in which an MR signal can be generated and received.

When RF is pulsed into the patient, the protons individually flip into the negative Z direction while continuing to precess. Then, one by one, these protons flip back to their normal state in the positive Z direction. The normal state is called the *equilibrium state* because the protons are at **equilibrium** in the B_0 magnetic field. As the individual protons return to equilibrium, the net magnetization precesses around the Z-axis and slowly returns (relaxes) to equilibrium (Figure 1-13).

To a disinterested observer, such as the RF receiving coil shown in Figure 1-13, such precession is not obvious. Only a magnetic field that first approaches and then recedes harmonically is observed.

With any moving magnetic field, an electric current can be induced in a properly designed coil. The induced current represents a radio signal

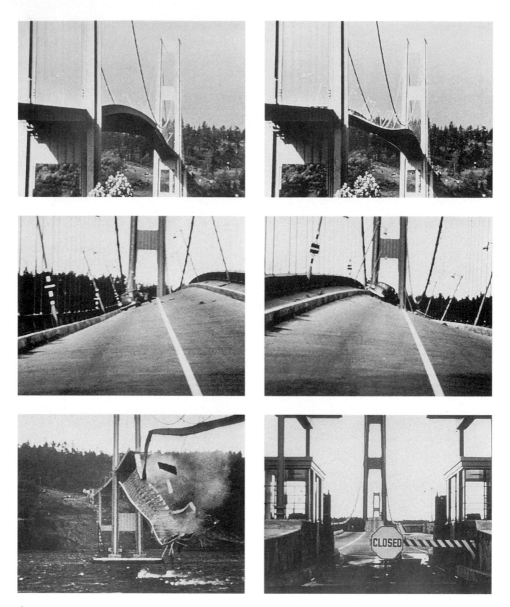

Figure 1-10 The Tacoma Narrows suspension bridge collapsed in buffeting gale force winds that set up a resonant oscillation. (Courtesy Civil Engineering Department, Rice University, Houston.)

emitted by the patient. This signal is called a *free induction decay* (FID). The RF coil surrounding the patient receives an oscillating signal that decreases with time (Figure 1-14). The signal decreases with time as the proton spins relax back to equilibrium. This time is known as a *relaxation time*. Two such relaxation times, T1 and T2, exist, and they are independent of one another and represent two different processes occurring at the same time.

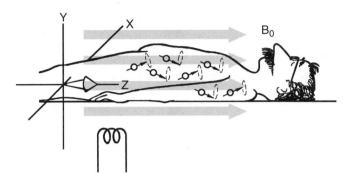

Figure 1-11 Placing a patient in a magnetic field (B_0) polarizes the patient and causes each proton dipole to precess randomly.

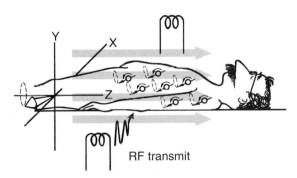

Figure 1-12 Net magnetization changes along the Z direction and the protons precess in phase when a proper radiofrequency *(RF)* pulse is transmitted into the patient.

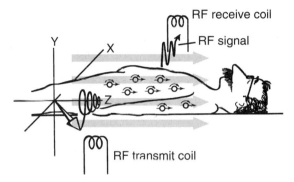

Figure 1-13 Precessing net magnetization induces a radiofrequency *(RF)* signal in a receiving coil. That RF signal is called a free induction decay.

Fourier Transformation

The FID is a plot of MR signal intensity as a function of time (see Figure 1-14). If a mathematical operation called a Fourier transformation (FT) is performed on the FID, the result appears as an NMR spectrum (Figure 1-15).

Whereas the FID is a graph of signal intensity versus time, the NMR spectrum is a graph of signal intensity versus inverse time (s^{-1}), or hertz (Hz). Therefore the NMR spectrum is signal intensity versus frequency. Each of the peaks in the NMR spectrum represents one characteristic of the tissue under investigation.

How is an image obtained from an NMR spectrum? The following is a simplistic expla-

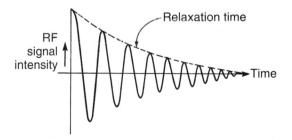

Figure 1-14 The free induction decay is a decreasing harmonic oscillation of the Larmor frequency.

nation. Figure 1-16 presents a transverse cross section through the trunk of the body. The patient lies in a uniform B_0, and two pixels are

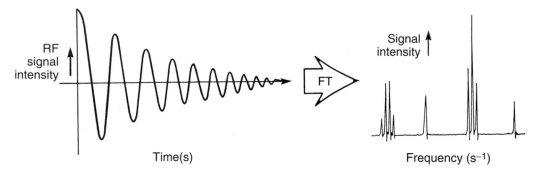

Figure 1-15   When a Fourier transformation *(FT)* is performed on the free induction decay, a nuclear magnetic resonance spectrum results.

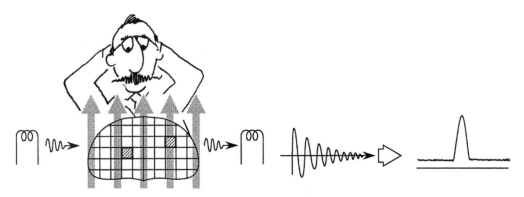

Figure 1-16   If the same tissue were in the two highlighted pixels, both pixels would be represented by the same peak in the nuclear magnetic resonance spectrum.

highlighted. If both pixels contain the same tissue, the peak in the NMR spectrum represents both pixels. One can tell by looking at the spectrum what is in both pixels but cannot determine their respective location.

If in addition to the uniform (B_0) magnetic field, a gradient magnetic field (B_x) is superimposed across the patient that varies in field strength, spatial localization is possible (Figure 1-17). Even though they represent the same tissue, the tissue in the pixel at the lower magnetic field strength has a lower Larmor frequency than the one located at the higher magnetic field.

The FID in this situation is considerably more complex. After FT, this spectrum has two

peaks instead of one. These two peaks carry spatial information. One represents the pixel at the lower magnetic field; the other represents the pixel at the higher magnetic field.

A uniform magnetic field is required for NMR spectroscopy; gradient magnetic fields are required for MRI.

Multiple projections can be obtained in MRI by electronically rotating the gradient magnetic fields around the patient to produce a set of projections (Figure 1-18). Then back projection reconstruction can be used to produce an image as in CT. The earliest MR images were created in this manner.

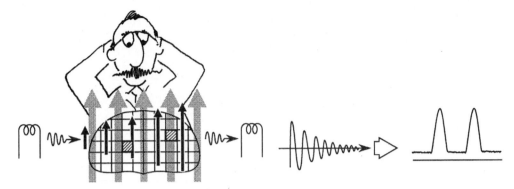

Figure 1-17 In the presence of a gradient magnetic field, B_x, the nuclear magnetic resonance spectrum provides information on pixel location.

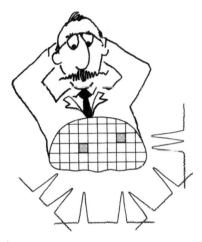

Figure 1-18 Projections can be obtained by rotating the gradient magnetic field around a patient. An image can be reconstructed from these projections by backprojection.

MR images are reconstructed differently now. The spatial information still comes from the application of gradient magnetic fields superimposed on the B_0; however, the reconstruction of an image occurs through a process called *two-dimensional Fourier transformation* (2DFT) or *three-dimensional Fourier transformation* (3DFT). This is a special application of higher mathematics that will be developed conceptually later.

CHALLENGE QUESTIONS

1. What three windows in the electromagnetic spectrum are available for the production of medical images?
2. What type of energy is involved in making MR images, and how would you describe that energy?
3. Isaac Newton is credited as the father of classical physics; Wilhelm Roentgen, the father of x-ray imaging; and Max Planck, the father of quantum mechanics. Who is considered the father of MRI and why?
4. What is contrast resolution?
5. What is spatial resolution, and why is it important in medical imaging?
6. Why does MRI exhibit superior contrast resolution?
7. The terms *sensitivity* and *specificity* are frequently used to describe imaging modalities. How do they differ?
8. State the Larmor equation and identify each parameter.
9. The description of the physical basis for MR imaging relies heavily on vector diagrams. What is a vector diagram?
10. Why does a toy top wobble when spun, and what is that wobble called?

Chapter 2

Electricity and Magnetism

OBJECTIVES

At the completion of this chapter, the student should be able to do the following:

1. Discuss the roles of the following: Franklin, Coulomb, Tesla, Faraday, and Oersted.
2. Describe the nature of the electric field.
3. List the four laws of electrostatics.
4. Describe the nature of magnetism.
5. Distinguish between magnetic susceptibility and magnetic permeability.
6. Examine the role of electromagnetism in magnetic resonance imaging (MRI).
7. Define imaging window.

OUTLINE

ELECTROSTATICS
 The Coulomb
 Electrification
 The Electric Field
 Electrostatic Laws
 Electric Potential Energy

ELECTRODYNAMICS
 Electric Current
 Ohm's Law
 Electric Power

MAGNETISM
 Magnetic Domains
 The Laws of Magnetism
 The Magnetic Field

ELECTROMAGNETISM
 Oersted's Experiment
 Faraday's Law

ELECTROMAGNETIC RADIATION
 Maxwell's Wave Equation
 The Electromagnetic Spectrum

Both electric and magnetic fields and electromagnetic radiation are used in magnetic resonance imaging (MRI). These are not unlike the physical agents used in x-ray imaging, although their method of use is vastly different.

Electricity is used to produce the primary static magnetic field (B_0) and the secondary gradient magnetic fields (B_X, B_Y, B_Z). These magnetic fields interact with the intrinsic nuclear magnetism of tissue, the proton dipoles. The tissue is excited with a radiofrequency (RF) pulse produced by an electrically stimulated coil, which usually also receives the magnetic resonance (MR) signal emitted from the body.

A modest understanding of the fundamental physical concepts of electricity and magnetism is necessary for an understanding of MRI. A logical sequence for dealing with such subjects is to discuss electrostatics and electrodynamics to develop an understanding of electricity. This is followed by a discussion of the phenomenon of magnetism, which leads into electromagnetism and electromagnetic radiation.

ELECTROSTATICS

The smallest unit of electric charge is contained in the electron, and it is negative. The proton likewise contains one unit of positive electric charge. Electric charge, unlike other fundamental properties of matter such as mass, cannot be subdivided. Furthermore, larger quantities of charge can only be multiples of the unit charge.

Although the magnitude of the electric charge of an electron and proton is the same, the mass of the proton is approximately 1840 times the mass of the electron. Protons are relatively fixed by virtue of their position in the nucleus of an atom, whereas electrons are free to migrate from atom to atom under some circumstances.

 Electrostatics deals with stationary electric charges.

It was not until the 1750s that Benjamin Franklin first described the nature of electric charge. Franklin's experiments have been popularly associated with flying kites, which is indeed true (Figure 2-1). However, he was and is also credited with being a laboratory scientist. Nevertheless, Franklin erroneously assumed that positive charges were migrating down his kite string.

Franklin called this migration of charge **electricity** and therein lies the origin of a confusing convention: that electric current (I) in a conductor flows opposite to electron movement. Franklin is also credited with much of the current terminology dealing with electricity: charge, discharge, battery, shock, positive, negative, plus, and minus among others. Not until the work of J.J. Thompson in the 1890s was the electron identified as the fundamental charged particle responsible for electricity.

The Coulomb

The unit of electric charge is the coulomb (C), with 1 C consisting of 6.24×10^{18} electronic charges, a sizable number of electrons. This definition, adopted in 1910, is such a strange number because the system for electrical measurement had already been established before the discovery of the electron. Ideally, the electron should be the smallest unit of

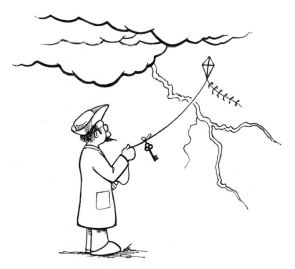

Figure 2-1 Benjamin Franklin described electricity as the flow of positive electrification rather than electrons.

electric charge. Instead, the charge on an electron is 1.6×10^{-19} C.

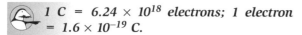 *1 C = 6.24 $\times$ 10^{18} electrons; 1 electron = 1.6 $\times$ 10^{-19} C.*

The coulomb is an unfamiliar quantity to most people. The lightning associated with a thunderstorm shown in Figure 2-2 ranges from perhaps 10 to 50 C. The shock experienced when grasping a doorknob in the dry air of winter is measured in microcoulombs (μC), a mere 10^{12} electrons.

Electrification

Whenever electrons are added to or removed from material, the material is said to be *electrified*. Electrification can occur by contact, friction, or induction.

Electrification by **contact** occurs when an object having an excess number of electrons contacts a neutrally charged object or an object with a deficiency of electrons. Rubbing a balloon over your hair to make it stick to the wall is an example of electrification by **friction**. The loosely bound electrons of hair are mechanically transferred so that the balloon becomes electrified.

 Induction refers to the transfer of mass or energy between objects without actual contact between the objects.

Electrification by **induction** occurs when a highly electrified object comes close to a neutral object so that the electrons are transferred by spark. Lightning bolts jump from cloud to cloud or cloud to earth to shed themselves of excess electrons. The earth is the ultimate sink for excess electrons and is called an *earth ground* or just *ground* in engineering terms.

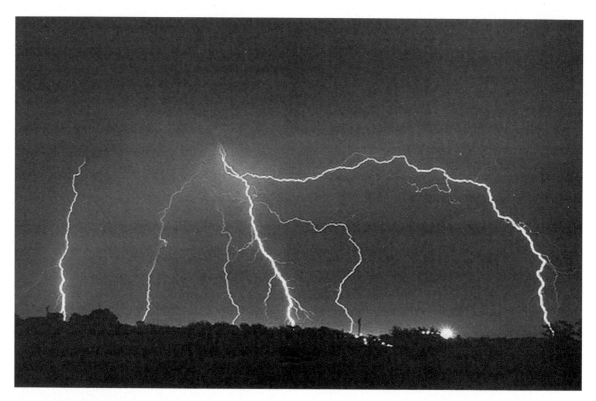

Figure 2-2   Lightning is the migration of electrostatic charge usually from cloud to cloud but also from cloud to ground.

The Electric Field

Charge cannot be destroyed by conversion to another form. In the universe, the total number of negative charges equals the total number of positive charges, and the net charge is always the same—zero. Furthermore, charge is quantized; it comes in discrete bundles rather than in a continuum of values.

A force field called the *electric field* (E) is associated with each charge. The proof of the electric field is much the same as that of a gravitational field—the exertion of a force.

The gravitational field produces a force that causes one mass to be attracted to another. Similarly, the electric field creates a force between one charge and another. Although the gravitational force is always attractive, the force of the electric field can be attractive or repulsive, depending on the nature of the charges involved.

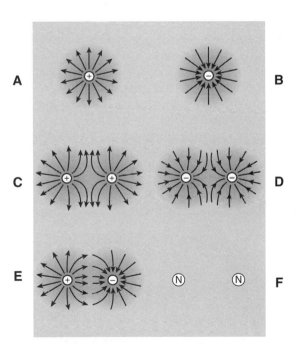

Figure 2-3 Electric fields radiate out from a positive charge (**A**) toward a negative charge (**B**). Like charges repel one another (**C** and **D**). Unlike charges attract one another (**E**). Uncharged particles do not have an electric field (**F**).

The electric field is most easily visualized as imaginary lines radiating from an electric charge (Figure 2-3). The intensity of the electric field is proportional to the concentration of lines, and therefore the electric field decreases as the square of the distance from the charge.

The electric field is a vector quantity; that is, it has not only magnitude but also direction. The direction of the electric field is determined by the movement of a positive charge in the electric field. In the presence of an electron, the positive charge is attracted, and therefore the imaginary lines of the electric field are directed toward the electron.

 In an electric field the lines of force begin on positive charges and end on negative charges.

Alternatively, if the positive charge is in the field of a proton, the positive charge will be repelled, and the imaginary lines will radiate from the proton (see Figure 2-3). Neutral objects, such as a neutron, do not have an electric field.

The magnitude of the electric field is defined as the force on a unit charge in the field as follows:

Electric Field

$E = F/Q$
where E is the electric field intensity (newton/coulomb), F is the force on the charge (newton), and Q is the electric charge (coulomb).

Although electric charge is discrete, its associated electric field is continuous, and this is a fundamental characteristic of field theory. Particles add in a quantized fashion; fields add in a continuum by superposition. For example, the force on an electric charge is determined by not only the movement of that charge but also the electric fields produced by all other electric charges near and far. That is **field superposition**.

Electrostatic Laws

The nature and intensity of the electric field form the basis for the four principal laws of electrostatics:

Unlike Versus Like Charges. Because of the vector nature of the electric field, like electric charges repel, and unlike electric charges attract. Particles having no electric charge, such as neutrons, are not influenced by an electric field.

Coulomb's Law. The force of attraction or repulsion between electrostatic charges was first described by Charles Coulomb in the 1780s. Coulomb noted that the force was proportional to the product of the two charges and inversely proportional to the square of the distance separating them. Coulomb's law can be stated as follows:

Coulomb's Law
$E = F/q = k\ Q/d^2$
or
$F = k\ q\ Q/d^2$
where F = the force (newton)
q and Q = the charges (coulomb)
d = the distance between them (meter)
k = a constant

The electrostatic force is one of the five fundamental forces in nature. It is 10^{37} times stronger than the gravitational force, 100 times as strong as the weak interaction, about equal to the magnetic force, and about $1/100$ of the strong nuclear force.

An electrified balloon will attract paper or repel a small stream of water. The electrostatic force of attraction holds electrons in orbit in an atom. The electrostatic force of repulsion among protons limits the size of the nucleus.

Charge Distribution. Because protons are fixed, whereas electrons are free to move, the remaining discussion of electrostatic phenomenon concerns electrons. Because the electric field associated with each electron radiates uniformly, electrons on any electrified object tend to be separated uniformly and to the maximum dimensions possible (Figure 2-4).

Free electrons are distributed on the surface of the object, not inside it.

Charge Concentration. If the electrified object is regularly shaped, such as a sphere or wire, the distribution of electrons on the surface will be uniform. On the other hand, if the surface is irregularly shaped (for example, has a point as in an electrified cattle prod or a microfocus field-emission x-ray tube) electrons will be concentrated at the sharpest region of curvature.

Electric Potential Energy

When two like charges are pushed together or two unlike charges are pulled apart, work is required. The resulting system has the ability to do work and therefore has electric potential energy.

The work done to create electric potential energy comes from an **energy source**, and the work obtained from the potential energy is deposited in an **energy sink**. A hydroelectric generator and a steam generator are common energy sources that convert mechanical energy into electric potential energy. Energy sinks, such as motors, lamps and heaters, abound.

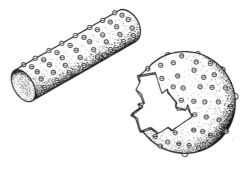

Figure 2-4 Electrons are distributed on the surface of electrified objects.

The electric potential energy of a charge, q, is converted to kinetic energy when the charge is in motion and work is done. The electric potential energy of a charge influenced by the electric field of other charges is given by the following:

Electric Potential Energy

$E = QV$

or

$W = QV$

or

$V = W/Q$

where E is the potential energy (joule), Q is the electric charge (coulomb), V is the electric potential (volt), and W is work (joule).

Electric potential has units of joule per coulomb, and it is not a force at all but rather

a force used to do work. Therefore electric potential is given a special name, volt, and is commonly called *voltage*.

ELECTRODYNAMICS

Electrodynamics involves what is commonly called an *electric current* or *electricity*. Electricity deals with the flow of electrons in a conductor.

 The science of electric charge in motion is electrodynamics.

A Houston freeway at rush hour is analogous to an electric current (Figure 2-5). Normally, about 10,000 cars (electrons) each hour will pass any given point on a six-lane freeway. If there is a wreck or construction, the speed of each car is reduced (resistance) at that point and the flow of traffic restricted. At an interchange, some cars may exit onto alternate routes. This allows those cars remaining on the main freeway and those that exited to travel

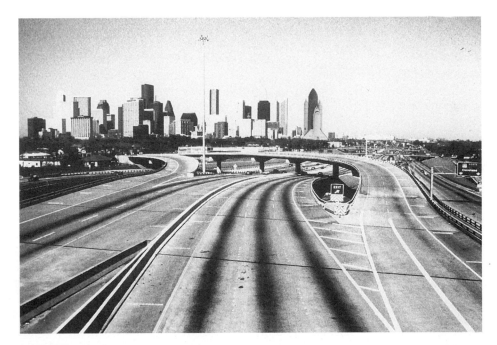

Figure 2-5 This Houston freeway at rush hour is analogous to an electric current, with the cars serving as electrons.

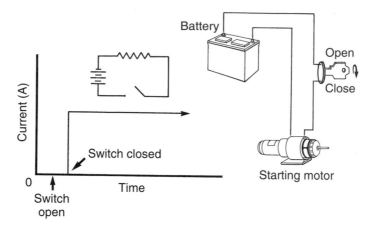

Figure 2-6   The electric circuit in an automobile is an example of direct current.

faster (parallel circuit). The traffic flow in each branch is reduced because there are fewer cars in each route, but the total flow will remain constant.

Electric Current

The electrons flowing in a conductor behave like the automobiles on the freeway. For an electric current to exist, a closed circuit is necessary. Each electron must have a place to go. If there is a barricade in a conductor, such as an open switch, electron flow ceases.

The reason for investigating electricity is that work can be extracted from the kinetic energy of electrons moving in a conductor. The number of electrons involved is given a special name, the ampere (A), which is equal to the flow of 1 C each second (1 A = 1 C/s).

An ampere is a rather large electron flow, 6.24×10^{18} electrons each second. Electrons cannot be counted that fast, so electric current is measured by the associated magnetic field.

Electric currents range from thousands of amperes in lightning bolts to picoamperes in electronic equipment. Household current can be up to approximately 30 A on any circuit. A current of only 100 milliamperes (mA) at 110 volts is almost always fatal, which is the reason grounded circuits and ground fault circuit interrupters are necessary elements in home wiring.

Direct Current.   If the energy source propels electrons in only one direction, as with an automobile battery, the form of electricity is direct current (DC) (Figure 2-6). At time zero, when the switch is open, no current flows. The instant the switch is closed, electrons flow but only in one direction.

Alternating Current.   On the other hand, if the energy source is of an alternating form (Figure 2-7), alternating current (AC) is produced. When the switch is open no current flows. When the switch is closed, electrons first flow in one direction and then reverse direction and flow oppositely.

When electrons begin flowing in the positive direction, they begin slowly at first and speed up to a maximum, represented by the first peak of the current waveform (see Figure 2-7). Then they begin to slow down, still traveling in the same direction, until they momentarily come to rest. This moment of rest occurs 120 times each second and is represented by the zero crossing of the waveform. Then the electrons reverse direction, first speeding up to a maximum, then slowing down to zero again.

The number of electrons in the circuit remains constant, and their net movement is zero. Both AC and DC are used to great advantage in MRI.

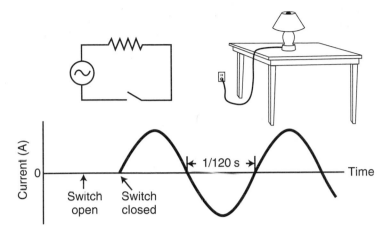

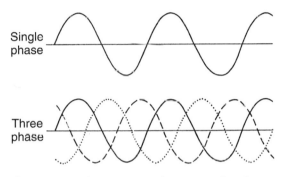

Figure 2-7   Normal household current is provided as an alternating current.

Figure 2-8   Electric power is generated and transmitted in three-phase form.

Phase. The current waveform shown in Figure 2-7 illustrates that at any instant, all electrons are moving in the same direction with the same velocity. They are said to be in phase, and the electricity is commonly called *single-phase current*.

Actually, commercial electric power is generated and transmitted as three-phase current. A three-phase waveform is shown in Figure 2-8. At any instant, not all electrons are moving in the same direction, and those that are have different velocities. They are out of phase with one another. The concept of phase is important to the understanding of the way an MR image is produced.

Ohm's Law

Electrons do not flow unimpeded in a circuit. They behave much like an individual walking along a crowded sidewalk, bumping into people. Electrons bump into other electrons of the conductor. This property of any electric device is called *impedance*, and it is a function of the size, shape, and composition of the conductor or circuit element.

There are three types of electric impedances: capacitive, inductive, and resistive. If the work done on the device changes the electric energy into heat, the impedance is resistive, and it is equal to the electric potential divided by the current.

Such heating may be a problem with a resistive electromagnet-type MRI system. The heating can require a closed cooling system incorporating a high-efficiency heat exchanger. Superconducting MRI magnets do not have this difficulty because the resistance-to-electron flow is zero. The electrons are basically walking along empty sidewalks.

The resistance of a conductor or circuit element is usually a fixed quantity and follows a simple relationship first described by George Ohm in the 1840s.

Ohm's Law

R = V/I
where R is the resistance in ohm (Ω), V is the electric potential in volt (V), and I is the electric current in ampere (A).

Although Ohm's law is fundamental to electronics, many electric devices are used because they do not obey Ohm's law. Vacuum tubes, transistors, and the integrated circuits of computer chips are prime examples.

Materials used in electric circuits are sometimes classified by their resistance. Those with low resistance, such as copper, aluminum, and seawater, are called **conductors.** Those with high resistance, such as quartz, rubber, and glass, are called **insulators.**

Some materials that lie between conductors and insulators are called **semiconductors.** Silicon, selenium, and germanium are semiconductors used extensively in fabricating diodes, radiation detectors, and all types of computer chips.

If the electric resistance of a material is zero, that material is a **superconductor.** However, to behave as a superconductor, as niobium and titanium do, a material must be in an extremely cold or **cryogenic** environment. This electric classification of material is summarized in Table 2-1.

Electric Power

When an electric current flows, it will do so because of an electric potential (volt). Because of the impedance of circuit elements to electron flow, energy must be supplied. Energy is required to move a charge, Q, through an electric potential, V. Power (P) is the rate at which energy (E) is used or work (W) is performed.

Electric Power

P = E/t = W/t (joule/second)
therefore

P = QV/t = IV
Alternatively, with application of Ohm's law

P = I^2R = V^2/R

The quantity for power, joule per second, is given a special name in physics, the watt (W). Therefore the watt is the unit of electric power.

 Energy and work are measured in joule. Power is joule per second.

In terms of human activity, the watt is very large. A construction worker may be able to work sufficiently hard to power a few 100-W light bulbs. In terms of human consumption, the watt is a small quantity. In the United States about 6 kilowatts (kW) per person is required continuously. In many of the developing nations, the figure is less than 500 W.

Resistive electromagnet-type MRI systems require considerable amounts of power. Some may require as much as 100 kW, and with the cost of electric power now running close to 10¢ per kilowatt per hour, it is obvious that this

---

TABLE 2-1	**The Four Electrical States of Matter**	
Class	**Property**	**Material**
Insulator	Resists the flow of electrons	Rubber, glass, plastic
Semiconductor	Can behave as an insulator or a conductor	Silicon, germanium
Conductor	Allows the flow of electrons with difficulty	Copper, aluminum
Superconductor	Freely allows the flow of electrons	Titanium, niobium

portion of the operating expense can be substantial.

MAGNETISM

Like mass and charge, magnetism is a fundamental property of matter. All matter is magnetic to some degree. For example, an iron magnet picks up a steel paper clip but not a copper penny. Steel is ferromagnetic and copper diamagnetic.

Even subatomic particles such as protons have magnetic properties. Basically, magnetism is a field effect associated with certain types of material said to be magnetic. The magnetic field is similar in many ways to the electric field, but its manifestation is different.

The earliest magnets were described 2000 years ago as naturally occurring black stones that attracted iron. These "leading stones," or lodestones, were thought to be magic by the natives in a region of present-day western Turkey, then known as Magnesia in the Greek language. The term *magnetism* was adopted and persists today.

Magnetic Domains

The smallest region of magnetism is called a *magnetic domain*. Most materials have their magnetic domains randomly oriented (Figure 2-9, *A*) and therefore exhibit no magnetism. Some materials, however, have their magnetic domains aligned and therefore become magnets (Figure 2-9, *B*).

The strength and number of magnetic domains in materials are associated with its

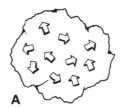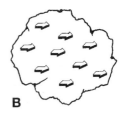

Figure 2-9 A, In most matter, magnetic domains are randomly oriented. **B,** Magnets exist when magnetic domains are aligned.

electron configuration. As discussed later, an electric charge in motion creates a magnetic field. In the case of common magnetic materials and electromagnetism, the magnetism is related to moving electrons. In the case of nuclei, the magnetism is related to the much weaker magnetic properties of the spinning electrically positive nucleus.

The magnetic fields of paired electrons cancel; therefore atoms with even numbers of electrons in shells exhibit little magnetism. Atoms with unpaired electrons produce strong magnetic domains. Atoms with nearly half-filled shells have the strongest magnetism because electrons generally will not begin pairing spins until a shell is half full.

 Electron configuration determines the three types of magnetism: ferromagnetism, paramagnetism, and diamagnetism.

Table 2-2 summarizes these types of magnetism. Materials with such properties are distinguished from each other according to the strength and alignment of their magnetic domains in the presence of an external magnetic field.

TABLE 2-2	The Three Magnetic States of Matter		
Class	**Property**	**Susceptibility**	**Material**
Ferromagnetism	Easily magnetized	>1	Iron, nickel, cobalt
Paramagnetism	Very weakly magnetized	0–1	Aluminum, platinum, manganese, gadolinium
Diamagnetism	Unaffected by a magnetic field	<0	Copper, silver, mercury, carbon

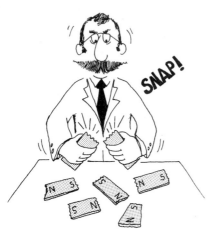

Figure 2-10 If a magnet is broken into smaller pieces, baby magnets result.

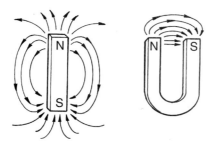

Figure 2-11 The imaginary lines of the magnetic field leave the north pole and enter the south pole.

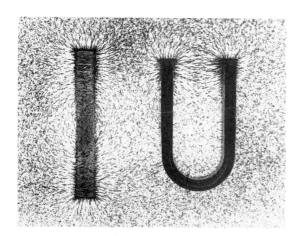

Figure 2-12 Demonstration of magnetic lines of force with iron filings. (Courtesy Robert Waggener, San Antonio, TX.)

Ferromagnetic materials are easily magnetized and have a magnetic susceptibility greater than 1. Such materials include iron, cobalt, and nickel. These materials make the strongest magnets and are used singly and in combination with the many MRI permanent magnets. Perhaps the most common permanent magnet is one made of an alloy of aluminum, nickel and, cobalt—alnico.

Paramagnetic materials include platinum, oxygen, tungsten, manganese, and gadolinium. These materials have a magnetic susceptibility less than 1. They are weakly influenced by an external magnetic field but do not exhibit measurable magnetic properties of their own.

Diamagnetic materials have negative magnetic susceptibility and in fact are slightly repelled by magnets. Such materials include mercury, silver, copper, carbon, and water.

 Magnetic susceptibility relates the relative ease that a material can be made magnetic.

The Laws of Magnetism

Dipoles. Unlike the situation that exists with electricity, there is no smallest unit of magnetism. Because each magnetic domain exists with two poles, a north pole and a south pole, it is commonly called a *dipole.* Unlike electric charge, a magnet cannot exist with a single pole. Dividing a magnet simply creates smaller magnets (Figure 2-10).

Attraction/Repulsion. As with electric charges, like magnetic poles repel and unlike magnetic poles attract. In addition, by convention the imaginary lines of the magnetic field leave the north pole of a magnet (Figure 2-11) and return to the south pole. How do scientists know that these imaginary lines exist? They can be demonstrated by the action of iron filings near a magnet (Figure 2-12).

The polar convention of magnetism actually has its origin in the compass. The end of a compass needle that points to the Earth's North Pole (actually, the Earth's magnetic south pole)

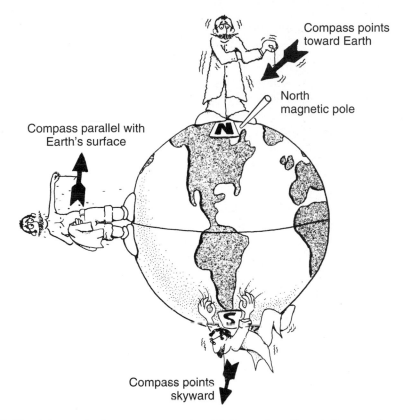

Figure 2-13   A free-swinging compass reacts with the earth as though it were a bar magnet.

is the north pole of the compass. If a compass were taken to the North Pole, it would point into the earth (Figure 2-13). At the South Pole, it would point to the sky.

Magnetic Induction.   Just as an electrostatic charge can be induced from one material to another, nonmagnetic material can be made magnetic by induction. The magnetic field lines just described are called *magnetic lines of induction,* and the density of lines is proportional to the intensity of the magnetic field.

When ferromagnetic material such as a piece of soft iron is brought into the vicinity of an intense magnetic field, the lines of induction are altered by attraction to the soft iron (Figure 2-14), and the iron will be made magnetic. If copper, a diamagnetic material, were to replace the soft iron, there would be no such effect. This

property of matter is called **magnetic permeability.**

This principle is used with many MRI systems that use iron as a magnetic shield to reduce the level of the fringe magnetic field. This is also the basis of antimagnetic watches, although the effect is not guaranteed near the strong field of an MRI system.

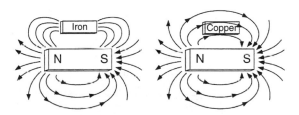

Figure 2-14   Ferromagnetic material such as iron attracts magnetic lines of induction, whereas nonmagnetic material such as copper does not.

Ferromagnetic material has high magnetic permeability and acts as a magnetic sink by drawing the lines of induction into it.

When ferromagnetic material is removed from the magnetic field, it usually does not retain its strong magnetic property. Therefore soft iron makes an excellent temporary magnet. It is a magnet only while its magnetism is being induced. If properly tempered by heat or exposed to an external magnetic field for a long period, however, ferromagnetic materials retain their magnetism when removed from the external magnetic field and become permanent magnets.

Another type of magnet is the electromagnet. It owes its magnetism to an electric current, which induces magnetism (Figure 2-15), but only while the electric current is flowing. The MRI systems use permanent magnets, resistive electromagnets, or superconductive electromagnets.

Magnetic Force.   The force created by a magnetic field behaves similarly to that of the electric field. The electric and magnetic forces were joined by Maxwell's field theory of electromagnetic radiation into a unified explanation.

Table 2-3 summarizes some of the similarities of these three fundamental forces. The defining equation is precisely the same among the three; however, the magnitudes are different.

The gravitational force is a long-range force. If it is assigned a relative value of 1, the electric and magnetic forces have a value of 10^{37} times its magnitude.

The equation of interacting magnetic fields is named for Karl Gauss, who used Coulomb's law to explain magnetism in the 1840s. The magnetic force obeys the inverse square law principle, and its magnitude is proportional to the product of the two interacting magnetic poles. Its formulation is as follows:

Gauss's Law
$F = k\ pP/d^2$ where F = the force in newton (N)   p and P = the relative pole strengths in ampere meter (Am)   d = the separation distance in meter (m)   k = a constant

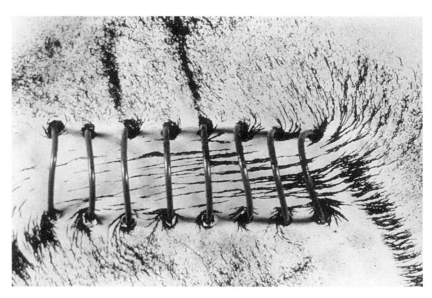

Figure 2-15   Iron filings show the magnetic field lines of an electromagnet. (Courtesy Murray Solomon, San Jose, CA.)

As with the gravitational force and the electric force, the magnetic force does not need a conducting medium. It acts through space.

The Magnetic Field

The imaginary lines of magnetic induction create a field effect. The strength of the magnetic field is defined by placing an imaginary north pole in it and measuring the force on the pole. This is similar to the definition of the electric field by its force acting on a positive charge. Therefore the magnetic field B is given by the following:

Magnetic Field

$$B = F/p$$

where B is the field strength in tesla (T), F is the force in newton (N), and p is the pole strength in ampere meter (Am).

The tesla (T) is the standard international (SI) unit for the magnetic field. An older unit still very much in use is the gauss (G); 1 T equals 10,000 G. As with other types of fields, the strength of magnetic fields ranges over many orders of magnitude.

ELECTROMAGNETISM

A motionless electron has an electric field associated with it. An electron in motion has both an electric and a magnetic field. The interaction between the electric field and the magnetic field is the basis for electromagnetism.

Oersted's Experiment

Until the 1820s, electricity and magnetism were considered two separate, unrelated, and independent manifestations. As with many great discoveries, Hans Christian Oersted accidentally noted that a compass was deflected by a DC current.

When no current exists in the circuit, the compass needle placed close to the conductor will point to the earth's North Pole (Figure 2-16). Once the switch is closed and current flows, the compass immediately aligns itself

TABLE 2-3	Three Fundamental Forces		
	Gravitational	**Electric**	**Magnetic**
The force is:	Attractive only	Attractive and repulsive	Attractive and repulsive
Acts in:	Mass, m	Charge, q	Pole, p
Through an associated field:	Gravitational field, g	Electric field, E	Magnetic field, B
With intensity:	$F = mg$	$F = qE$	$F = pB$
The source of the field is:	Mass, M	Charge, Q	Pole, P
The intensity of the field at a distance from the source is:	$g = \dfrac{GM}{d^2}$	$E = \dfrac{kQ}{d^2}$	$B = \dfrac{kP}{d^2}$
The force between fields is given by:	Newton's law $F = G\dfrac{Mm}{d^2}$	Coulomb's law $F = k\dfrac{Qq}{d^2}$	Gauss's law $F = k\dfrac{Pp}{d^2}$
Where:	$G = 6.678 \times 10^{-11}\ \dfrac{Nm^2}{C^2}$	$k = 9.0 \times 10^9\ \dfrac{Nm^2}{C^2}$	$k = 10^{-7}\ \dfrac{W}{A^2}$

perpendicularly to the current-carrying wire. If the electron flow is as illustrated in Figure 2-16, the north pole of the compass is attracted to the wire as shown. Reversing the current causes the south pole of the compass to point to the wire.

Oersted's observation demonstrated that a magnetic field is always associated with a moving charged particle. Furthermore, if either the electric field or magnetic field is time variant, that is, changing in intensity with time, profound interactions can occur.

The magnetic field induced by a moving electron is illustrated in Figure 2-17. The magnetic field lines exist radially from the axis of motion.

How is it known that moving charged particles create a magnetic field? This cannot be shown in an isolated frame of reference. Such a demonstration requires another magnetic field so that the interaction between the two magnetic fields can be observed.

An electron is shown moving out of this page between the poles of a magnet (Figure 2-18); this electron direction is indicated by the (⊙), which represents the head of an arrow. If the electron were moving into the page, (X), representing the tail of an arrow, would be shown.

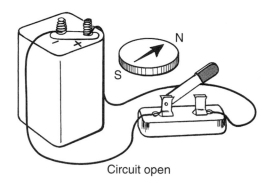

Circuit open

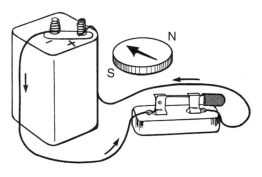

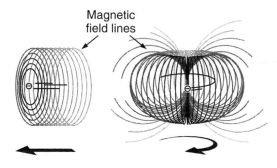

Figure 2-17   A moving charged particle induces a magnetic field in a plane perpendicular to its motion.

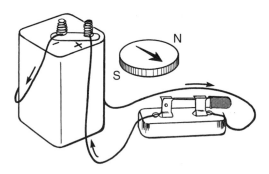

Figure 2-16   A compass is deflected by a direct current, and the direction of deflection depends on the direction of the electric current.

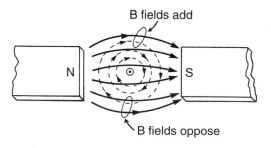

Figure 2-18   An electron moving in a magnetic field experiences a force causing it to curve. The force results from the interaction between the electron's magnetic field and the external magnetic field.

The electron moving in the magnetic field experiences a force that is at right angles to both its velocity and the external magnetic field. This force tends to deviate the electron in its motion, causing it to follow a curved path.

The direction of the force is given by the left-hand rule (Figure 2-19). With application of the left-hand rule, it can be concluded that the electron in Figure 2-18 should move down the page. This is so because the external magnetic field and that of the electron reinforce one another above the path of the electron and oppose one another below that path. The magnitude of this force is the following:

Magnetic Force

$F = qvB$

where F = the force in newton (N)
  q = the charge in coulomb (C)
  v = the electron velocity in meter per second (m/s)
  B = the magnetic field in tesla (T)

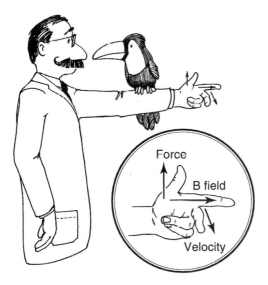

Figure 2-19 The left-hand rule demonstrates the directional relationships among force, velocity, and external magnetic field.

This expression is yet another approach to the definition of the magnetic field. A magnetic field of 1 T exists when 1 C traveling at 1 m/s is acted on by a force of 1 N (1 T = 1 N/Am).

 One tesla is equal to one newton per ampere-meter.

The total force on a moving electron is the sum of the forces caused by external electric and magnetic fields.

Lorentzian Force

$F = qE + qvB$

This is called the Lorentzian force, and it is the basis for such diverse yet readily recognizable phenomena as the aurora borealis (northern lights), the cathode-ray tube, and the operation of a cyclotron for positron-emission tomography (PET).

When electrons move in a conductor, the Lorentzian force determines their use in electromechanical devices such as motors and generators. In an MRI system, this force can be used to explain the operation of the primary magnet, the gradient coils, and the RF coils.

The Solenoid. Still another method for defining a magnetic field is based on the force on a long section of current-carrying wire (Figure 2-20). The external magnetic field B could be

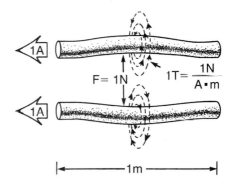

Figure 2-20 Parallel current-carrying wires repel each other. This forms the basis for the definition of the tesla.

created by a permanent magnet or an adjacent current-carrying wire. The defining equation for the strength of the magnetic field is the following:

Magnetic Field

$B = F/Idl$

where F is force in newton (N), I is the current in ampere (A), and dl is an incremental length (m) of a long wire.

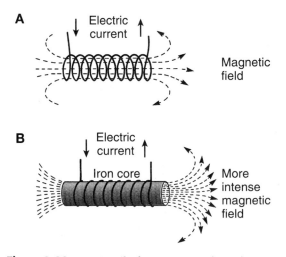

Figure 2-21   A magnetic dipole is produced by a current-carrying loop of wire.

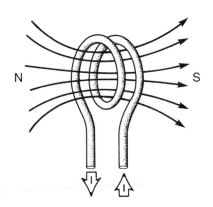

Figure 2-22   **A,** A coil of current-carrying wire produces a magnetic field. This is called a *solenoid*. **B,** With an iron core, it is called an *electromagnet*.

   If the force on a 1-m section of wire conducting 1 A is 1 N, the magnetic field has a strength of 1 T.

If the straight length of wire is shaped to form a loop, a magnetic dipole is produced (Figure 2-21). If the current is reversed, the polarity of the dipole is reversed.

If a series of loops is formed from a current-carrying wire, a more intense magnetic field is produced (Figure 2-22, *A*). Such a helically wound coil of wire is called a **solenoid.**

The Electromagnet.   If a rod of ferromagnetic material is inserted inside the solenoid (Figure 2-22, *B*), the intensity of the induced magnetic field is greatly strengthened because of the concentration of magnetic field lines. The device described is an electromagnet, and it is the basis for switches, large industrial magnets, and one type of MRI magnet. It is also the foundation for more complicated electromagnetic devices such as motors, generators, and transformers. All these devices function because coils of current-carrying wire are wrapped around ferromagnetic cores and magnetic fields are induced.

A motor is a device that converts electric energy into mechanical energy. A generator does the opposite; it converts mechanical energy into electric energy. A transformer alters the magnitude of electric current and voltage.

The intermediate step in each of these devices is the induced magnetic field. Mechanical motion can be extracted from electric power or supplied to produce electric power because of the force on a current-carrying wire in the presence of a magnetic field.

Faraday's Law

A force is exerted on a length of current-carrying wire when a magnetic field is present. The force is perpendicular to both the magnetic field and the direction of electron flow.

If a loop of wire is connected to an ammeter to produce a closed circuit with no source of electric potential, such as a battery, there is no electric current in the loop (Figure 2-23, *A*). If a permanent magnet is moved through the loop, as in Figure 2-23, *B*, a current will flow. If the movement of the permanent magnet is reversed, the electric current is reversed (Figure 2-23, *C*).

The changing magnetic field created by the moving permanent magnet induces a voltage in the circuit, causing electrons to flow. This phenomenon was demonstrated by Michael Faraday in the 1830s and is stated as Faraday's law of electromagnetic induction.

Faraday's Law

$$V = -dB/dt$$

where V is the induced voltage (V), dB represents the changing magnetic field, and dt is the time taken for that change.

The negative sign in Faraday's Law is a consequence of Lenz's law. The direction of the induced electron flow, and therefore the

induced voltage, is such that it opposes the agent inducing the flow.

The electron flow induced by moving the north pole of the permanent magnet towards the loop is in such a direction that the north pole of the induced magnetic field opposes a further push of the magnet (Figure 2-23, *B*). If the permanent magnet is pulled away from the loop (Figure 2-23, *C*) or the south pole of the magnet is pushed toward the loop, the induced electron flow is reversed, and the polarity of the induced magnetic field is reversed. Regardless of whether the magnetic field or the loop of wire is moved, a current is induced, which in turn induces a secondary magnetic field to oppose the inducing field.

If an opposing loop of wire is used instead of a permanent magnet as the inducing agent, a simple transformer is made (Figure 2-24). If the first coil is energized by a source of AC power, the magnetic field associated with the first coil alternates in polarity. This primary alternating magnetic field interacts with the second coil as though one alternately pushed and then pulled a permanent magnet along the axis of the second coil. The induced electron

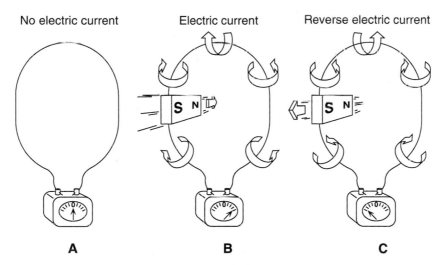

No electric current   Electric current   Reverse electric current

A   **B**   **C**

Figure 2-23 **A,** No electric current exists in a closed circuit that has no source of electric potential. **B,** When a magnetic field moves through a closed coil of wire, an electric potential is created and an electric current induced. **C,** Reverse the magnet, and the electric current reverses.

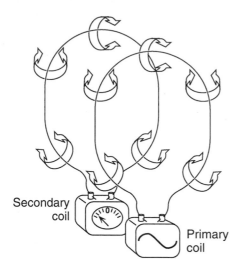

Secondary coil

Primary coil

Figure 2-24 An alternating current in one coil creates an alternating magnetic field that can induce an alternating current in a nearby second coil.

flow in the secondary coil is AC, and the induced magnetic field always opposes the action of the primary field.

The Transformer. This principle is the basis for the transformer. A transformer incorporates hundreds of loops of wire coiled on a ferromagnetic core. The core concentrates and intensifies the magnetic field. Because a moving magnetic field is required, a transformer will not work on DC, only on AC.

The RF Coil. The current in a primary coil induces a current in a secondary coil through magnetic induction but only when the primary current varies in intensity (Figure 2-24). However, the phenomenon of Faraday induction can be carried one step further. If electrons are not only varying in intensity but also accelerating and decelerating alternately, electromagnetic radiation is emitted.

This is the principle of the radio, in which case the electromagnetic radiation is called RF (Figure 2-25). Oscillating electrons in the transmitting antenna (coil) produce RF, which in turn induces a signal in the receiving antenna (coil). This is similar to MRI.

ELECTROMAGNETIC RADIATION

As previously discussed, a resting electric charge radiates an electric field. When the charge is in motion, a magnetic field is generated.

When the moving electric charge slows down (decelerates), a photon of electromagnetic radiation is emitted. Radiologists and radiographers know that bremsstrahlung x-rays are produced by the deceleration of a projectile electron in the vicinity of the nucleus of an atom in the anode of an x-ray tube.

Electrons decelerated or accelerated within the conducting element of a radio coil emit photons of RF. This phenomenon was described

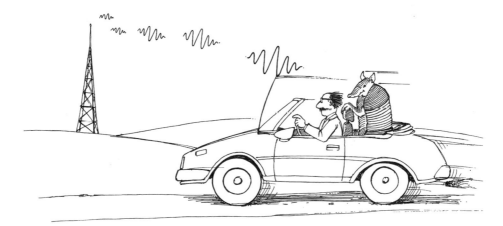

Figure 2-25 Magnetic resonance imaging has several characteristics of a radio.

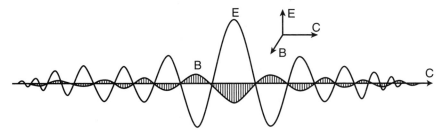

Figure 2-26 An electromagnetic photon consists of electric and magnetic fields oscillating at right angles to one another and traveling at the speed of light.

mathematically in the 1860s by James Clerk Maxwell.

Maxwell's Wave Equations

Maxwell synthesized the then-known laws of electricity and magnetism into what is now known as *Maxwell's wave equations of electromagnetic fields*. At that time, the only electromagnetic radiation recognized was visible light.

Maxwell described light mathematically in terms of oscillating electric and magnetic fields and showed that the interaction of these fields caused a wave to be propagated in free space at a direction 90° to the fields. Furthermore, the velocity of propagation, c, was later shown to be 3×10^8 m/s.

Maxwell's mathematical equations describe a photon of electromagnetic radiation (Figure 2-26). The electric and magnetic fields are at right angles to one another and are also at right angles to the velocity vector, c.

When the field disturbance is perpendicular to the direction of propagation, such radiation is known as a **transverse wave**. In contrast with an ultrasound wave, tissue molecules oscillate in the direction of the velocity vector. Consequently, ultrasound is known as a **longitudinal wave**. The terms *transverse* and *longitudinal* are used later to describe the two MRI relaxation times; however, when so used in MRI, they are not related to waves.

The intensity of each photon begins at zero, increases rapidly to a maximum, and decreases

to zero again. Consequently, each photon does have an origin and a termination. The energy of the electromagnetic photon is determined by the amount of kinetic energy lost by the charged particle.

Maxwell's equations also demonstrated that electromagnetic photons obey the classical wave equation.

Wave Equation
$v = f\lambda$ where λ is the photon wavelength (m), f is the photon frequency (Hz), and v is the velocity (m/s).

The Electromagnetic Spectrum

Mention of Albert Einstein's 1905 theory of relativity and Max Planck's 1915 formulation of quantum mechanics is required to complete a discussion of electromagnetic radiation. Einstein showed that electromagnetic photons behaved relativistically; that is, if two electrons are decelerated together, stationary observers would observe the emission of two photons. However, if observers were on one of the electrons, they would be able to verify that the neighboring electron had only an electric field; no electromagnetic radiation would be detected.

Furthermore, Einstein showed not only that energy was conserved by the conversion of kinetic energy into electromagnetic energy but also that electromagnetic energy could represent the conversion of energy into matter, according to his famous equation.

Relativity

$$E = mc^2$$

where E is the energy in joule (J), m is the particle mass (kg), and c is the photon velocity (m/s).

By the time of Max Planck, the various forms of electromagnetic energy were recognized as being different manifestations of a similar fundamental disturbance. The great body of physical measurements resulting from the previous 100 years' experience with light and optics held that the interaction of electromagnetic radiation with matter was wavelike.

Planck's quantum theory quantized electromagnetic radiation into photons and showed the way such radiation could behave as a particle during its interaction with matter. The proof of this is the photoelectric effect described by Einstein and the fundamental equation underlying Planck's theory.

Plank's Quantum Theory

$$E = hf = hc/\lambda$$

where E is the energy of the photon (J); h is Planck's constant, 6.63×10^{-34} Js; f is frequency; c is the velocity of light; and λ is the wavelength (m).

Planck further showed that electromagnetic radiation indeed actually possessed a duality of nature insofar as its interaction with matter was concerned. Electromagnetic radiation does interact as a particle or a wave, depending on the photon energy.

Electromagnetic radiation extends over an enormously wide range (see Figure 1-1). This span of electromagnetic radiation is known as the *electromagnetic spectrum,* and it extends from radio emissions on the low-energy side through microwaves, infrared, visible light, and ultraviolet to high-energy x-radiation and gamma-radiation.

This representation of the electromagnetic spectrum contains three scales, E, λ, and f, each of which is equivalent according to Planck's quantum theory. In addition, each scale has some historical interest, because it reflects the manner in which the photons are produced and interact with matter.

Light was the earliest electromagnetic radiation to be studied. It was shown to interact primarily as a wave and therefore was usually characterized by its wavelength.

Radio emissions are produced by oscillating electrons energized by a special electric circuit called an **oscillator.** This was first demonstrated by Heinrich Hertz in the 1880s. Because the oscillation of emission is the principal design parameter, these waves are identified by their frequency.

Roentgen discovered x-rays in 1895, and they were characterized by the voltage of production. When Einstein and Planck explained x-ray interaction with matter as particles, it became convention to identify such photons by their energy.

Interest in diagnostic imaging lies in these three distinct regions of the electromagnetic spectrum called **imaging windows.** Each of the three windows is described by one of the three scales.

 An imaging window is a range within the electromagnetic spectrum used to produce images.

The Visible Window.   Visible light interacts with matter more like a wave than a particle. Diffraction, refraction, reflection, and interference are all properties of wavelike interactions, and they all apply to visible light.

Visible light photons range from approximately 400 to 700 nm. Visible light is produced essentially by electron shifts from an excited energy state to the ground state of the outermost shell of an atom. Its wavelength allows it to interact with the receptor cells of the retina, but its quantum energy is too low to ionize matter.

Imaging with visible light occurs by sensing the reflection of light from a patient. Therefore the image of the patient is a surface image and not an image of interior structures. Individual light photons are detected by specially evolved optical light sensors, the rods and cones, of the human eye or by the special molecules in the emulsion of a photographic film.

The X-ray Window. X-rays are produced by changes in the kinetic energy of fast-moving electrons. Bremsstrahlung x-rays can be viewed simplistically as being created by the deceleration of a high-velocity electron in the vicinity of the nucleus of a target atom. Characteristic x-rays are produced when the outer-shell electrons are decelerated at an inner shell. The energy of photons used for x-ray imaging ranges from approximately 20 to 150 kiloelectron volts (keV).

X-rays are used to image the body in much the same way a shadowgram is produced with light (Figure 2-27). Of course, in a shadowgram, only the outline of the figure is imaged. During x-ray examination, not only the outline but also the internal structures are imaged.

X-ray imaging is possible because of the particle-like interactions between x-rays and tissue atoms. These interactions occur principally by way of photoelectric effect and Compton scattering, although at low energies, coherent scattering may also contribute to the attenuation of the x-ray beam. Therefore a radiograph represents the pattern of x-ray attenuation while passing through the patient. The resulting image is a function of the x-ray attenuation coefficient.

The MRI Window. Electromagnetic radiation with frequencies of approximately 10 to 200 MHz is used in MRI. This radiation is in the RF portion of the electromagnetic spectrum.

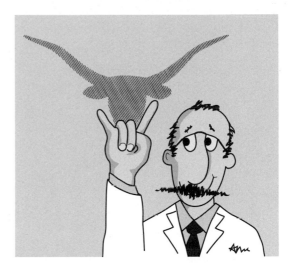

Figure 2-27 X-ray images are similar to a shadowgram except that they provide outlines of internal structures as well as the surface. (Dedicated to Xie Nan Zhu, Guangzhou, People's Republic of China.)

RF is used extensively in communications (television, radio, and microwave). Standard commercial AM broadcast operates from approximately 540 to 1640 kHz. FM radio and television occupy a band of frequencies from approximately 50 to 100 MHz. This range overlaps with the range used in MRI.

Many sources of RF radiation exist in this frequency range, all of which can interfere with the MRI signal. Measures usually must be taken to ensure that these extraneous sources of RF are attenuated or entirely excluded from the coil used to receive the MRI signals.

This presents a problem similar to that encountered in x-ray imaging. An x-ray examination room is shielded to ensure that x-radiation does not escape from the room and create a radiation hazard to persons nearby. An MRI room may require shielding to exclude extraneous RF from the imaging system. Such a shielded room, called a Faraday cage, is discussed in Chapter 13.

CHALLENGE QUESTIONS

1. In an MRI system, what produces the static magnetic field (B_0) and the gradient magnetic fields, (B_{XYZ})?
2. X-ray imaging rooms must be shielded (usually with lead) to reduce the radiation exposure of persons outside of the room. Why are MRI rooms shielded?
3. Who is considered the father of the study of electrostatics, and precisely what is electrostatics?
4. X-rays resemble RFs used in MRI in many ways. What are the similarities and differences?
5. The physical basis for MRI is electromagnetic induction. Just what does the word *induction* mean in this sense?
6. What is the underlying equation that describes quantum mechanics?
7. The electric field is force exerted per electrostatic charge. What are the units of the electric field, and what does each unit represent?
8. The universal wave equation applies to all harmonic motion and in particular to diagnostic ultrasound, x-ray imaging, and MRI. State the wave equation and the units for each parameter.
9. State the four principal laws of electrostatics.
10. How is a magnetic field defined and measured?

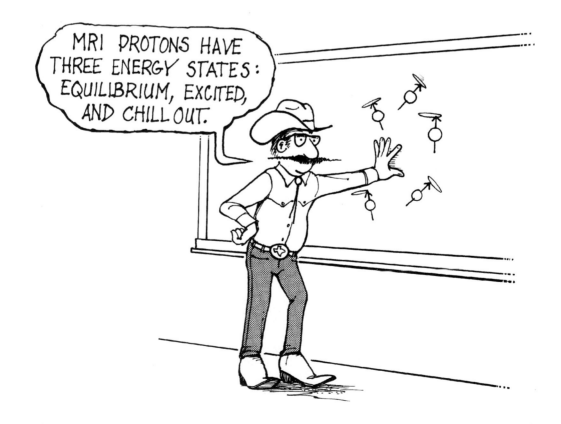

Chapter 3

Nuclear Magnetism

OBJECTIVES

At the completion of this chapter, the student should be able to do the following:

1. Distinguish between classical mechanics and quantum mechanics.
2. State the Larmor equation and relate its importance to magnetic resonance imaging (MRI).
3. Describe the appearance of net magnetization on a vector diagram.
4. Discuss the factors that influence the magnitude of net magnetization.
5. Distinguish between stationary frame and rotating frame and state which is used in MRI.

OUTLINE

QUANTUM MECHANICAL DESCRIPTION
CLASSICAL MECHANICAL DESCRIPTION
    Net Magnetization
    Vector Diagrams
    Control of Net Magnetization

REFERENCE FRAMES
    Stationary Frame
    Rotating Frame

As the name nuclear magnetic resonance (NMR) indicates, the magnetic resonance imaging (MRI) signal originates from the nuclei of atoms resonating in a patient in the presence of a magnetic field. Because this is a nuclear phenomenon, an accurate and complete description requires the use of quantum mechanics.

Quantum mechanics is the branch of physics that describes the behavior of very small objects, such as x-rays, protons, neutrons, and electrons. This branch of physics evolved in the first quarter of the twentieth century and is the basis for contemporary investigations into the structure of matter.

Quantum mechanics, though, is complex and does not provide an intuitive understanding of what is really happening during an MRI examination at the subatomic level. It is highly mathematical and abstract, and although it most accurately describes MRI, it will be avoided here.

> *Classical mechanics deals with large objects; quantum mechanics deals with subatomic particles and photons.*

MRI can mostly be understood in terms of classical mechanics. *Classical mechanics* is the branch of physics that describes the behavior of large objects like rockets, automobiles, and Ping-Pong balls. It has its origins in the seventeenth-century ideas of Sir Isaac Newton.

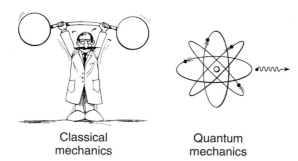

Classical   Quantum
mechanics   mechanics

Figure 3-1 The motion of large objects is described by classical mechanics, that of subatomic particles and photons by quantum mechanics.

The differences between these two branches of physics are demonstrated in Figure 3-1. For many cases, the statistical averaging that occurs over a patient reduces the quantum mechanical description to a classical mechanical description. One quantum mechanical concept, however, that cannot be overlooked or avoided is **nuclear spin.**

QUANTUM MECHANICAL DESCRIPTION

According to quantum mechanics, every nucleus has a quantity called *spin.* This quantity is not exactly what is normally thought of as spin, but it is close enough.

There is one anomaly, though; this spin is quantized into units of half-integer values and called the *spin quantum number.* There are only certain precisely allowed states of spin. The allowed values are 0, ½, 1, ³⁄₂, and so on.

Each nucleus has its own characteristic spin quantum number. For example, all hydrogen atoms of atomic mass 1 have a spin quantum number of ½. All carbon atoms of atomic mass 12 have a spin quantum number of 0. All carbon atoms of atomic mass 13 have a spin quantum number of ½.

The spin quantum number dictates many of the magnetic resonance (MR) properties of a given nuclear species. Table 3-1 presents some nuclei of interest to MRI and their respective spin quantum numbers. Once this quantum mechanical premise is accepted, it is easy to use classical mechanics to describe the way the MR signal is generated.

One result of the spin being quantized is that there are a limited number of ways a nucleus can spin. Each of these ways is called a *spin state.* For a spin ½ nucleus, there are only two allowed spin states, $+\frac{1}{2}$ and $-\frac{1}{2}$.

In general, for a particle with spin S, there are 2S possible spin states, and each spin state is one integer value separated from the next. Thus for a nucleus such as ^{23}Na with a spin quantum number of ³⁄₂, the allowed spin states are $+\frac{3}{2}$, $+\frac{1}{2}$, $-\frac{1}{2}$, and $-\frac{3}{2}$.

A fundamental law of physics states that a spinning mass induces a magnetic field about itself. Earth is one such example. In general, a spinning mass with charge induces an even stronger magnetic field.

The nucleus is a spinning charged particle and therefore has an associated magnetic field. This field is given the special name of **nuclear magnetic moment,** and its intensity is related to the mass, charge, and rate of spin of the nucleus.

 A spinning proton induces nuclear magnetism.

Thus each spin state has a different nuclear magnetic moment. In the absence of an external magnetic field, each spin state has the same energy, but in the presence of an external magnetic field, each spin state has a different energy.

A nucleus in the presence of an external magnetic field prefers to be in the lower energy state than in the higher energy state. Therefore the lower energy state has more nuclei than the higher energy state. Such a system of nuclear spins is said to be at **equilibrium** with the external magnetic field.

With the use of electromagnetic radiation that has an energy exactly equal to the energy difference between two nuclear energy states, this population difference can be disturbed by causing some nuclei of a lower energy state to absorb energy and join the higher energy nuclei (Figure 3-2). The system of energized nuclear spins slowly returns to its original population difference while emitting a signal that can be observed. This is the MRI signal.

CLASSICAL MECHANICAL DESCRIPTION

From the classical mechanics point of view, the nucleus is simply a charged particle that is spinning. The spinning motion generates a magnetic field parallel to the axis of spin.

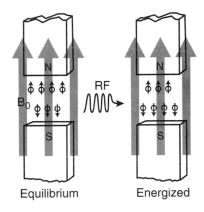

Figure 3-2 At equilibrium, more proton spins are aligned with the magnetic field and said to be in the low-energy state. When energized, more proton spins are aligned against the field.

TABLE 3-1	Magnetic Resonance Imaging Properties of Medically Important Nuclei		
Isotope	**Spin Quantum Number**	**Gyromagnetic Ratio (MHz/T)**	**% Abundance**
^1H	½	42.6	99
^{12}C	0	0	98
^{13}C	½	10.7	1.1
^{16}O	0	0	99
^{17}O	5/2	5.8	0.1
^{19}F	½	40.0	100
^{23}Na	3/2	11.3	100
^{25}Mg	5/2	2.6	10
^{31}P	½	17.2	100
^{33}S	3/2	3.3	0.7
^{57}Fe	½	1.4	2.2

This magnetic field is given the same name of **nuclear magnetic moment** (μ) that was described in quantum mechanics (Figure 3-3). It is referred to with the Greek letter mu (μ). For any individual nucleus, the orientation of the axis of rotation and therefore the direction of the nuclear magnetic moment is random.

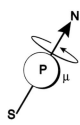

Figure 3-3 A representation of the nuclear magnetic moment (μ) of a hydrogen nucleus.

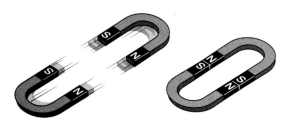

Figure 3-4 The behavior of horseshoe magnets is to align parallel with opposing polarity.

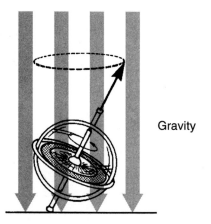

Gravity

Figure 3-5 The motion of a spinning gyroscope in the presence of gravity.

For MRI, the question is how this nuclear magnetic moment will interact with an externally applied magnetic field (B_0). Classically, when two magnets are near, a force is generated that tends to make the two magnetic fields become parallel and pointed in the opposite direction. For horseshoe magnets, this force is manifested by the magnets' aligning in opposition to each other (Figure 3-4).

However, the nucleus is a spinning particle, and thus its actual movement in response to an applied force such as the external magnetic field, B_0, is the same as that produced by a gyroscope; it moves perpendicular to the applied force (Figure 3-5). In the case of the gyroscope, the interaction is mass-mass: the mass of the earth and the mass of the gyroscope.

Similarly, when a nuclear magnetic moment is placed in the presence of an intense static magnetic field, B_0, its axis of rotation precesses about the magnetic field (Figure 3-6).

The exact frequency of precession by such a nucleus can be calculated with the Larmor equation.

Larmor Equation

$f = \gamma B_0$
where f is the frequency of precession (MHz), γ is the gyromagnetic ratio (MHz/T), and B_0 is the strength of the external magnetic field (T).

This equation demonstrates that there is a strictly linear relationship between the frequency of precession, f, and the strength of the external magnetic field, B_0. The gyromagnetic ratio is unique for each type of nucleus and must be measured for each. Thus it is an empirically determined factor used to convert field strength to precessional frequency. The values vary widely and can be found in Table 3-1 for several nuclei of interest to MRI.

This important relationship is used to explain many phenomena for both MRI and

NMR spectroscopy. The key factor is not what the strength is of the external magnetic field but what magnetic field is experienced by the nucleus as modified by many other environmental influences.

For spectroscopy this includes the contribution from the magnetic fields generated by the motion of the bonding electrons, which results in chemical shifts. It also includes time-varying magnetic fields that contribute to T2 relaxation and gradient magnetic fields that result in T2* relaxation. Each of these parameters is dealt with later (see Chapter 7).

For high-resolution NMR spectroscopy, magnetic field strengths are often described in terms of the Larmor frequency at which hydrogen atoms resonate. Thus a 2.35-T magnet is often referred to as a 100-MHz magnet, and an 11.7-T magnet is a 500-MHz magnet. Such odd-numbered field strengths are often used to get the resonant frequency of hydrogen atoms to multiples of 50 or 100 MHz.

For the imaging world, this convenience has not yet been achieved. Field strength values such as 0.5, 1.0, 1.5, and 3.0 T are common, although they result in approximate hydrogen resonant frequencies of 21, 42, 63, and 126 MHz, respectively.

Net Magnetization

Because measuring the action of individual nuclei is impossible, any signals received or data collected during MRI are the result of a bulk phenomenon from perhaps as many as 10^{26} nuclei. This is the approximate number of nuclei in a patient.

 Individual nuclei precess in the presence of an external magnetic field.

A single, isolated nucleus is never observed, just collections of similar nuclei as an aggregate. This aggregate of spins is sometimes called an **ensemble of spins** to emphasize the bulk of the signal-producing nuclear spins. Fortunately the signal from a spin ensemble accurately reflects the behavior of each of the individual nuclei, and therefore the net magne-

tization (M) can be used. M is simply the sum of the individual nuclear magnetic moments, μ.

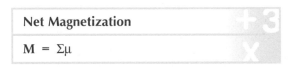

Net Magnetization
$M = \Sigma\mu$

With this equation, the properties of net magnetization during various circumstances can be considered. Because M is just the sum of many μ's, the general behavior of M is identical to the behavior of the individual μ's.

Consider the armadillo shown in Figure 3-7 crossing a highway outside of College Station, Texas, where the Earth's magnetic field is negligible. The orientation of the spin axis of each nucleus is random. Therefore the orientation of an individual nuclear magnetic moment pointing in any given direction is canceled by another nucleus, with its magnetic moment pointing exactly opposite to the first. Consequently, the sum of a large number of nuclear magnetic moments averages out to zero, or M = 0. This agrees with the everyday observation that armadillos are totally nonmagnetic.

Vector Diagrams

Also shown in Figure 3-7 are three axes (X, Y, and Z) drawn perpendicular to one another to

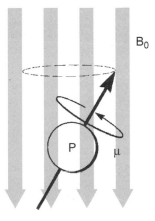

Figure 3-6 Precession of a nuclear magnetic moment in the presence of an external magnetic field.

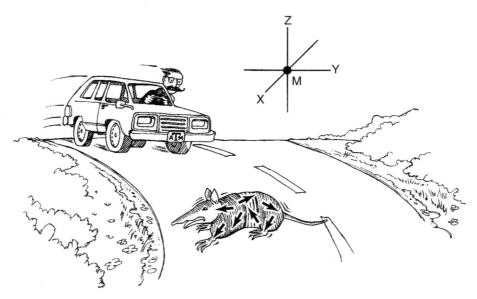

Figure 3-7   The net magnetization of an armadillo in the absence of an external magnetic field is zero.

describe a coordinate system. The illustration shows the Cartesian coordinate system used by mathematicians to diagram phenomena in space. For MRI, such a coordinate system is used to construct vector diagrams.

A *vector* is a quantity that has direction. If a speed of 50 mph is discussed, that is a *scalar* quantity. If traveling 50 mph in a northerly direction is discussed, that is a vector quantity. The net magnetization, M, in Figure 3-7 is a vector quantity with a magnitude of zero. Vector diagrams are extremely helpful in describing MRI phenomena.

When the armadillo is brought to the laboratory and placed in an external magnetic field, something different happens (Figure 3-8). Classically, all the nuclei should precess about the applied field, and the net magnet moment should remain zero.

Quantum mechanics predicts that more nuclei will be in one state rather than in another. This nuclear alignment does not occur instantly but rather over a period of time determined by the molecular nature of the tissues of the armadillo. Some tissues align quickly and others more slowly. One result of this alignment is that the net magnetization will not be zero.

The external magnetic field provides a small preference for the spins to align with the field. This is a small force compared with normal thermal interactions, and only a small number

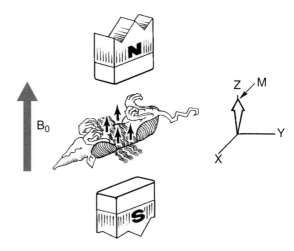

Figure 3-8   The net magnetization of an armadillo resting in a laboratory magnet has magnitude and direction.

of spins align with the external magnetic field. The result can be illustrated as the vector in Figure 3-8, which shows that net magnetization exists along the Z-axis, parallel to the external field.

If the armadillo is left in the magnet for a sufficiently long time, the number of spins oriented with the field stabilizes to an equilibrium value. This value is referred to as M_0 or the **net magnetization at equilibrium,** and it is the largest possible value of M.

By convention, the external magnetic field is parallel to the Z-axis of the Cartesian coordinate system; therefore this magnetization can also be referred to as M_Z or the Z component of the net magnetization. At equilibrium the X and Y components of net magnetization are zero, so $M_X = M_Y = 0$ because all of the equilibrium magnetization is along the Z-axis.

 At equilibrium, $M_Z = M_0$; $M_X = M_Y = 0$.

The intensity of the MR signal is related to the value of M_0. The larger the M_0, the stronger the MR signal. The number of nuclei contributing to M_0 is small (only about one of every 1 million nuclei contribute to M_0), and MRI is therefore a technique that has a poor signal-to-noise ratio. In addition to the number of contributing nuclei, other factors affect the amount of signal available for MRI. These factors can be summarized by the following:

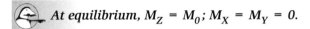

Net Magnetization at Equilibrium
$M_0 \propto \dfrac{PD\gamma^2 \, B_0}{T}$

where α = symbol meaning proportional to
PD = the number of nuclei (proton density) in the volume of interest
T = the temperature of the material under investigation
γ = the gyromagnetic ratio
B_0 = the strength of the external magnetic field

Thus as the concentration of the nuclear species or the volume of tissue being sampled increases, the MR signal increases because the proton density (PD) is greater.

Hydrogen has the highest γ of any nucleus other than tritium (^3H) and has the second largest signal per number of nuclei. Tritium would therefore make an excellent MRI agent, but patients would frown on its use because it is radioactive. For ^{13}C, γ is about one fourth the value for ^1H, and for an equal number of nuclei, the signal available is much less.

At higher magnetic field strength (B_0), the increase in net magnetization results in a stronger MR signal and therefore improvement in any MR image. This is the major reason for going to higher magnetic fields for human imaging systems and spectroscopy. It is only one factor, albeit a very important one.

As the temperature (T) of tissue decreases, the net magnetization increases. However, because this is temperature in Kelvin (K), drastic cooling must be used to obtain any significant increase in the MR signal.

Control of Net Magnetization

Unfortunately, the net magnetization along the Z-axis, M_Z, is invisible. From the quantum mechanical point of view, directly measuring this magnetization is impossible; from the classical point of view, this magnetization, M_Z, is so small relative to B_0 that it cannot be measured.

This fact will become more apparent later. Essentially, it is not possible to measure M_Z; only M_X and M_Y, which are collectively represented by M_{XY}, can be measured.

M_{XY} is net magnetization in the transverse plane (XY plane) and called transverse magnetization.

For M_Z to be observed, the net magnetization must be flipped off the Z-axis and onto the XY plane. M, the net magnetization, is the sum of many nuclear moments and behaves in the same way that the individual nuclear magnetic moments behave. Therefore if the net magnetization is pointing anywhere except exactly along the Z-axis, it precesses about the Z-axis with the same frequency that the individual nuclear magnetic moments precess, the Larmor frequency.

Precession is a form of change of the magnetic field, and this changing magnetic field induces an electric current in a loop of wire or coil placed nearby. The signal can be detected, measured, and recorded.

How is the net magnetization flipped off the Z-axis, and what precisely does this mean? Flipping the net magnetization describes the

direction in which the net magnetization of the patient is altered. Instead of pointing straight up, it will now point somewhere else, actually anywhere else. It is just as big as it was before but has a new direction.

REFERENCE FRAMES

The concept of a **frame of reference** is necessary to follow the motions of the individual nuclear magnetic moments and the net magnetization vector. The frame of reference used is the standard three-dimensional Cartesian coordinate system shown in Figure 3-9.

One convention within this system is that the applied magnetic field is always parallel to the Z-axis. Although the Z-axis is always drawn as up, its actual orientation is determined by the direction of B_0 in the particular magnet system (Figure 3-10).

The B_0 field for a permanent magnet is vertical and therefore passes through the supine patient in the anterior-posterior direction. For some resistive and most superconducting electromagnets, however, the B_0 is horizontal and parallel with the axis of the body and therefore passes through the patient from head to toe.

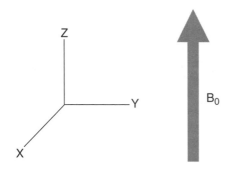

Figure 3-9 The conventional three-dimensional coordinate system used to describe the motion of the net magnetization vector.

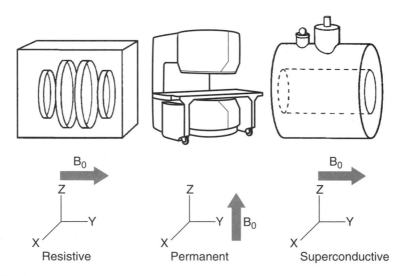

Figure 3-10 The orientation of B_0 and the stationary frame of reference in three types of magnetic resonance imaging systems.

Stationary Frame

The view of someone standing next to the magnet is referred to as the *stationary frame of reference* because all motions are compared with someone standing still in the imaging room.

A second magnetic field with special properties must be used to flip the net magnetization off the Z-axis. The second magnetic field must precess about the B_0 magnetic field with the same frequency as the nuclei, which is the Larmor frequency.

If it does not precess at the Larmor frequency, no interaction between the second magnetic field and the nuclear spins is produced. This phenomenon is called *resonance* because of the requirement that the second magnetic field precesses at exactly the correct frequency or else nothing will happen to the net magnetization vector.

 The second magnetic field must precess with the frequency of the precessing nuclear magnetic moments.

Locating such a magnetic field may seem difficult, but it is not. An electromagnetic emission such as a radiofrequency (RF) is composed of an oscillating electric field positioned 90° to an oscillating magnetic field (see Figure 2-26).

The magnetic field component of an RF emission at the Larmor frequency is effectively a magnetic field rotating at the Larmor frequency. The precessing nuclear magnetic moments interact with the magnetic field component of the RF. Thus through irradiation of the sample with an RF emission, a rotating magnetic field is produced to flip the net magnetization vector into the XY plane.

Rotating Frame

Because the net magnetization is precessing so fast, visualizing its motion is difficult. A trick is used to make it easy to follow the motion of the net magnetization. An example of this can be found in an amusement park.

If someone is in line to go on a carousel and a friend is already on the carousel, it is the same problem presented by the precession of the net magnetization in the stationary frame of reference (Figure 3-11). The rotation of the friend on the carousel relative to the person on the ground makes it difficult to carry on a conversation. However, if the person steps onto the carousel, the friend is stationary relative to the person who can now converse easily. The rest of the world is rotating "backwards" relative to them.

The solution is to use a frame of reference that exactly matches the motion of the net magnetization. This is a reference frame precessing about the Z-axis of the stationary frame of reference and has the same Z-axis. This new frame of reference is called the **rotating frame.**

The stationary frame of reference has axes labeled X, Y, and Z; the rotating frame uses axes X′, Y′, and Z′ to avoid confusion.

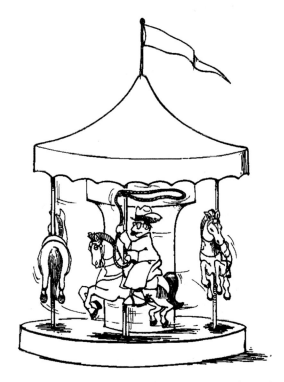

Figure 3-11 The carousel serves to explain the rotating frame. The only way to carry on a conversation with a friend is to jump on the carousel and rotate too.

Unfortunately, because essentially all MRI vector diagrams use the rotating frame of reference, most authors leave the primes off the axes for the rotating frame. This convention is followed in the remainder of this book.

Within the rotating frame of reference, the net magnetization does not precess and is thus easier to follow. The motion of the net magnetization when the second magnetic field is turned on can now be followed.

In the rotating frame of reference, the second magnetic field, B_X, is stationary and is usually aligned along the X-axis (Figure 3-12). It can, however, be aligned along the Y-axis just as easily.

This new magnetic field causes the net magnetization to precess around in the YZ plane with a frequency of γB_X. B_X can be turned off when the net magnetization has reached any given location in the YZ plane. One such point is the XY plane. At this point, all of the net magnetization has been moved into the horizontal plane and will generate the maximum MR signal possible.

The conditions of strength of B_X used to accomplish this are called a *90° RF pulse* because the net magnetization moved through

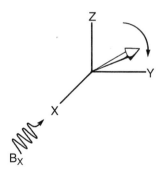

Figure 3-12 In the rotating frame, a secondary magnetic field (B_X) from an radiofrequency emission causes net magnetization to rotate in the YZ plane.

an arc of 90°. These conditions are determined by the time and intensity of the RF pulse.

Each imaging system has its own combination of RF time and intensity; this is related to the RF power and pulse duration used. Another interesting stopping point for the flipped net magnetization is −Z or rotation of the net magnetization through an arc of 180°. The combination of RF power and duration of the pulse that does this is called a *180° RF pulse.*

CHALLENGE QUESTIONS

1. Discuss the differences between the two principal areas of physics, classical mechanics and quantum mechanics.
2. What frame of reference is used when describing MRI vector diagrams?
3. What is a magnetic moment?
4. If hydrogen nuclei, protons, precess at a frequency of 42 MHz, where could one possibly find another alternating field of the same frequency?
5. When an ensemble of proton spins is placed in an external magnetic field, some align with the external field; others align against. Which has more aligned spins, and which spins are in a higher energy state?
6. How are longitudinal magnetization and transverse magnetization symbolized?
7. What is meant by the term *equilibrium?*
8. Precisely, what determines the value of net magnetization at equilibrium, and how is this value symbolized?
9. Nuclear magnetic spectroscopy is usually identified by the frequency of analysis not the magnetic field intensity. Why?
10. Relate the equation that describes net magnetization and identify each parameter.

Chapter 4

Equilibrium–Saturation

OBJECTIVES

At the completion of this chapter, the student should be able to do the following:

1. Define net magnetization and its relationship to equilibrium, partial saturation, and saturation.
2. Distinguish between a hard and a soft radiofrequency (RF) pulse.
3. Identify the primary magnetic resonance (MR) signal.
4. Draw a two-line RF pulse sequence and label all of its components.

OUTLINE

Chapter 3 concluded with an explanation of net magnetization, vector diagrams, and reference frames. Some of this discussion is repeated to properly develop the origin of the radio signal that results in the magnetic resonance image. Furthermore the discussion involves the rotating frame of reference, not the stationary frame.

It is first necessary to consider more closely the way the magnetic resonance imaging (MRI) signal arises. The two basic properties of a nucleus that are important to this signal are the nuclear magnetic moment and spin.

When a sample is placed in an external magnetic field, as indicated by B_0 in Figure 4-1, the nuclei attempt to align with this field. The nuclei act like tiny bar magnets, each seeking to orient itself with the external magnetic field.

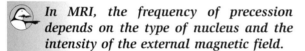 *In MRI, the frequency of precession depends on the type of nucleus and the intensity of the external magnetic field.*

The spin of the nucleus adds a complicating factor. Instead of each nucleus acting like a simple bar magnet, it behaves like a spinning bar magnet. Rather than just aligning with the external field, the nucleus precesses around the axis of the external magnetic field, as described by the Larmor equation.

NET MAGNETIZATION

A patient placed in an MRI system consists of a multitude of proton spins. Many of these protons attempt to align with the external field and precess at the Larmor frequency (Figure 4-2). Although all the protons shown are oriented in an upward direction, the exact direction to which they point at any instant is slightly different because they are at random positions in their precession. The net result is that the individual magnetizations sum to a net magnetization (M) parallel to the direction of the external magnetic field.

Equilibrium

In the preceding situation, the net magnetization does not precess but is a vector of constant magnitude pointed in the direction of the external magnetic field, which is the Z direction. Because they are randomly oriented, the horizontal or X and Y components of all the individual nuclear spins are out of phase, and therefore there is no net magnetization in the XY plane.

This state of the net magnetization is called **equilibrium**. The proton spins are said to be at equilibrium with the external magnetic field.

The magnitude of the net magnetization at equilibrium along the Z-axis, symbolized as M_0, is determined by several physical factors. The more protons available for alignment, the larger M_0 will be.

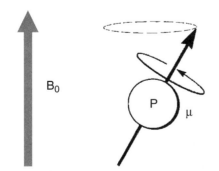

Figure 4-1 In the presence of an external magnetic field, protons align with the field and precess at the Larmor frequency.

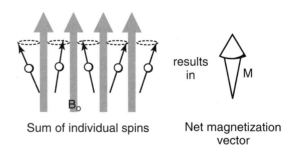

Sum of individual spins

Net magnetization vector

Figure 4-2 The protons aligned with the external magnetic field precess randomly at the same frequency. This results in the net magnetization represented by the vector M.

The number of nuclei available that do align is determined by the intensity of the external magnetic field. Finally, a large gyromagnetic ratio results in a large M_0. Therefore N (the number of nuclei available), B_0, and γ contribute to M_0.

> 🐢 *The larger the M_0, the stronger the MR signal will be.*

Unfortunately, the component of M along the Z-axis cannot be measured directly. It is much too weak compared with B_0 to be detected. Only components of the net magnetization vector in the XY plane, that is, M_{XY}, can be detected by the MRI receiving coil.

The magnetization in the XY plane, M_{XY}, is rotating at the Larmor frequency; therefore it makes no sense to refer to stationary magnetization along either the X- or Y-axis. At equilibrium, no signal is received from the patient because the net magnetization vector, M, points only in the Z direction, M_Z, and has no component in the XY plane, M_{XY} (Figure 4-3).

For a signal to be received from a patient, the magnetization vector must be rotated from the Z-axis so that it has some nonzero component in the XY plane. This rotation follows a pulse of radiofrequency (RF) tuned to the nuclei's Larmor frequency. If the RF is not at this frequency, the nuclei do not absorb energy, and the net magnetization is not rotated.

For typical magnetic fields and nuclei of interest, such as hydrogen, the Larmor frequency corresponds to electromagnetic radiation in the RF range. Thus if the MRI technologist sends a pulse of RF tuned to the precessional frequency of hydrogen, some hydrogen nuclei absorb energy from the RF, and the magnetization vector flips away from the Z-axis (Figure 4-4).

Flip Angle

The net magnetization vector has been rotated an angle α from the Z-axis because individual nuclei have absorbed RF energy and are now in a high-energy state. The high-energy state is opposite the direction of the external magnetic

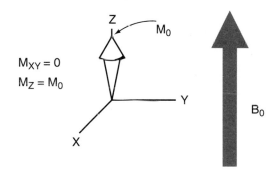

Figure 4-3 At equilibrium, there is no XY component to net magnetization, and the Z component is at its maximum value, M_0.

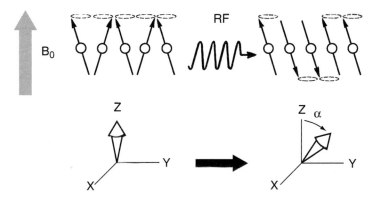

Figure 4-4 A radiofrequency *(RF)* pulse at the Larmor frequency causes the net magnetization vector to flip through the angle α.

field. As long as the RF is energized, the net magnetization vector continues to rotate.

 The net magnetization vector can be rotated to any angle by application of a designed time/intensity RF pulse.

RADIOFREQUENCY PULSES

Hard and Soft Pulses

The angle through which the net magnetization vector is rotated is controlled by two factors. The speed of rotation is controlled by the strength of the RF pulse. A strong RF pulse rotates net magnetization rapidly, whereas a weak RF pulse rotates it more slowly.

The final angle of rotation is controlled by the duration of the RF pulse. It is the product of these two factors—the RF pulse intensity and duration—that determines the final angle of rotation.

 Strong, very short RF pulses are called **hard pulses;** *weaker but longer RF pulses are called* **soft pulses.**

Thus, for example, a 90° RF pulse can be achieved by either a strong RF pulse of short duration or a weak RF pulse lasting a longer time. Regardless, the duration of even the longest RF pulse used in practice is still very short, rarely exceeding 10 ms; this is the reason for calling the burst of RF radiation a *pulse.*

XY Magnetization

Regardless of whether the RF pulse is hard or soft, what is important is how far the net magnetization vector has been rotated—the flip angle. For this reason, both hard and soft pulses are most commonly labeled not by their strength and duration but by the angle through which they rotate the net magnetization vector.

Net magnetization can be rotated through any angle. A 90° RF pulse and 180° RF pulse are most often used in MRI (Figure 4-5).

A 90° RF pulse rotates the net magnetization vector from equilibrium onto the XY plane. Similarly, a 180° RF pulse rotates the net magnetization vector from equilibrium to the −Z-axis. Many fast MRI techniques use so-called alpha (α) pulses. The alpha pulse is identified by a rotation angle less than 90° (e.g., a 10° RF pulse, a 30° RF pulse).

The use of RF pulses in MRI produces an XY component to the net magnetization. When the net magnetization vector is rotated, M_Z shrinks and M_{XY} grows. As previously mentioned, the net magnetization in the XY plane (M_{XY}) is the only magnetization that can be detected as an MR signal from the patient.

 Spins are saturated after a 90° RF pulse so that $M_Z = 0$, $M_{XY} = M_0$.

The net magnetization vector shown in Figure 4-6 has absorbed energy from an RF pulse and is no longer at equilibrium. The components of the net magnetization vector are different from

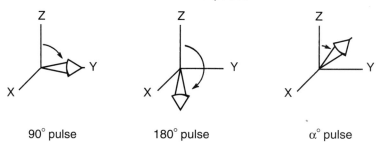

Nomenclature of pulses

90° pulse   180° pulse α° pulse

Figure 4-5   In MRI, 90° and 180° radiofrequency pulses are often used. Smaller flip angles may be used for fast imaging.

those at equilibrium. M_Z is smaller than M_0 and M_{XY} is no longer zero. When this occurs, the nuclear spins are said to be **partially saturated**. If the net magnetization were totally in the XY plane, then the spins would be **saturated**.

M_{XY} Precession

After excitation by an RF pulse, the net magnetization vector does not remain stationary but undergoes a complex motion made up of two parts. First, the magnetization vector begins to precess, just as if it were an individual nucleus. This occurs because the individual nuclear magnetic moments that were precessing randomly are caused to precess **in phase** (see Figure 4-4). This precession is also at the Larmor frequency. Thus if M_{XY} is looked at from above, it would be seen rotating at the Larmor frequency (Figure 4-7).

Return to Equilibrium

Immediately after RF excitation, the net magnetization vector seeks to realign itself with the external magnetic field. That is, the magnetization vector M_Z slowly returns to its equilibrium position as the saturated nuclear spins individually flip back to their normal state of alignment with the external magnetic field. This is shown in Figure 4-8 as the regrowth of M_Z along the Z-axis.

The net result of these two motions, precession and return to equilibrium, can be thought of as a spiral pattern (Figure 4-9). The spiral pattern is a graphic simplification because the two processes are independent. The XY component precesses at the Larmor frequency and shrinks until it disappears. The Z component gradually grows until it reaches its maximum value at equilibrium, M_0.

Both of these changes in component magnitude, the shrinking of the XY component and growth of the Z component, are independent processes that are linked through the Bloch equations. The net magnetization vector is not rigid like a pencil. Rather, it changes size as it rotates, resulting in a complex motion. The XY

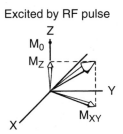

Figure 4-6 Flipping net magnetization from the Z-axis reduces M_Z and increases M_{XY}.

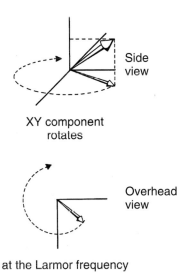

Figure 4-7 After a radiofrequency pulse that flips net magnetization from the Z-axis, the XY component, M_{XY}, rotates at the Larmor frequency.

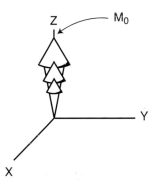

Figure 4-8 After a radiofrequency pulse, the Z component of net magnetization, M_Z, relaxes to equilibrium, M_0, along the Z-axis.

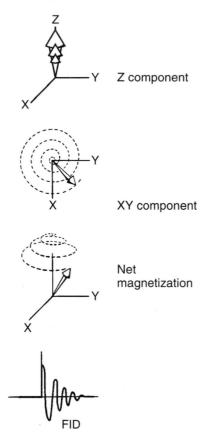

Z component

XY component

Net
magnetization

FID

Figure 4-9 Relaxation of M_Z and precession with relaxation of M_{XY} bring about a complicated corkscrewlike motion that results in return to equilibrium and the MR signal, a free induction decay *(FID)*.

component shrinks at a much faster rate than the Z component returns to equilibrium. The decreasing M_{XY} is **transverse relaxation (T2)**; the increasing M_Z **is longitudinal relaxation (T1).**

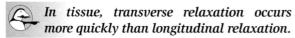 *In tissue, transverse relaxation occurs more quickly than longitudinal relaxation.*

Only M_{XY}, however, is responsible for the MR signal. A receiving coil outside the patient views the precessional motion as an oscillating magnetic field alternately approaching and receding. The coil is unaware of the return of net magnetization along the Z-axis to M_0.

The electric current induced in the coil by the oscillating magnetic field has a waveform

like that shown in Figure 4-9. This is the primary MR signal: the free induction decay. Secondary MR signals, the spin echo and the gradient echo, are discussed later.

FREE INDUCTION DECAY

With all this complex motion of the net magnetization occurring, what can be observed? The only part of the net magnetization that can be observed is the XY component. As long as M_{XY} precesses with spins in phase and is not zero, an oscillating signal is received. The strength of the signal received is proportional to the size of the XY component. As M_{XY} relaxes to zero, the MR signal is reduced to zero. This decreasing MR signal, which is received after an RF pulse, is called a **free induction decay (FID)**. The free induction decay is the primary MR signal.

When the net magnetization vector is at equilibrium, there is no signal. The effect of the 90° RF pulse is to rotate the net magnetization vector onto the XY plane. At this point an oscillating MR signal is received, because there is now a large XY component to the net magnetization vector (Figure 4-10).

 The oscillation of the signal is at the same frequency as the rotation of M_{XY}, namely, the Larmor frequency.

As the net magnetization returns to equilibrium, the XY component shrinks rapidly, and the Z component increases but less rapidly. When M_{XY} relaxes to zero, the MR signal is again zero. This sequence of events is shown in Figure 4-10 and, when repeated many times, constitutes the simplest MRI RF pulse sequence, which is called **saturation recovery.**

RADIOFREQUENCY PULSE DIAGRAMS

In the macroscopic world, two events occur during an MRI sequence. First, an RF pulse, for example, a 90° RF pulse, is transmitted into the patient. The transmitted RF pulse is symbol-

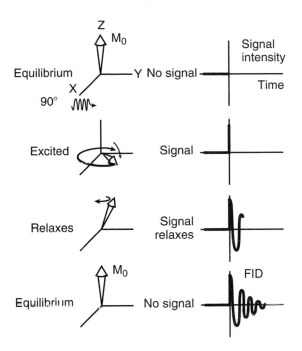

Figure 4-10 Equilibrium followed by excitation followed by relaxation to equilibrium with emission of a radiofrequency (RF) signal is the simplest magnetic resonance imaging RF pulse sequence.

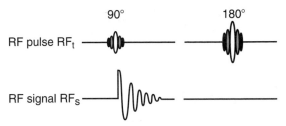

Figure 4-11 Simple radiofrequency (RF) pulse diagrams for a 90° and a 180° RF pulse. The top line represents the transmitted RF pulse *(RF_t)*, and the bottom line represents the RF signal received *(RF_s)*.

The signal from the patient is indicated by a plot of the intensity of the signal versus time. For the simple case given here, the diagram is correspondingly simple. In more complicated situations involving many pulses and signals, such diagrams are complicated but can be extremely descriptive.

Additional lines are added to indicate excitation of the gradient magnets necessary for spatial localization of the RF_s. For now, it is sufficient to become familiar with this simple two-line form of an RF pulse diagram. This is the forerunner of the musical score to be discussed in Chapter 16.

What about the amplitude and shape of the FID? The amplitude of the FID is equal to the amplitude of M_Z at the start of the RF pulse sequence. This amplitude is often equal to and always dependent on M_0, the equilibrium value. Therefore the amplitude of the FID is determined by the same parameters that influence M_0, namely, the number of spins involved (the proton density), B_0, and γ.

CHALLENGE QUESTIONS

1. Why do different nuclear species (e.g., hydrogen, sodium, fluorine) precess at a different frequency in the presence of the same magnetic field?
2. How does one indicate and symbolize an RF pulse that is transmitted into the patient?

ized as RF_t. Second, an RF signal symbolized as RF_s is received from the patient. This signal is the FID, and these two events are diagrammed in Figure 4-11.

There are two lines of information on the diagram. The horizontal axis in both cases is time. The top line, or RF_t, is the RF signal transmitted into the patient. The bottom line, or RF_s, is the FID, the MR signal received from the patient.

RF pulses transmitted into the patient are usually indicated on the RF_t line by several ovals, as shown on the top line. The label above the smaller pulse indicates that it is a 90° RF pulse, and the label above the larger pulse indicates that it is a 180° RF pulse. After a 180° RF pulse, there is no FID because there is no XY component to the net magnetization.

3. At equilibrium, the net magnetization vector aligns with the external magnetic field rather than precesses as the proton spins do. Why?
4. What is the primary MR signal and its origin?
5. Why can the net magnetization at equilibrium, M_0, not be detected and generate an MR signal?
6. Which takes longer to relax to equilibrium value after excitation, longitudinal magnetization or transverse magnetization?
7. What is the value of M_Z and M_{XY} at equilibrium?
8. What MRI parameter ultimately determines the intensity of the MR signal?
9. What is M_Z and M_{XY} for an ensemble of proton spins that are saturated?
10. What is the flip angle in MRI?

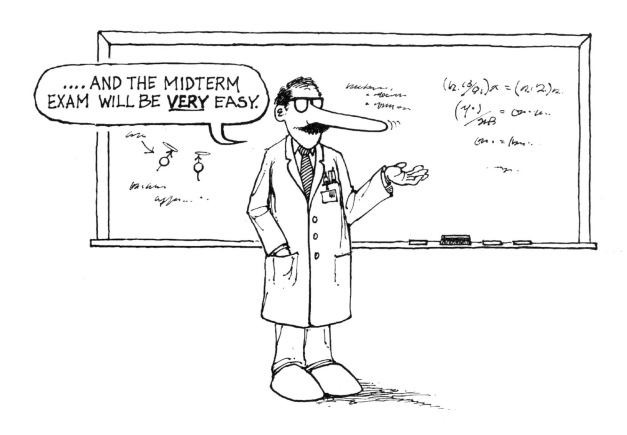

Chapter 5

Radiofrequency Pulse Sequences

OBJECTIVES

At the completion of this chapter, the student should be able to do the following:
1. Identify the components of a radiofrequency (RF) pulse sequence.
2. Draw and describe the saturation recovery pulse sequence.
3. Draw and describe the spin echo pulse sequence.
4. Draw and describe the inversion recovery pulse sequence.
5. Draw and describe the gradient echo pulse sequence.

OUTLINE

Although the free induction decay (FID) is the primary magnetic resonance imaging (MRI) signal, it is difficult to use in practice. A hard radiofrequency (RF) pulse must be transmitted into the patient at the Larmor frequency to obtain the FID. The FID, which is a weak signal, also at the Larmor frequency, immediately follows this RF pulse.

The RF coil must listen for a very weak signal after a very strong excitation RF pulse. In most systems the RF transmitter and the signal receiver share the same electronics and frequently the same coil. This makes it necessary to switch quickly from transmit mode for the RF pulse to receive mode for the FID.

Although this switching is done electronically and is extremely fast, some finite delay is involved. This results in the loss of some of the initial part of the FID. Therefore, for the patient to provide additional signals, more than one RF pulse may be required.

This grouping of two or more RF pulses is called a **pulse sequence**. The term *pulse sequence* as used in MRI includes the RF pulses and excitation of gradient magnetic fields.

MRI involves three basic pulse sequences (saturation recovery, spin echo, and inversion recovery) and several fast imaging pulse sequences (gradient echo and echo planar). This chapter introduces the reader to the nomenclature that accompanies these pulse sequences. Later chapters detail what these pulse sequences do and how they affect the magnetic resonance (MR) image.

SATURATION RECOVERY

Saturation recovery (SR) is the simplest of pulse sequences. It consists of a string of 90° RF pulses and is sometimes indicated as 90°-90°-90° . . . (Figure 5-1). An FID is produced after each 90° RF pulse.

 When $M_Z = 0$ and $M_{XY} = M_0$, the spins are said to be saturated.

In MRI, except for some fast imaging techniques, the data from one pulse sequence are not sufficient to generate an image; rather the sequence must be repeated many times. A sequence may need to be repeated 256 times to obtain data for a 256 × 256 image.

These repetitions are usually spaced by a sizable delay. The time from the start of one pulse sequence to the start of the next pulse sequence is the repetition time (TR).

If the TR is long, the amplitude of the second and successive FIDs equals the amplitude of the first FID. If the TR is short, M_Z will not have relaxed to equilibrium, M_0. The spins remain partially saturated, resulting in a smaller-intensity FID for the second and successive FIDs. This pulse sequence is a **partial saturation** pulse sequence.

SPIN ECHO

MRI does not use the FID except for very fast techniques. The first part of the FID is difficult to detect because of the simultaneous need for gradient magnetic fields and slice-selective RF

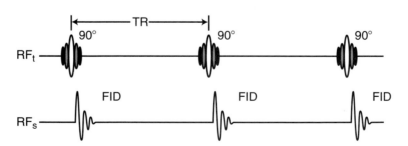

Figure 5-1 The saturation recovery pulse sequence.

pulses. If a 180° RF pulse follows the 90° RF pulse at some later time, an echo signal of the FID can be generated.

This echo signal, called a **spin echo (SE),** does not follow the 180° RF pulse immediately. Thus switching the coil from the transmit-mode to the receive-mode does not cause any of the SE to be missed (see Chapter 6 for further discussion).

 The time between the initial 90° RF pulse and the SE is called time-to-echo (TE).

The time between the 180° RF pulse and the SE equals the time between the 90° and the 180° RF pulses. By controlling the time for the 180° RF pulse, the MRI technologist can control TE. The SE pulse sequence is indicated as 90°-180° . . . 90°-180° . . . .

If another 180° RF pulse follows the SE, an additional SE can be generated with a TE that once again is measured from the initial 90° pulse (Figure 5-2). This pulse sequence is a SE pulse sequence.

INVERSION RECOVERY

Another common pulse sequence is inversion recovery (IR). The IR RF pulse sequence adds a 180° RF pulse before the 90° RF pulse. This 180° RF pulse rotates the net magnetization vector through 180° onto the –Z-axis; that is, it inverts the net magnetization.

 No MR signal is generated after a 180° RF pulse.

After a delay called *inversion-delay-time* (TI), a 90° RF pulse is applied to rotate the net magnetization onto the XY plane where it can be detected and produce a signal. Once again, SEs are created by adding one or more 180° RF pulses (Figure 5-3).

As with the SE pulse sequence, the FID produced by the 90° RF pulse is disregarded. Only SEs are used to make an image. The IR pulse sequence is indicated as 180°-90°-180° . . . 180°-90°-180° . . . 180°-90°-180° . . . .

GRADIENT ECHO

Some fast imaging techniques use a gradient echo (GRE) pulse sequence. An RF pulse of less than 90° called an α *RF pulse* is applied, which results in an FID that is manipulated. The signal intensity of the FID is lower with lower flip angle RF pulses.

Gradient magnetic fields, rather than additional RF pulses, cause the spins to dephase and rephase forming the signal echo within the FID, which is a **GRE.** The GRE, like the SE, is a secondary MR signal that has lower intensity with lower α flip angle RF pulses. However, even with α as low as 10°, a sufficient signal is produced to provide quality images.

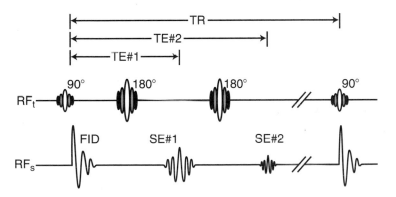

Figure 5-2 When the 90° radiofrequency *(RF)* pulse is followed by an 180° RF pulse, a spin echo *(SE)* results. This is an SE pulse sequence.

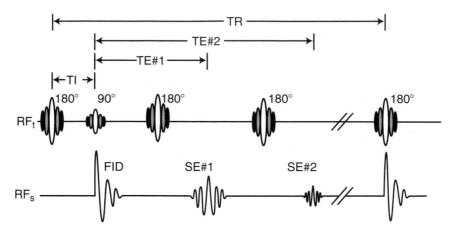

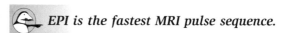

Figure 5-3 The inversion recovery pulse sequence also produces spin echoes *(SEs)*.

This pulse sequence is indicated as $\alpha°$-$\alpha°$-$\alpha°$ . . . . The GRE pulse sequence is shown in Figure 5-4 without the gradient magnetic fields. Subsequent chapters will expand on the importance of TR, TE, and TI in image production and contrast rendition.

ECHO PLANAR IMAGING

The fastest MR RF imaging sequence is echo planar imaging (EPI); this pulse sequence produces complete images in as little as 50 ms. EPI is used for MR fluoroscopy and functional imaging.

EPI involves a 90° RF excitation pulse, which may be followed by a 180° RF refocusing pulse, which creates a conventional SE. However, if the phase-encoding and read gradient is cycled 64 times during the SE, 64 GREs will be created and detected (Figure 5-5).

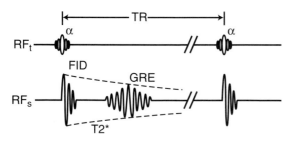

Figure 5-4 The gradient echo *(GRE)* pulse sequence.

EPI is the fastest MRI pulse sequence.

The following summarizes these principal MRI RF pulse sequences:

MRI RF Pulse Sequences
SR 90° . . . . . . 90° . . . . . . 90° . . . . . .
SE 90°-180° . . . . . . -90°-180° . . . . . . 90°-180° . . . . . .
IR 180°-90°-180° . . . . . . 180°-90°-180° . . . . . .
GRE $\alpha°$ . . . . . . $\alpha°$ . . . . . . $\alpha°$ . . . . . .
EPI 90°-180° . . .

CHALLENGE QUESTIONS

1. What makes the FID more difficult to detect than an SE?
2. Describe the RF pulse sequence used for SE imaging.
3. What does the term *pulse sequence* mean when applied to MRI?
4. Of all the available MRI pulse sequences, which provides the fastest imaging?
5. When does an SR pulse sequence become a partial saturation pulse sequence?

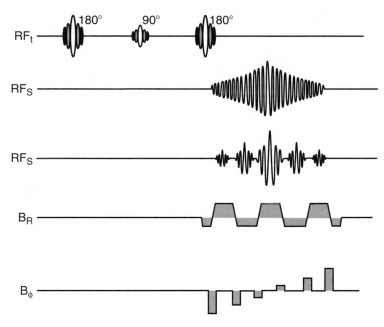

Figure 5-5 The echo planar imaging pulse sequence.

6. How is the RF pulse indicated for a GRE echo pulse sequence?
7. What is the TE in SE imaging?
8. Diagram the transmitted and received signals for a double echo, SE pulse sequence.

9. What is the inversion time in an IR pulse sequence?
10. What is the MRI signal called when it is obtained during an IR pulse sequence?

Magnetic Resonance Imaging Parameters

It is essential to understand the following three principal parameters of magnetic resonance imaging (MRI): proton density (PD), T1 relaxation time, and T2 relaxation time. Each is fundamentally different from and independent of the others.

Images of each of these parameters cannot be produced directly. Images weighted by each of these parameters can be produced by carefully selecting the type of radiofrequency (RF) pulse sequence and the RF pulse times, which include repetition time (TR), time-to-echo (TE), and inversion-delay time (TI). Such images are identified as proton density weighted (PDW), T1 weighted (T1W), and T2 weighted (T2W) according to which parameter is emphasized.

PROTON DENSITY

The amplitude of the net magnetization is related to several parameters as previously described in Chapter 3. It is reasonable to expect that one of the parameters that affects the amplitude of the magnetic resonance (MR) signal might be the number of hydrogen nuclei within the volume of the sample. If no hydrogen nuclei are present, no signal should be expected. Conversely, if the sample is rich in hydrogen, a strong MR signal may be expected. Voxels with high hydrogen concentration or PD appear bright. This reasoning holds true only to a certain extent.

 MR signal intensity is proportional to PD, γ^2, and B_0.

MRI signal amplitude depends on the presence or absence of hydrogen nuclei and is also sensitive to the environment of the hydrogen nuclei. How hydrogen is bound within a molecule also influences the amplitude of the MR signal.

Tightly bound hydrogen creates a weak signal. Therefore the MR signal received originates from loosely bound hydrogen nuclei, which are called **mobile hydrogen**. Hydrogen nuclei found in liquids are mobile.

An example of this effect is bone. Cortical bone appears black on an MR image because it does not emit an MR signal. This is not due to the absence of hydrogen; rather, the hydrogen nuclei are tightly bound to the molecule. As a result, bone looks like air, which has a low hydrogen concentration. However, medullary bone is visible because of the fat located in the spaces between the trabeculae and in the marrow cavities.

PD is the measure of the concentration of mobile hydrogen nuclei available to produce an MR signal. The higher the concentration of mobile hydrogen nuclei, the stronger the net magnetization at equilibrium (M_0) and the more intense the MR signal. A strong MR signal results in a better MR image.

Figure 6-1 shows three pixels highlighted in the cross section of the patient. Each represents a voxel containing different tissue with different concentrations of mobile hydrogen nuclei. The tissue with the highest proton density (PD) also has the largest value M_0. Table 6-1 shows averages of relative values of PD for several tissues.

Although a large M_0 is necessary for a strong MR signal, the M_Z is undetectable. In an MRI system, the receiver detects only the XY component of net magnetization—M_{XY}. Because M_{XY} is zero at equilibrium, no MR signal is received. Patients whose nuclei are at equilibrium do not emit an MR signal. The net magnetization must have a component in the XY plane to produce an MR signal.

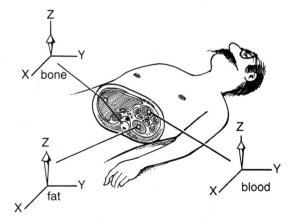

Figure 6-1 M_0 and signal intensity are proportional to mobile hydrogen concentration or proton density (PD). These three voxels each have different PDs.

TABLE 6-1	Approximate Values of Mobile Hydrogen Nuclei Spin Density for Various Tissues

Tissue	Relative Spin Density
Muscle	90
White matter	60
Fat	95
Cerebrospinal fluid	100
Kidney	95
Gray matter	70
Spleen	90
Liver	90
Blood	85
Cortical bone	1-10
Lung	1-5
Air	<1

T1 RELAXATION TIME

When a patient is positioned in the magnetic field of an MRI system, the net magnetization of the patient does not change instantly. In fact, the M_Z changes rapidly at first and then relatively slowly (Figure 6-2; Appendix A). The longitudinal magnetization, M_Z, reaches equilibrium after approximately five T1 relaxation times.

 One T1 relaxation time results in relaxation to 63% of M_0.

Once equilibrium is reached and M_Z equals M_0, this condition of net magnetization continues indefinitely unless the spins are disturbed. If the magnet is turned off or the patient is removed from the magnetic field, the individual nuclear magnetic moments reposition randomly. This causes the net magnetization along the Z-axis to disappear, so M_Z returns to zero (Figure 6-3).

The time constant that describes the rate at which M_Z returns to M_0 is the *T1 relaxation time*. For tap water, T1 is about 2500 ms. For tissue in vivo, T1 can be as short as 100 ms for fatty tissues and as long as 2000 ms for bodily fluids such as cerebrospinal fluid (Table 6-2).

 Generally, the T1 of diseased and damaged tissue is longer than that for corresponding healthy tissue.

An equation describing how M_Z relaxes toward equilibrium has an exponential form. The further M_Z is from M_0, the faster it approaches M_0. As the ensemble of nuclear spins gets closer to M_0, M_Z approaches more slowly.

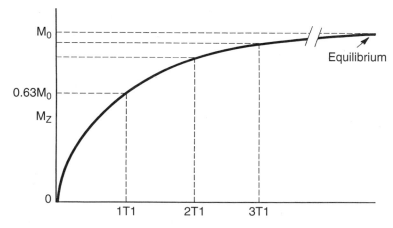

Figure 6-2   The relaxation of M_Z with time after positioning a patient in a strong magnetic field depends on the T1 relaxation time.

The ensemble of nuclear spins relaxes to $0.63\ M_0$ in one T1. As a result, it takes approximately five T1 for a spin ensemble to return to M_0 once it has been disturbed. When repetitive MR signals are sampled for imaging, the amount of magnetization available for the next sampling is limited.

T1 is also called the *longitudinal* or *spin-lattice relaxation time*. The term *longitudinal* refers to events occurring along the axis of the net magnetization vector, which is parallel to B_0. T1 relaxation describes the growth and decay of M_Z; therefore it is longitudinal in nature.

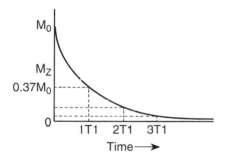

Figure 6-3 M_Z shrinks with time constant T1 when the patient is removed from an external magnetic field.

TABLE 6-2	Approximate T1 Relaxation Times at a Field Strength of 1.0 T for Various Tissues

Tissue	T1 (ms)
Fat	180
Liver	270
Renal cortex	360
White matter	390
Spleen	480
Gray matter	520
Muscle	600
Renal medulla	680
Blood	800
Cerebrospinal fluid	2000
Water	2500

 T1 relaxation time is the same as longitudinal relaxation time or spin-lattice relaxation time.

When a patient is in the magnet at equilibrium, the net magnetization is constant and of maximum amplitude, M_0. If the nuclei become disturbed by directing an RF pulse at the Larmor frequency into the patient, the nuclei absorb energy, and the net magnetization is rotated and changed in magnitude.

This new magnetization state of the patient is unstable because the nuclei want to realign with the external magnetic field and return to equilibrium. The regrowth of M_Z is the T1 process and represents the spin's return to equilibrium.

Nuclei must give up the energy gained from the transmitted RF pulse to return to equilibrium. The hydrogen nuclei are bound with other atoms to form a molecule. This arrangement is called a **lattice**. The regrowth of M_Z is accomplished by transferring energy to other atoms in the molecule or to the molecule as a whole; that is, the energy is released by an interaction between the individual hydrogen nuclei (spin) and the surrounding molecule or other molecules (lattice).

Pixel intensity in an MR image is a complicated function of the T1 relaxation time. Whether a pixel appears bright or dark depends on the RF pulse sequence.

 Generally, for T1W images, tissue with short T1 appears bright; tissue with long T1 appears dark.

T2 RELAXATION TIME

The magnitude of M_Z and M_{XY} after the application of a 90° RF pulse is shown in Figure 6-4. They are similar in shape. Much like radioactive decay, they are both exponential in form. The T1 relaxation time is much longer than the T2 relaxation time. Just as T1 relaxation controls M_Z, T2 relaxation controls M_{XY}. The constants T1 and T2 control the rate of relaxation of M_Z and M_{XY}, respectively. Each is a fundamental property of tissue.

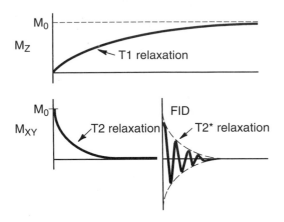

Figure 6-4 After a 90° radiofrequency pulse, M_Z relaxes to M_0. M_{XY} relaxes to zero more quickly because T2 relaxation times are considerably shorter than T1 relaxation times. T2* relaxation is the envelope of the free induction decay *(FID)*.

 T2 relaxation never exceeds T1 relaxation time for any given tissue.

A large value for T1 or T2 indicates a long, gradual relaxation; a small value indicates a rapid relaxation. For example, the T1 and T2 for water are approximately 2500 ms, indicating that the signal would take several seconds to relax. This occurs much like a struck bell, which reverberates for several seconds.

Because the relaxation of M_Z is independent of M_{XY}, T1 and T2 are also independent. T2 is always less than T1. Because the MR signal received is proportional to M_{XY}, it also relaxes according to T2, and the envelope of the free induction decay (FID) is exponential in T2 (Figure 6-4).

It may seem strange that T1 relaxation is represented by an increasing value with time, whereas T2 relaxation is represented by a decreasing value. This happens because the relaxation of M_Z to M_0 is actually a relaxation from the excited state to the equilibrium state, whereas M_{XY} is relaxation to zero.

Analogous to T1, T2 is called the *transverse relaxation time*. Because T2 relaxation represents a loss of XY magnetization, it represents the loss of phase coherence in a plane perpendicular to or transverse to M_0. M_0 lies along the Z-axis.

 T2 relaxation time is the same as transverse relaxation time or spin-spin relaxation time.

T2 relaxation also involves the exchange of energy among the nuclei. The M_{XY} vector shrinks because the nuclei are interacting with each other, and this causes spin dephasing.

In any material above absolute zero in temperature, molecules and atoms are in constant motion. At room temperature, this motion is so rapid that the nuclei continually bounce into each other. This continual jostling allows one nucleus to lose energy to other nuclei. This is the principal mechanism for the relaxation of M_{XY}—the transfer of energy from one spin to another.

Pixel intensity in an MR image is also a complicated function of T2 relaxation time. The pulse sequence that is used determines the T2-related brightness of pixels. Table 6-3 presents approximate values of T2 relaxation times for various tissues.

TABLE 6-3	Approximate T2 Relaxation Times at a Field Strength of 1.0 T for Various Tissues
Tissue	**T2 (ms)**
Muscle	40
Liver	50
Renal cortex	70
Spleen	80
Fat	90
White matter	75
Gray matter	90
Renal medulla	140
Blood	180
Cerebrospinal fluid	200
Water	2500

Generally, with T2W images, tissue with long T2 appears bright; tissue with short T2 appears dark.

Phase Coherence

With the three fundamental MRI parameters known, a simple experiment can be done to see whether the effects of each can be observed. After a 90° RF pulse, the net magnetization is rotated onto the XY plane. A large M_{XY} will be detected as a signal. As a result of T2 relaxation, M_{XY} shrinks and the signal shrinks, too. Before equilibrium is reached, the signal has relaxed to zero.

The T2 can be calculated directly, because the shrinking of the MR signal follows the relaxation of M_{XY} exactly. However, unexpected results are obtained when the experiment is performed.

After excitation with a 90° RF pulse, the FID shrinks more rapidly instead of lasting for several seconds. The T2 obtained from such a measurement is called *T2 star* (*T2**). T2* is much shorter than T2 (Figure 6-5).

T2 must be determined indirectly. Consider the nuclei in the B_0 magnetic field of a patient who is approximately 50 cm long. Divide that length into three regions and consider the nuclear spins that lie within each of these three regions (Figure 6-6). After the 90° RF pulse at time zero, the net magnetization vectors of the three regions are flipped onto the XY plane along the Y-axis (Figure 6-7).

Even though the patient is considered to be divided into three regions, the received MR signals still come from throughout the patient. Therefore the signal is the vector sum of the net magnetization of the three regions. Because the magnetization vectors in the three regions all point in the same direction, they add maximally and produce a large signal.

At some later time (time A), the three net magnetization vectors of Figure 6-7 have changed. They are shorter because of T2 relaxation. They have rotated and now point in a new direction (i.e., they are precessing). The rate of precession is the same for each net magnetization vector because this is controlled by the magnetic field strength in the three regions and B_0 is the same in each region.

The net result is that each M_{XY} is smaller and changed direction, but they all still point in the same direction. Their sum is smaller than at time zero because of T2 relaxation.

At some later time (time B), the net magnetization vectors have continued to decrease because of T2 relaxation. Now they point in another direction as a result of precession, but they still all point in the same direction. Once again, their sum has decreased.

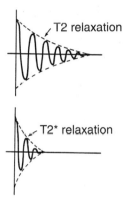

Figure 6-5 Theoretically, M_{XY} should relax as T2. The actual relaxation is much shorter and is called T2*.

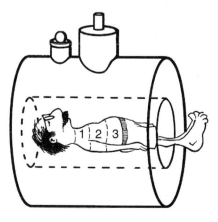

Figure 6-6 To visualize T1 and T2*, consider a patient in a magnet whose trunk is divided into three regions.

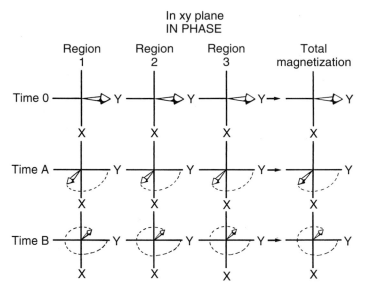

Figure 6-7   In a perfect magnet, loss of M$_{XY}$ is the same throughout a homogeneous tissue.

The dotted line in Figure 6-8 represents the envelope of the decreasing, precessing signal, which results in an FID. The envelope is reduced with a time constant T2. This condition in which all the spins precess together so that they are always pointing in the same direction is termed **in phase.** The spins have maintained **phase coherence.**

Frequency and phase are sometimes confused. For example, a saloon in Houston has five clocks above the bar (Figure 6-9). Each indicates the same time. They each have the same frequency (i.e., one revolution per hour for the minute hand) and the same phase, because all hands point in the same direction. A reception desk in a fancy San Francisco hotel also has five clocks (Figure 6-10). These clocks indicate the time in various cities around the world. The clocks have the same frequency, but they are out of phase.

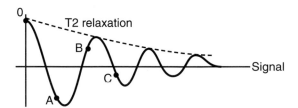

Figure 6-8   The envelope of the free induction decay obtained from a perfect magnet describes T2 relaxation. Times *0* (zero), *A*, *B*, and *C* refer to Figure 6-7.

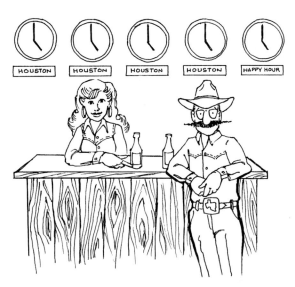

Figure 6-9   The five clocks above the bar in a Houston saloon have the same frequency. They are also in phase.

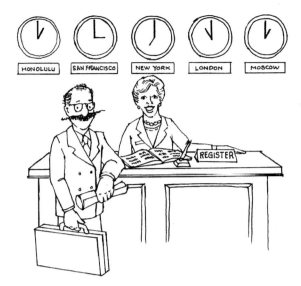

Figure 6-10 The five clocks above the reception desk of a fancy San Francisco hotel have the same frequency, but they are out of phase.

The key assumption in the earlier description is that the magnetic field in the three regions of the patient is the same. Such B_0 field uniformity causes all net magnetization vectors to rotate at precisely the same frequency and remain in phase.

It is impossible to build such a perfect magnet in real life. Although the magnets used in MRI are high quality, the magnetic fields are not perfectly uniform. The field strength varies slightly from place to place in the imaging aperture. Even this small nonuniformity in magnetic field intensity greatly affects the MR signal.

T2* Relaxation

A different FID results if the earlier MRI experiment is repeated with a less-than-perfect magnet. Once again, a 90° RF pulse is transmitted into the patient, and the net magnetization vectors in the three regions flip together onto the XY plane along the Y-axis, as shown at time zero in Figure 6-11. At this point, the magnetization vectors are all parallel and add maximally as before. However, as time progresses, something different occurs. The magnetization vectors will be different at time A.

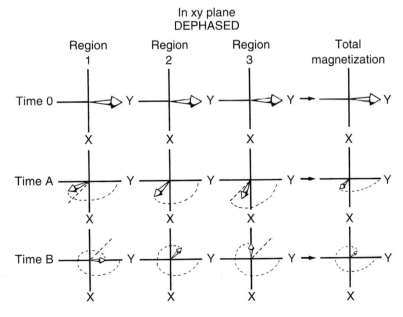

Figure 6-11 In a magnetic resonance imaging system, inhomogeneity of the magnetic field causes M_{XY} to relax more rapidly than expected. The result is T2* relaxation.

Each vector shrinks by the same amount as a result of T2 relaxation, so they remain at equal but reduced length. Each has also precessed in the magnetic field. However, because the magnetic field is slightly different in the three regions, each vector rotates differently so that they now point in slightly different directions. For example, the magnetization vector in region 1 is in a slightly higher field and precesses at a slightly faster rate; therefore, at time A, it has rotated a little further than its neighbor in region 2. In contrast, the magnetization vector in region 3 is in a slightly lower magnetic field and therefore has precessed more slowly. It points in yet another direction.

When these three magnetization vectors are added together, the total net magnetization vector is smaller for two reasons. First, T2 has shortened all three magnetization vectors equally. Second, the vectors no longer point in the same direction because of inhomogeneities in the B_0 magnetic field. Therefore the total net magnetization vector is shorter than that for the perfect magnetic field.

At time B, the effect of the variations in the magnetic field on the direction of the magnetization vectors is even more pronounced. The higher-field magnetization vector on the left is farther ahead, and the lower-field magnetization vector on the right falls farther behind. The sum is almost zero.

The resulting MR signal relaxes more rapidly than that caused by T2 alone (Figure 6-12). The small variations in the magnetic field cause the magnetization vectors in different regions to precess at different frequencies; that is, the spins in different regions rapidly lose their phase coherence—they dephase.

Although this discussion has used a three-compartment model, the actual situation involves a multicompartment model. The scale of the magnetic field inhomogeneity is not regional but intravoxel.

 The inhomogeneity in the magnetic field causes each spin to precess differently so that T2* is significantly shorter than T2.

The T2* measured in such an MRI experiment combines two factors: the real T2 of tissue and the magnetic field inhomogeneities. Unfortunately, in practical magnets, the effect of magnetic field inhomogeneities outweighs that of relaxation. The imperfections of the magnet, rather than the T2 of the tissue, end up being measured.

CHALLENGE QUESTIONS

1. Name the three principal MRI parameters characteristic of each tissue.
2. Arrange the three MRI relaxation times, T1, T2, and T2*, from shortest to longest for soft tissue.
3. Which MRI characteristic of tissue principally determines the intensity of the MR signal?
4. What is the principal reason that the T2* is always shorter than T2?
5. How much longitudinal relaxation occurs during one T1, and approximately how many relaxation times are needed for complete relaxation to reach equilibrium?
6. Distinguish between frequency and phase.
7. T1 relaxation is spin-lattice relaxation. To what does lattice refer?
8. What does the envelope of an FID represent?
9. In a T1W image, which tissues appear bright and which dark?
10. When a T2W image is presented, what tissues will appear bright?

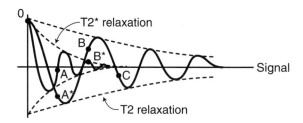

Figure 6-12 The envelope of the free induction delay obtained from an imaging magnet describes T2* relaxation. T2* is considerably less than T2 because of magnetic field inhomogeneities.

How to Measure Relaxation Times

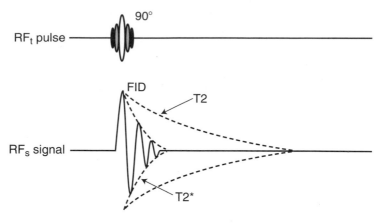

Figure 7-1   After a 90° RF pulse, T2*, rather than T2, relaxation is observed.

Many quantities in science, such as distance, mass, and time, can be measured directly. Other quantities rely on multiple observations followed by a computation. The determination of radioactive half-life from sequential counts of a radionuclide is one such example that requires multiple observations. Likewise, magnetic resonance imaging (MRI) relaxation times cannot be measured directly but must be computed after multiple observations.

Although the following section describes methods for measuring relaxation times, keep in mind that in the clinical setting this is never done. Clinically, relaxation times are not measured or calculated; they are referred to as *relative weighting* of an image.

HOW TO MEASURE T2

The radiofrequency (RF) pulse sequence shown in Figure 7-1 results in a magnetic resonance (MR) signal, the free induction decay (FID). The dotted line indicates the FID in a perfect magnet. A more realistic, shorter FID is also shown.

If, in real-world magnets, the FID does not relax according to the T2 of the sample because of B_0 inhomogeneity, how can the true T2 be measured? Several methods have been developed, all of which use additional pulses after the initial 90° RF pulse. The most common of

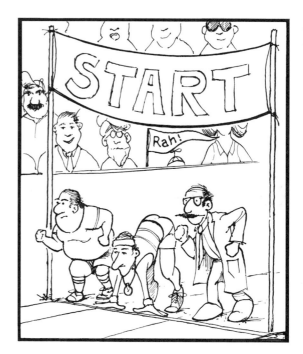

Figure 7-2   Immediately after a 90° radiofrequency pulse, all spins begin at the same starting line, just like runners in a race.

these is the spin echo pulse sequence (see Chapter 4).

In Figure 7-2, the net magnetization in the three regions of the patient is represented by three runners on an oval track. At time zero, they all leave the starting line together. A perfect magnet system is represented by runners moving at exactly the same speed, so that at some later time the runners are still exactly together and in step (Figure 7-3).

However, in a real magnet the net magnetization in the three regions dephases because spins are precessing at slightly different rates (Figure 7-4). The runners start together but now each runs at a slightly different speed, so that after some point in time, they are no longer together.

Is there some way to cause the runners to come back together even though they each run at a different speed? It is possible if a new rule is introduced to the race. For example, at the time in Figure 7-4, a whistle is blown, and all the runners immediately have to turn around, reversing their direction and run back toward the starting line.

If the race is now run making use of this rule, the scene will change. The runners start out together but soon begin to separate, that is,

dephase. Now at time A, the whistle is blown, and all the runners reverse and start running back toward the starting line. Suddenly the fastest runner, who was far ahead, is behind, and the slowest runner, who was behind, is in the lead. Even though they have changed directions, they have not changed speed. Therefore even though the faster runner is now behind, he will catch up with the others.

 A 180° RF pulse causes spins to rephase and form a spin echo.

Running toward the starting line is exactly the reverse of the start, when the runners ran from the starting line. This means that as the runners cross the starting line (Figure 7-5), they will again be precisely together; they are in phase again. They will cross the starting line at a time exactly twice that when the whistle was blown. For example, if the whistle was blown at 20 seconds, "rephasing" of the runners occurs at 40 seconds.

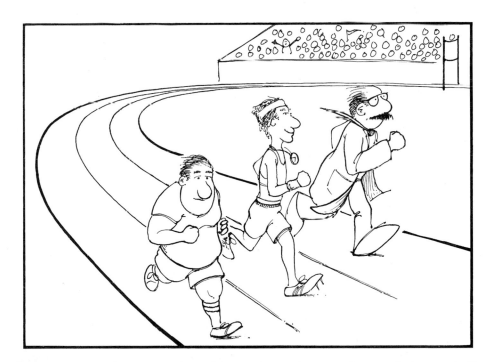

Figure 7-3 A perfect magnet is analogous to a perfect race. In a perfect magnet, M_{XY} remains in phase. In a perfect race, the runners remain in step.

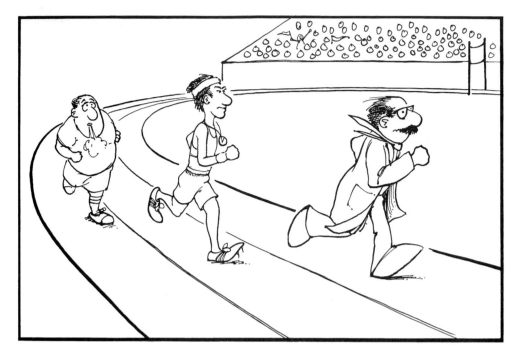

Figure 7-4   In an imaging magnet, M_{XY} dephases rapidly. In a real race, competitors run at different speeds.

If the race continues, the runners again dephase (Figure 7-6). However, they can then be forced to rephase by blowing the whistle at a later time, which will cause them to reverse direction again and come together at the starting line.

This process can be repeated any number of times. Each time the runners will rephase, and the information lost because of the difference in runners' speeds is recovered. The difference in the runners' speeds is analogous to the dephasing that occurs as a result of magnetic field inhomogeneities.

In a magnet, these reversals of the runners are accomplished with a 180° RF pulse. Such a pulse causes all the net magnetization vectors to flip 180°, in essence, reversing their direction. The spins then begin to rephase, and as they do, a signal is generated. The maximum signal occurs at the point where they are again in phase. If the 180° RF pulse were at time t, the maximum rephasing would occur at time 2t.

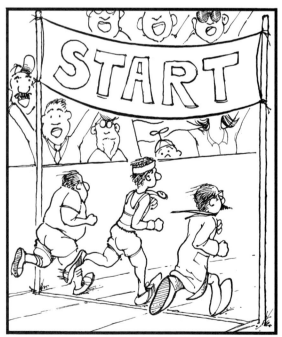

Figure 7-5   If the runners in Figure 7-4 reverse direction, they will cross the starting line at precisely the same time. They are back in phase.

During imaging, the spin ensemble begins at equilibrium. A 90° RF pulse rotates the net magnetization onto the XY plane, that is, the starting line (Figure 7-7). The spins precess at the Larmor frequency, but because this is illustrated in the rotating frame, the precession is not shown. The dephasing (varying speed of the runners) is illustrated by the shrinking and spreading arrows. Figure 7-7 also has vector diagrams showing the relaxation of the MR signal during this time. The dephasing results in a decreasing signal intensity until there is no signal. This is the FID.

Now a 180° RF pulse is applied, and the result flips all spins, which then rephase to form a spin echo with a maximum amplitude at exactly the time the spins rephase (runners cross the starting line). Additional 180° RF pulses can be applied to the spin ensemble to produce additional spin echoes. Each additional spin echo will be reduced in amplitude.

The spin echo first increases in intensity to a maximum and then relaxes back to zero (Figure 7-8). The first half of the spin echo is a mirror image of the second half.

 __The second half of the spin echo is an FID, and the first half is a mirror image of an FID.__

The key point that allows rephasing of the runners is that even though the runners' speeds are different, the speed of each runner is constant. There is a systematic difference among the runners, and the effect of this difference can be detected by reversing direction. In the same way, the loss of signal due to magnetic field inhomogeneities can be recovered because the inhomogeneities are constant. A region of the magnetic field that is slightly lower in field strength will remain so throughout an imaging sequence.

However, any random changes cannot be recovered in this manner. For example, if the

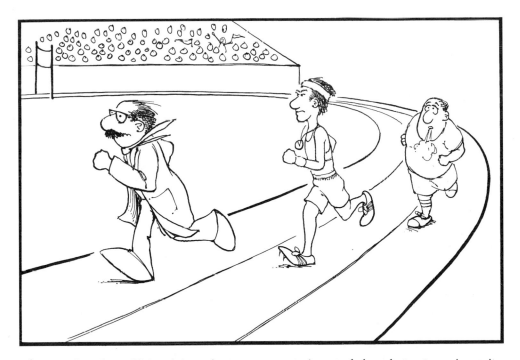

Figure 7-6 After additional time, the runners are again out of phase but not running quite so fast. A whistle blown at this time causes the runners to reverse direction again and rephase at the starting line.

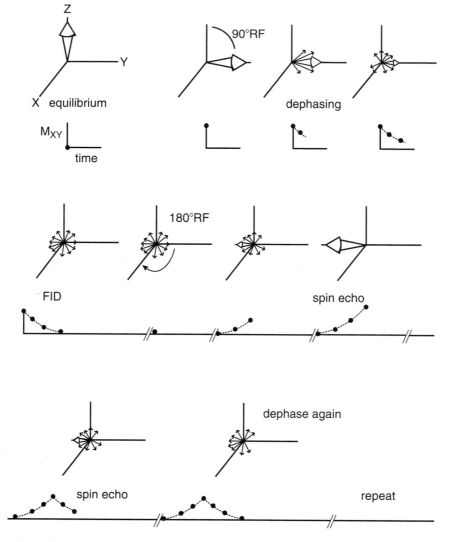

Figure 7-7 Vector diagram showing the formation of multiple spin echoes and the associated graph of transverse relaxation.

runners bump into each other momentarily on the track, the distance lost is not recoverable by reversing directions; the runner still ends up a little behind or "out of phase" when the runners "rephase."

In a similar manner, the effects of true T2 relaxation are not recovered by the 180° pulses. Thus the spin echoes reflect a removal of magnet inhomogeneity but not the removal of true T2 relaxation. Subsequent amplitudes of the

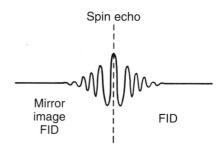

Figure 7-8 The spin echo consists of a free induction delay *(FID)* and its mirror image.

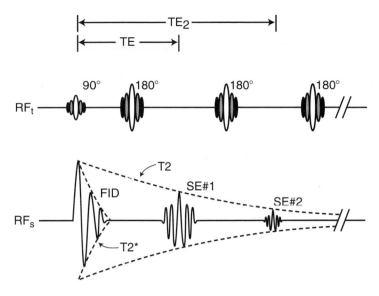

Figure 7-9 T2 relaxation time is measured from the envelope of multiple spin echoes.

spin echoes are smaller because of true T2 alone, and this leads to a method to calculate true T2 (Figure 7-9).

If the maximum amplitude of multiple spin echoes are plotted over time (Figure 7-10), the result is a curve that reflects true T2 relaxation (see Appendix A). Each time a 180° RF pulse is used a spin echo results, and each spin echo is smaller than the previous one and reversed in polarity. The time from the 180° RF pulse to the echo is always equal to the time from the 90° RF pulse to the 180° RF pulse.

 The envelope of the amplitude of multiple spin echoes describes the true T2 relaxation time.

HOW TO MEASURE T1

T1 is not so easily measured because it represents magnetization along the Z-axis. Such magnetization cannot be detected because it is exceedingly small compared with the static B_0 magnetic field.

Consider a 180° RF pulse that is transmitted into the patient so that the net magnetization is inverted. Once again this is an unstable state, and the net magnetization seeks to realign with the external magnetic field. It does this by shrinking in the −Z direction until it disappears and then grows in the +Z direction until it finally relaxes to equilibrium. This process happens because individual proton dipoles are flipping back to the low-energy state (Figure 7-11).

A plot of the net magnetization vector versus time results in a curve (Figure 7-12) that can be fitted by an equation containing the T1

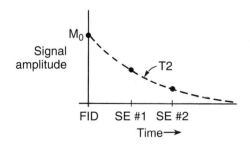

Figure 7-10 A plot of the amplitude of multiple spin echoes allows determination of the T2 relaxation time.

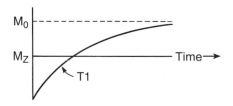

Figure 7-11 A 180° radiofrequency *(RF)* pulse inverts the net magnetization along the Z-axis so that $M_Z = -M_0$. With time, M_Z relaxes along the Z-axis to its equilibrium state of $M_Z = M_0$.

relaxation time (Appendix A). The problem with this approach is that after the 180° RF pulse, a signal is never detected because the net magnetization is completely along the Z-axis.

 The net magnetization must have a component in the XY plane to detect a signal.

For a signal to be detected, the 180° RF pulse must be followed by a 90° RF pulse to flip the net magnetization onto the XY plane where it can be detected. If the 180° RF pulse is immediately followed by a 90° RF pulse (Figure 7-13), the net magnetization is rotated onto the XY plane along the −Y-axis, and a signal is received.

The situation is now exactly the same as described previously, and the signal is an FID that begins in the negative direction and relaxes according to T2*. The initial magnitude of the FID is exactly equal to the length of the net magnetization vector after the 180° RF pulse.

The situation must be changed slightly to estimate the T1 relaxation time. Instead of the 90° RF pulse being given immediately after the 180° RF pulse, a short time is allowed. This results in the situation shown in Figure 7-14.

The delay time between the 180° and 90° RF pulses is the TI or **inversion-time** (see Chapter 5). Because there is now a little time before the net magnetization vector is rotated onto the XY plane, the net magnetization has a chance to shrink somewhat because of T1 relaxation. Although still starting out negative, the FID received is smaller than that in Figure 7-13. The initial magnitude of the FID is once again equal to the size of the T1 relaxed net magnetization vector.

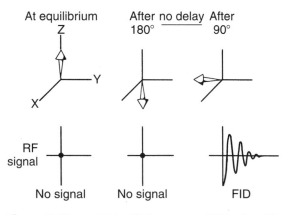

Figure 7-13 A 180° radiofrequency *(RF)* pulse followed immediately by a 90° RF pulse produces a free induction decay *(FID)* whose amplitude is equal to M_0. This is equivalent to a single 270° RF pulse.

Figure 7-12 If the value of M_Z is plotted at various times during relaxation to equilibrium the T1 relaxation time can be obtained.

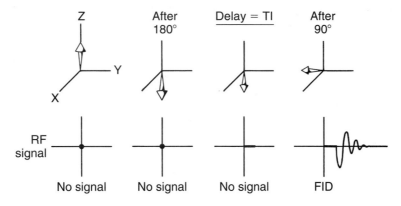

Figure 7-14 If a short time is allowed between the 180° and 90° radiofrequency *(RF)* pulses, a reduced amplitude free induction decay *(FID)* is produced.

If this process is continued, with longer and longer TIs, MR signals that can be interpreted for T1 are received (Figure 7-15). In Figure 7-15, *c,* the inversion time (TI) is just long enough to sample the net magnetization at a time when it is zero, switching from –Z to +Z, so that when the 90° RF pulse is emitted, there is no signal. In Figure 7-15, *d,* TI is long enough that the net magnetization is back along the +Z-axis, and the FID has a positive initial magnitude.

The results of this type of sequential experiment are used to determine T1. A curve like that in Figure 6-2 is obtained by plotting the initial magnitude of each FID versus the TI (Figure 7-16).

This should be no surprise. As was pointed out, the initial height of the FID is exactly the same as the length of the net magnetization vector after a delay of TI. Thus the plot is actually the length of the net magnetization vector at the various times chosen by TI. A value for T1 can be obtained by fitting these points to the curve given by the equation in Appendix A.

This RF pulse sequence, a 180° pulse followed by a 90° pulse after delay of TI, is called an **inversion recovery** pulse sequence because it inverts the net magnetization vector and then allows it to recover before measurement. As before, the discussion has been simplified with the assumption that an FID is the measured MR signal. Actually, spin echoes are measured.

T1 VERSUS T2 MEASUREMENTS

There are several differences in the techniques used to measure T1 and T2. The T2 relaxation time can be obtained by the use of a multiple echo, spin echo pulse sequence. A minimum of two inversion recovery pulse sequences are required to determine T1. Furthermore, for this technique to be applied accurately, the net magnetization must start out at equilibrium. Because of this, the T1 measurement often requires a significantly longer time than the T2 measurement.

For the T2 measurement, a sufficient number of points must be obtained along the T2 relaxation curve. Because the T2 relaxation time of most tissues is approximately 30 to 300 ms, enough data can easily be obtained to fit the T2 curve in less than 1000 ms.

On the other hand, the inversion recovery pulse sequence must be repeated at least twice, with two different TI times to obtain a value for T1. Between these two different TI times, enough time must pass for the net magnetization to relax to equilibrium. If enough time is not allowed between the two inversion recovery sequences, the net magnetization of the second sequence will not have recovered completely after the first sequence. Thus the net magnetization starts lower than it should for the second sequence, and the MR signal is correspondingly smaller.

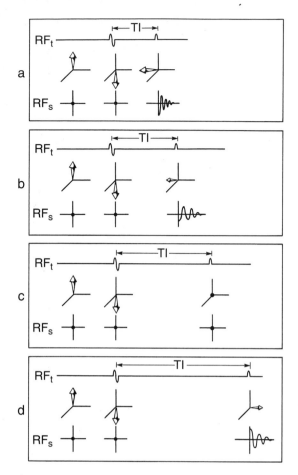

Figure 7-15 As inversion-time *(TI)* is increased, the magnitude of the free induction decay (FID) is reduced by T1 relaxation until it is zero. With still longer TIs, the FID amplitude increases as M_Z relaxes to M_0.

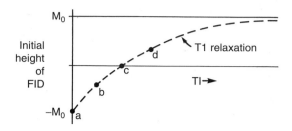

Figure 7-16 A plot of free induction decay *(FID)* amplitude versus inversion time can be used to determine T1 relaxation time. The letters of each data point correspond to Figure 7-15.

This results in an erroneous value for T1. The repetition time (TR) between the inversion recovery pulse sequences must be at least five times T1 to allow the net magnetization to relax to equilibrium. Most tissues have T1s of several hundred milliseconds. This means that several seconds are required to obtain two T1 points. Furthermore, more points must be added to the T1 curve to increase accuracy; each repetition requires another wait of five T1s.

However, several points for the T2 curve can be obtained with little increase in time with the spin echo sequence. Thus from a time standpoint, it is easier to obtain data for an estimate of T2 than for a T1 determination.

CHALLENGE QUESTIONS

1. What is the principal reason that MRI relaxation times cannot be measured directly?
2. What pulse sequences can be used to determine T1 relaxation time?
3. At what time after the 180° RF refocusing pulse is the MR signal most intense?
4. What is the MR signal used to make an inversion recovery image?
5. If one conducted a spin echo pulse sequence in an absolutely uniform B_0 magnetic field, what would be the results?
6. During inversion recovery imaging, why is a signal not detected after the initial 180° RF pulse?
7. Diagram the difference in transverse relaxation representing T2 and that representing T2*.
8. What would result from the following RF pulse sequence: 90° . . . 180° . . . 180° . . . 180° . . . ?
9. Describe the signal obtained during inversion recovery imaging when the inversion time equals the time that longitudinal relaxation passes through the origin.
10. Draw the vector diagram that represents tissue magnetization after a 90° RF pulse.

Chapter 8

Fourier Transforms in Magnetic Resonance Imaging

OBJECTIVES

At the completion of this chapter, the student should be able to do the following:

1. Define mathematical transform.
2. Describe the use of the Fourier transform in magnetic resonance imaging (MRI).
3. Identify the following concepts: spatial domain, frequency domain, and spatial frequency domain.
4. Discuss how the magnetic resonance (MR) signal is located in the patient (spatial localization).
5. Define the Nyquist theorem and discuss its use in MRI.
6. Identify the MRI artifact aliasing and its cause.

OUTLINE

Jean Baptiste Joseph Fourier (1768-1830) was a French physicist and mathematician who lived at the time of the French Revolution. Among his many accomplishments is the derivation of the mathematical transform that carries his name, the Fourier transform (FT).

The FT has always played an important role in digital image processing. Until recently, this role was buried in the depths of the derivation of the computed tomography (CT) reconstruction algorithm or in more complex image quality specifications such as the modulation transfer function (MTF). However, with the advent of magnetic resonance imaging (MRI), the FT has been called to center stage.

FT is the mathematical mechanism for changing any of the magnetic resonance (MR) signals (free induction decay [FID], spin echo [SE], or gradient echo [GRE]) into a nuclear magnetic resonance (NMR) spectrum for chemical analysis or into a diagnostic image. Therefore an understanding of this transform is necessary, especially as it relates to MRI. Among other features, the FT provides an explanation of a type of artifact encountered in MR images (i.e., aliasing).

WHAT IS A TRANSFORM?

The FT is only one of many transforms in mathematics. For an understanding of what mathematicians mean by a transform, perhaps it is best to provide an analogy.

In nature, connections between numbers always occur. For example, the length of the side of a square affects the area of the square and vice versa. With the measurement of a few squares, a pattern of values begins to appear (Table 8-1).

It is obvious that the area of the square depends on the length of the side of the square. A general relationship between these quantities can be defined: to find the area of the square, multiply the length of the side of the square by itself. The area equals the square of the length of a side. This relationship between two sets of numbers is called a **function**. The relationship may be written as follows:

Transform

$2 — f(\text{area}) → 4$
where the notation $f(area)$ denotes the "area function"

Note that this area function includes the following important properties:

1. The function gives a unique result. A particular length for the side of a square results in only one possible value for its area.
2. The function possesses a unique inverse. Given the area of a square, the length of its side can be computed, and only one answer is possible. For example,

Inverse Transform

$4 — f(\text{area}^{-1}) → 2$
where the −1 superscript means *inverse*.

3. General rules regarding this function can be derived. For example, if the length of the side of the square doubles, then the area is multiplied by a factor of 4.
4. A mathematical formula can be written to represent this relationship.

TABLE 8-1	The Relationship between the Side and Area of a Square
Side of Square	**Area of Square**
1	1
2	4
4	16
8	64
10	100

Variable Transform
(area of square) = **(length of side)²** or with symbols instead of words: $A = s^2$

5. The units used are changed by the function. For example, if the length of the side is measured in centimeter (cm), then the area is measured in square centimeter (cm²).

 A function establishes a relationship between numbers; a transform establishes a relationship between functions.

WHAT IS THE FOURIER TRANSFORM?

The FT is only one of many transforms available; however, its properties make it uniquely useful in MRI. The FT can be presented in terms of graphs of functions to see how the FT changes the shape of these graphs. For example, the square wave function is transformed into the wavy function by Fourier transformation (Figure 8-1). The symbol *FT* in the figure indicates this mathematical formulation.

The FT has properties analogous to the area-of-a-square function discussed previously. The FT gives a unique result; for example, the square function of Figure 8-1 is Fourier transformed only into the wavy function shown. This wavy function is called a *sinc function* or *sin x/x*. The amplitude and width of the square function are related to the amplitude and wavelength of the sinc function.

Because the FT is unique, a unique inverse FT also exists. Only one function can produce the wavy function of Figure 8-1; that is, the FT can be undone so that the original function is produced (Figure 8-2). The symbol *FT⁻¹* represents the inverse Fourier transform.

A mathematical formula can be written to define the FT. The exact form of this formula is unimportant, except that it contains sines and cosines. Sines and cosines are oscillating functions whose effects are often seen in the FT. For example, the square function in Figure 8-1 is sharp edged, yet its FT has waves in it. These waves include sines and cosines.

The units of the source function and the resulting transformed function are different but related. If the source function is a plot of signal intensity versus time, then the Fourier transformed function is a plot of signal intensity versus 1/time (i.e., frequency).

 The FT of intensity versus time is intensity versus frequency.

WHY A TRANSFORM?

What is the use of a transform? The answer lies in the desire to solve problems. Physicists and engineers are always trying to understand the real world and how it reacts to changing situations. They write formulas to represent some part of the world then try to solve these formulas to see how that part will behave. For example, the response of a bridge to a crosswind can be predicted by setting up a set of equations that represent the properties of the bridge and by solving these equations in the

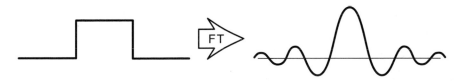

Figure 8-1   With Fourier transformation, a square wave results in a "wavy" pattern.

presence of a force that represents the wind. Unfortunately these equations are often extremely complicated, and their solution is not at all obvious (Figure 8-3).

Sometimes if a transform like the FT is applied to source equations, the solution of the transformed equations is easier to obtain than the solution of the source equations. The answer to the FT of the source equation is in **Fourier space**. If an inverse transform is applied to the Fourier space equation, the result is in real space (Figure 8-4). This result is the same as if the problem had been solved directly. In addition, viewing the problem in Fourier space sometimes gives unique insights to the situation, insights that are not obvious in real space.

The FT does not really change the information present in a function. Rather, it represents that information in a reorganized way, offering a new viewpoint on the data. Thus the situation is viewed in either real space or Fourier space. In both spaces the same real-world thing is represented (e.g., an image, an MR signal). The FT just offers a new and unique viewpoint of these data. For example, the MR signal is a function of intensity versus time (i.e., time domain). The FT gives a representation of those same data as intensity versus frequency (i.e., the frequency domain).

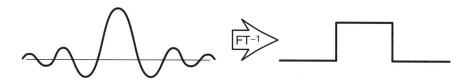

Figure 8-2   The inverse Fourier transform *(FT⁻¹)* of the wavy pattern is a square wave.

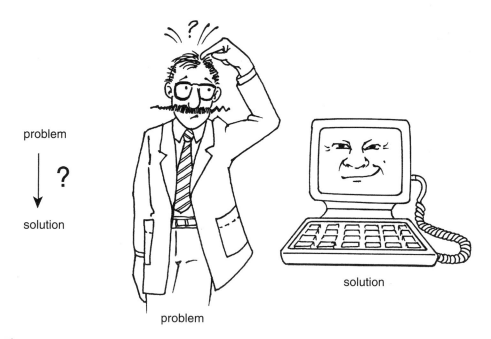

Figure 8-3   Mathematical formulas state problems. The solution often requires a transformation.

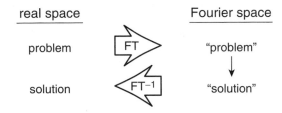

Figure 8-4 A magnetic resonance image is obtained by transforming a signal into Fourier space, reassembling the data, and computing the inverse transform.

THE FREQUENCY DOMAIN

Suppose that the real space function represents some sort of signal in time, that is, a representation of the signal intensity as it varies with time, like an MR signal. The Fourier space representation does not have the same units. The units on the horizontal axis in Fourier space are inverse of the units in real space. In this case, the horizontal real space unit is time (e.g., seconds). Therefore the unit in Fourier space is 1/time (e.g., 1/seconds).

The quantity 1/time (e.g., cycles/second, hertz) occurs often and is frequency. A plot of intensity versus frequency is a **spectrum**. The FT can take a picture of intensity versus time (i.e., the time domain) and create a picture of the same signal represented as intensity versus frequency (i.e., the frequency domain).

Once again, real space and Fourier space views are two different representations of the same real-world object. For example, the MR signal is a real space representation of how that signal varies with time. The FT shows how the same signal varies with frequency, that is, what frequencies are present in the signal.

The concept of frequency domain or **spatial frequency domain** is easy to recognize. For example, ears do a frequency transformation of the signals (i.e., sounds) that they receive. The time domain representation of the sound generated by a complex source such as a symphony orchestra can be represented by a rapidly varying oscillating signal. This signal alone conveys little meaning. However, human hearing takes this time-varying signal and transforms it into frequencies.

In the complex sound from a symphony, the ear can distinguish between the high treble pitch of a violin and the deeper bass pitch of a tuba. Indeed, a small percentage of people have absolute pitch, the ability to tell the precise pitches (i.e., frequencies) of the sounds they hear. In this sense, ears "view" the world in the frequency domain.

Too Small to See

On the left side of Figure 8-5 are three smooth, bell-shaped (i.e., Gaussian) functions in real space. On the right side are their corresponding Fourier transforms. If these real-space functions represent a signal (i.e., the representation of intensity with time), then the Fourier space representation is a frequency spectrum (i.e., representation of the frequencies present).

The time domain representation in the top pair of curves shows a wide curve that changes slowly over time. The corresponding Fourier space representation shows a narrow function in the frequency domain. This means that the signal contains only a narrow range of frequencies. As the time domain signal narrows (i.e., the signal is made to change faster in time), the curves in the frequency domain become broader, indicating that a wider range of frequencies is required.

In extreme cases where a sharp signal spike exists in the time domain, the range of frequencies contained in that spike approaches infinity. Thus the more localized a signal is in time, the wider the range of frequencies that must be handled. In other words, the sharp edges of objects contain more extremely wide ranges of frequencies and higher frequencies than smooth objects.

 A bone-soft tissue interface is a high spatial frequency object.

This simple fact has profound implications for viewing the world. Consider again the square wave of Figure 8-1. This sharp-edged object might be an MR signal of a fluid-filled cyst. In

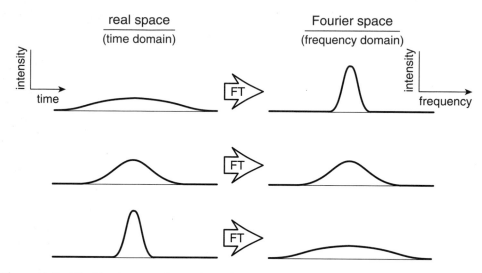

Figure 8-5   The Fourier transformation of a broad gaussian distribution results in a narrow frequency spectrum and vice versa.

Figure 8-1, the Fourier space representation shows what frequencies are present in the object as given by the wavy function to the right. Note that this representation only shows part of the Fourier space function; the ripples diminish in height to the right and left but never totally disappear until reaching plus and minus infinity. For this object to be truly represented, an infinite range of frequencies must be handled.

This is unfortunate because no system can handle an infinite range of frequencies. When an object is detected with the radio receiver of an MRI system, the frequencies inherent in the object must pass through the imaging system. If the electronics of the system do not pass all the frequencies in the object, then part of the structure of that object is lost.

The system could be designed more carefully, but there is always a finite limit to the range of frequencies that it allows to pass. Therefore some part of the information from the object (i.e., the part of the object contained in the high frequencies) is always lost. Various curves show the effect of this loss (Figure 8-6).

From a curve in Fourier space, the view of that curve in real space can be obtained by applying the inverse FT. In the top set of curves, the high frequencies have been abruptly chopped off. This is **truncation**, and the signal is said to be truncated. Truncation results in large oscillations at the sharp edges of the real space square wave.

If an MRI system has a sharp cutoff of frequencies, a false, sharp ringing will be detected every time the signal changes abruptly. Because this ringing is so objectionable, systems are designed so that they do not cut off sharply at the edge of their frequency range; rather, they fade away gradually. A sharp square wave received by such a system would come out with rounded edges. The information that forms the sharp edges of the object is lost, thereby causing the object to become blurred. Spatial resolution is reduced.

Consequently, there is a limit to the ability to image sharp edges and produce fine detail in that image. This situation can be improved by increasing the ability of the MRI system to handle high frequencies. Because there is always a limit to the frequencies that any MRI system can handle, there is always a limit to the object size that can be imaged.

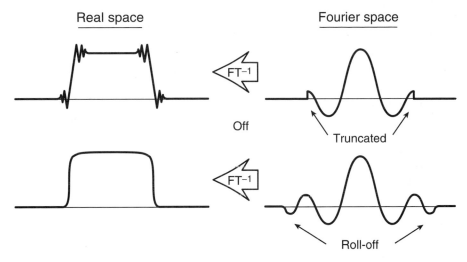

Figure 8-6 If the high frequencies of a signal in Fourier space are chopped off (i.e., truncated), the inverse Fourier transform *(FT⁻¹)* results in a ringing appearance at the sharp boundaries in an image.

 No imaging system can pass an infinite range of frequencies.

Chemistry's Signature

The MR signal is profoundly affected by the chemical bonding of the atoms generating the signal. If a complex molecule emits the MR signal, the signal would have a correspondingly complex structure.

A nucleus that is bound inside a complex molecule would resonate at a slightly different frequency than a nucleus in a simple water molecule. This is due to the magnetic fields of electrons in the atom shielding the nucleus from the B_0 field (see Chapter 9).

These changes in resonance are changes in frequency, but the signal received is changing in time. The FT is the bridge connecting the time domain signal to the frequency domain representation.

The sample FID is the plot of signal intensity versus time for a complex molecule (Figure 8-7). If an FT is applied to this signal, a plot of signal intensity versus frequency is obtained. The clear arrangement of sharp peaks of various heights should be noted because this particular arrangement of peaks is the unique chemical signature for that molecule.

A trained NMR chemist learns to recognize the standard arrangements of these peaks. The relationships of these peaks to one another and their widths and heights indicate the nature of the bonding between atoms. All this same information is contained in the original FID, although in an obscured form. The FT produces a new and useful view of the data.

SPATIAL LOCALIZATION AND THE FOURIER TRANSFORM

For an MR image to be made, the origin in space for each part of the signal must be known. Unfortunately, only one signal at a time is received from the patient. Therefore spatial information must be encoded into each such signal (see Chapters 15 and 16).

In a uniform external magnetic field, all nuclei resonate at the same frequency, called the **resonant frequency**. If a gradient magnetic field that varies uniformly in the Z direction is added to this primary magnetic field, the spins

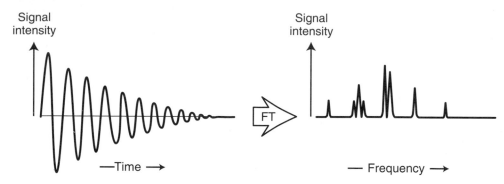

Figure 8-7   The Fourier transform *(FT)* of a free induction decay results in a nuclear magnetic resonance spectrum, which is in the frequency domain.

on the −Z-axis would be in a lower magnetic field than those on the + Z-axis. Therefore they will resonate at a lower frequency. This difference in frequency directly relates to the position of the spins along the Z-axis and the amplitude of the gradient magnetic field.

Two globs of fat are shown at different positions in the Z direction (Figure 8-8). With no Z gradient magnetic field, the two globs resonate at the same frequency and contribute to a single peak in the frequency domain. When a gradient magnetic field, G_Z, is added, this single peak splits into two peaks, one peak for each glob, each of which is now at a different frequency.

The frequency difference between the peaks directly relates to the distance between the globs of fat in the Z direction. The stronger the gradient magnetic field, the further apart the peaks in the frequency domain; thus it is easier to separate objects in space.

Gradient magnetic fields provide spatial localization of the MR signal.

This process relies on the FT. Because an MR signal is a variation of intensity as a function of time, an FT must be applied to the signal to view the frequency distribution that is related to the spatial distribution.

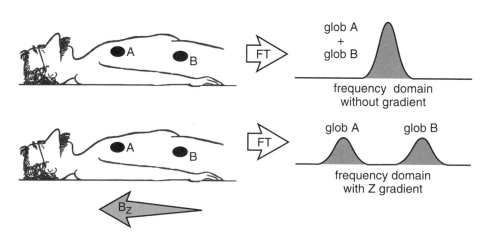

Figure 8-8   When a Z gradient magnetic field is applied, the same tissue results in different peaks in the frequency domain.

In the example found in Figure 8-8, each fat glob generated a signal. A gradient magnetic field was used to determine where along the Z direction the signal from each originated. Another approach can also be taken. Such a method would energize only one part of the object so that any signal received would only come from that part, rather than from the entire object.

This method uses the same gradient magnetic field system as seen in the previous methods. For a signal to be received from the spins in only one object, the initial RF pulse must only excite those spins. For example, if the spins in object B are energized and the spins in object A are left undisturbed, any signal received would come from object B alone.

For the precessing nuclei to absorb energy, the RF signal must exactly match the frequency of precession of the spins. Because objects A and B are in a gradient magnetic field, the spins in the objects have slightly different resonant frequencies. Therefore an RF pulse with a frequency distribution unique to object B, not that of object A, is required if object B is to be imaged (Figure 8-9).

For the RF signal to be actually generated, however, knowledge of the signal as a function of time is required. The FT allows a change between time and frequency. To go from the frequency domain to the time domain, one must apply the inverse FT. This exercise provides the shape of the RF pulse that must be used. If this shaped RF pulse were transmitted into a patient, only the spins in a chosen part of the patient would be excited. This isolates the MR signal in a narrow section of the patient.

In these simple examples, spatial information has been encoded in only one dimension. Similar methods, which are also heavily based on the use of the FT, are used to obtain spatial information in all three dimensions.

FLOW AND THE FOURIER TRANSFORM

A true FT generates two parts of the square wave function (Figure 8-10). These parts are called the **real part** and the **imaginary part**. These names are imaginative names traditionally used by mathematicians for these mathematical parts. Therefore the imaginary part is just as real as the real part. They could have been called anything: parts A and B, left and right, or Brenda and Fred, for that matter. Until now, the imaginary part of the transform has been ignored, because this part has been zero for the examples used. However, under certain circumstances, the imaginary part of the transform contains some useful information.

One general property of the FT is that if the real space function is an even function, then the FT of that function has an imaginary part

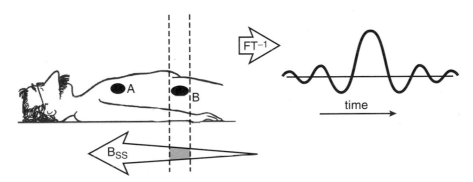

Figure 8-9   A radiofrequency pulse containing only the frequencies of tissue B is obtained from the inverse Fourier transform *(FT⁻¹)* of the frequency distribution.

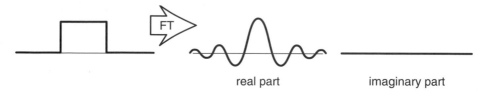

real part   imaginary part

Figure 8-10   The Fourier transform *(FT)* has two parts, real and imaginary.

that is zero, and the nonzero information is contained in the real part. An even function is one that is symmetrical around the vertical axis (i.e., the right and left halves of the function are mirror images). The simple functions considered to this point (i.e., the square-wave function and the bell-shaped Gaussian functions) have been even functions and therefore have had an FT with an imaginary part equal to zero.

In most cases the SE from an MRI system is also an even function. As the spins come back into phase, the signal intensifies to its maximum and then relaxes back to zero as the spins again dephase. The signal produced (i.e., the SE) is symmetrical because the process of rephasing and dephasing is symmetrical.

Theoretically, an image produced from a set of SEs actually results in two images: a real part image and an imaginary part image. However, because the SE is symmetrical, the imaginary part image contains noise but little useful information. As a result, most MRI systems use magnitude reconstruction in which both the real and imaginary moduli are used.

In some cases, however, the SE is not symmetrical, as when there is motion, for example, blood flowing in a vein. If the blood moves in the direction of one of the gradient magnetic fields, with time it experiences a different magnetic field as it moves from one position in the gradient magnetic field to another.

Thus when an SE is received from moving blood, the rising shape of the SE is not the same as the falling shape, and the SE can no longer be exactly an even function. Therefore when the image is formed, the imaginary part

of the image is not zero, and the real part has missing or distorted information. For simple imaging pulse sequences, this motion can generate artifacts in the image.

In practice there are sophisticated pulse sequences designed to suppress these motion artifacts. On the other hand, the detection of moving material, especially blood flow, is of special interest. Special pulse sequences designed to enhance and quantify this effect are continually under development (see Chapter 23).

SAMPLING AND ALIASING

In all MRI systems, the FT is performed by a computer. A computer does not deal with continuous curves like the graphs of signals presented earlier; rather, it manipulates individual (i.e., discrete) numbers. This has several important consequences. The data of the continuous MR signal must somehow be changed to individual numbers.

This change is done by a process called digitization or **sampling**. The intensity of the signal is sampled, measured, and stored at regular intervals. The results are a series of data points that give a representation of the original continuous signal when they are connected.

A form of the FT that handles discrete numbers rather than continuous curves must be available. This form of the FT is called the **discrete Fourier transform**. Because FTs are commonly implemented on computers, the discrete FT has been optimized for the binary architecture of such computers. This special optimized form is called the **fast Fourier transform (FFT)**.

When an RF signal is sampled, how much of the signal should be measured and stored?

How rapidly must the signal be sampled to give a good representation of it? If rapidly sampled, the data points are spaced extremely close to one another. This always provides a good representation of the signal.

Fast signal sampling creates practical problems. It is more difficult to design electronics to sample data quickly; therefore the equipment becomes more expensive and error prone. The more data sampled, the more there is to store. When there are more data to store, more computer memory is required, thereby making the process more expensive. As more data are collected, it takes more time to analyze it and longer to reconstruct the images.

On the other hand, if too little data are sampled, important parts of the signal may be missed, and important information may be lost. Therefore it is important to know whether there is an optimum rate at which to sample the data. The optimum rate is that which provides an adequate representation of the data. Oversampling is common and produces small signal-to-noise gain. The FT can help answer this question and explain what happens if too few points in the data are sampled.

When a real space function is Fourier transformed, only a finite range of frequencies are needed to represent this signal (i.e., frequencies up to some maximum value f_{max}) (Figure 8-11). The required range of frequencies is from $-f_{max}$ to $+f_{max}$. Therefore the width of the frequency band is $2f_{max}$ and symbolized as Δf. The electronics are then designed to handle only the range of frequencies up to and including this maximum frequency (i.e., up to and including f_{max} Hz). Any frequency above this limit cannot pass through the system, but because no such frequencies exist in the desired signal, this is irrelevant.

This real space curve is sampled with data points spaced at some fixed interval and sent through the system. Is the result of using the sampled data the same as if the continuous signal were Fourier transformed? The FT of the discrete sampled function is a continuous function, not discrete as may be suspected (Figure 8-11). The difference between the FT of the continuous and discrete functions is that the FT of the discrete function has additional clones of the desired FT.

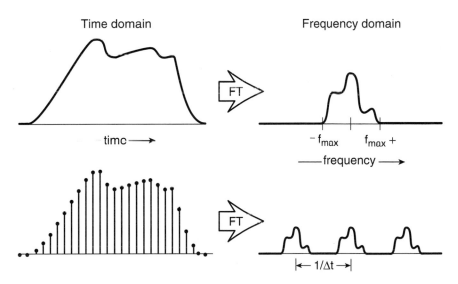

Figure 8-11 The Fourier transform *(FT)* of the discrete function of the sampled signal results in clones of continuous functions.

There are an infinite number of these clones of the desired FT spaced evenly up and down the frequency spectrum and extending to both plus and minus infinity. These clones do not matter. Because the system only passes frequencies up to f_{max} Hz, all the clones are cut off, provided they lie at frequencies beyond f_{max} Hz (i.e., the maximum frequency handled by the system).

This last condition is critical to the proper representation of the data. The clones are spaced apart in the frequency domain by $1/\Delta t$. As the sample points are moved in real space further apart, the clone curves in frequency space creep closer to the central curve. Trouble occurs when the bottom point of the first clone curve begins to touch the top point of the central curve. The sample points can be widened until this condition occurs and no farther.

More precisely, the sampling distance between the clone curve and the central curve ($1/\Delta t$) must always be greater than the frequency width of the curve itself ($-f_{max}$). This is mathematically expressed as follows:

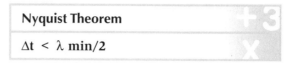

Sampling Theory

$1/\Delta t \ > \ -f_{max}$

The wavelength is 1/frequency and 1/maximum frequency is 1/minimum wavelength. Sampling theory can be rearranged to become the Nyquist sampling theorem.

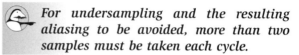

Nyquist Theorem

$\Delta t \ < \ \lambda \ min/2$

Therefore at least two points must be sampled within the smallest wavelength within an object.

For undersampling and the resulting aliasing to be avoided, more than two samples must be taken each cycle.

The wavelength of a simple oscillating signal is easy to determine (Figure 8-12). It is the distance between crests or valleys or any two similar points of the oscillation. According to the Nyquist theorem, a sample must be taken at least twice in that wavelength.

If more than two samples are taken in each wavelength, an attempt to redraw the curve by connecting the points is possible (Figure 8-12, *A*). The reconstructed curve matches the original signal through connection of the dots. If the Nyquist theorem is purposely disobeyed so that fewer than two points are sampled in

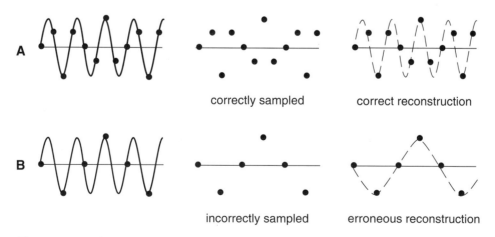

correctly sampled   correct reconstruction

incorrectly sampled   erroneous reconstruction

Figure 8-12 If the sampling frequency is too low, the reconstruction will be false and result in aliasing.

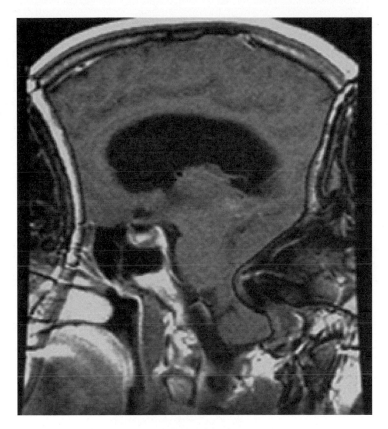

Figure 8-13 Signals from both the anterior and posterior of the head fall outside the prescribed FOV (field of view). The signals are thus undersampled and reconstructed as originating within the FOV but from opposite sides. (Courtesy Bill Faulkner, Chatanooga, TN.)

every wavelength, a false reconstruction of the signal results, (Figure 8-12, *B*).

The reconstructed signal has a longer wavelength. Not only does the original signal match these sampled points, but it also matches a longer wavelength signal. This second wavelength (i.e., frequency) signal is an **alias**.

 If the frequencies in a signal are undersampled, bogus frequencies result in the output and an aliasing artifact results.

Because MR images use frequencies to encode position information, aliasing usually results in the image appearing to be "wrapped around" another part of the image. For example, a por-

tion of the left part of the image appears as a ghost on the right part of that image and vice versa (Figure 8-13).

CHALLENGE QUESTIONS

1. The FT changes the MR signal from intensity versus time to what quantity?
2. What artifact results when the MR signal is not adequately sampled?
3. What is another name for spatial frequency domain?
4. What is the minimum sampling rate of an MR signal that will ensure aliasing does not occur?

5. Whose name is applied to sampling theory?
6. Identify three examples of tissue with high spatial frequency components.
7. Are there any other disadvantages to oversampling an MR signal?
8. Which component of the MRI system is principally responsible for locating the position of the MR signal in the body?
9. What is a FFT?
10. Graphically, show how the FT of a square wave and an SE should appear.

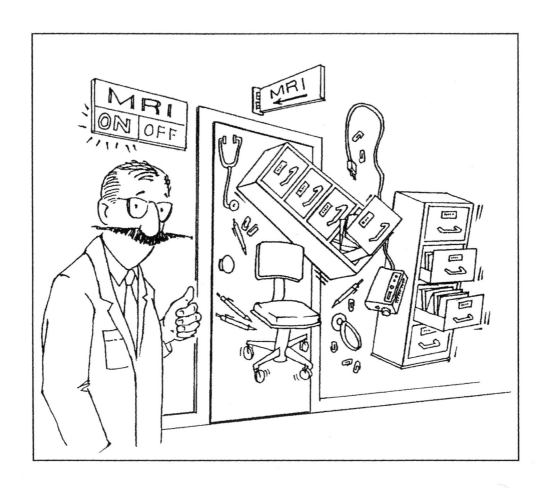

Nuclear Magnetic Resonance Spectroscopy

This chapter has several goals: to explain basic nuclear magnetic resonance (NMR) spectroscopy, to get the reader excited about the use of NMR in medicine, and to show that expert treatment of NMR spectroscopy is a specialty topic. The treatment is thus illustrative, not comprehensive. The scientific literature of NMR and its medical companion magnetic resonance spectroscopy (MRS) are extensive.

Magnetic resonance imaging (MRI), the principal subject of this book, evolved from the scientific application of NMR high-resolution spectroscopy. Knowledge of NMR spectroscopy is not essential for an understanding of MRI. Rather, it is an enhancement that should be in the tool chest of any serious MRI radiologist or technologist.

This chapter deals with NMR spectroscopy in simple terms. It should give the imaging physician and technologist a brief look into the history of NMR and a similar glance at the future. It should also give the chemical NMR spectroscopist an equally interesting view of the future. One principal aim of MRS use in MRI is the performance of in vivo analysis of pathologic conditions, which thereby increases the diagnostic value of MRI.

The first concept to remember is **spectrum**. A spectrum, sometimes referred to as a **frequency distribution,** is a convenient graphic means of presenting specific frequency or wavelength-related material. Two spectra that should be familiar are those associated with the emission of light from rare-earth radiographic intensifying screens and the absorption of that light in the emulsion of radiographic film (Figure 9-1).

Absorptiometry is an analysis of the absorption of ultraviolet (UV), visual, and infrared (IR) light transmission through a sample. If the measurement is made at many different wavelengths or frequencies, the resulting graph is reported as a spectrum. For NMR spectroscopy the X-axis defines the radiofrequencies (RFs) emitted by the patient, and the Y-axis is the intensity of the signal

produced by the patient at each frequency. Representative UV absorption, IR transmission, and NMR emission spectra are shown in Figure 9-2.

The line widths seen in Figure 9-2 are different in these three spectra. Those of the first two methods are "broad," whereas the NMR signals appear "sharp." Indeed, NMR is widely regarded as high-resolution spectroscopy.

 MRS line widths can be exceedingly sharp.

An NMR spectrum can be obtained from any free induction decay (FID). The FID is the NMR signal emitted at the Larmor frequency from an excited sample. The FID may be viewed as a plot of signal intensity versus time (Figure 9-3). If the FID results from the excitation of an NMR sample by a single RF pulse, a mathematical process called the Fourier transform (FT) can be used to convert the abstract FID to a readily interpreted spectrum. The NMR spcctrum is presented as signal intensity versus frequency.

Fourier transformation is used to analyze periodic (sine or cosine) wave functions mathematically. Knowledge of the operation or underlying mathematics of the FT is not required for the production of MR images or spectra. The reader can simply accept the FT as a black box that produces acceptable results from FID data sets.

Consider an analogy to poker strategies (Figure 9-4). One strategy is to make all moves on the basis of experience, the ability to keep a poker face, and a good feel for the game. Another, more technical, strategy is to factor in the role of probability in the construction of the hand and to discard and draw more cards to improve the chances of making a better hand. At the end of play, a player using the first strategy will probably admit that poker is fun but a little expensive. A more technical player may or may not enjoy the game as much but will probably have extra money.

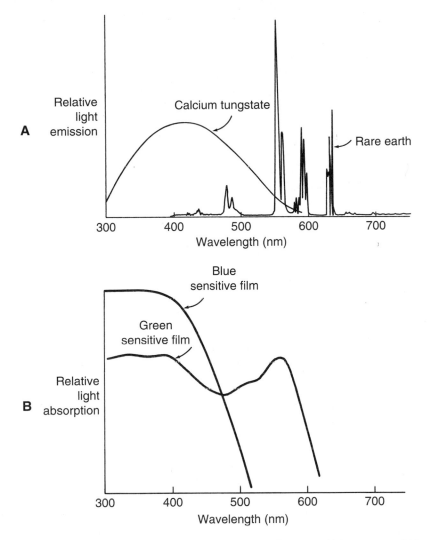

Figure 9-1 The spectrum of light emitted by radiographic intensifying screens (**A**) and that absorbed by a photographic emulsion (**B**) are familiar examples of spectra.

NUCLEAR SPECIES

Shortly after the discovery of NMR, one principle became well known: each nuclide in the periodic table has a unique resonance frequency at a given magnetic field strength. In the Larmor relationship the resonant frequency of any NMR signal depends only on the gyromagnetic ratio and the magnetic field strength. The value of gyromagnetic ratio varies by a factor of more than 100 among nuclides.

 Each nuclide has its own gyromagnetic ratio.

The gyromagnetic ratios of several nuclides of interest to MR in medicine are given in Table 3-1. If a total NMR spectrum of the body could be produced, it would include many nuclear species (Figure 9-5). This is a thought experiment only, so the scale is in reverse of that encountered in NMR spectroscopy.

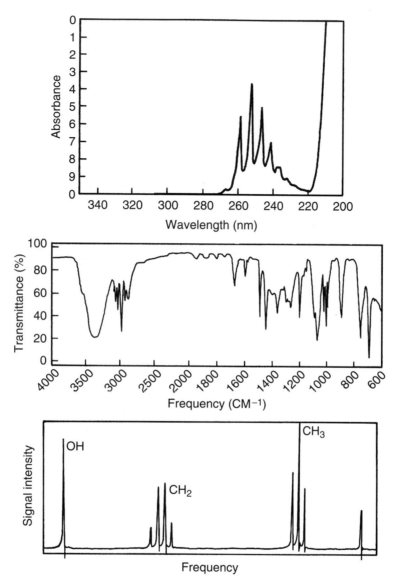

Figure 9-2   Three examples of a spectrum are ultraviolet absorption, infrared transmission, and nuclear magnetic resonance emission.

The spacing between the signals can be understood in the following manner. The gyromagnetic ratio for hydrogen is the largest of any nuclide normally observed. The gyromagnetic ratio for ^{13}C is about four times smaller, so the carbon resonance frequency is reduced four times. Other nuclides scale accordingly.

In any event the extremely large frequency separations between nuclides and the small range of chemical shifts for any given nuclide make it impractical to observe more than one

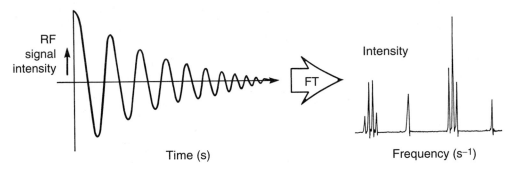

Figure 9-3   The nuclear magnetic resonance spectrum is the Fourier transform *(FT)* of the free induction decay.

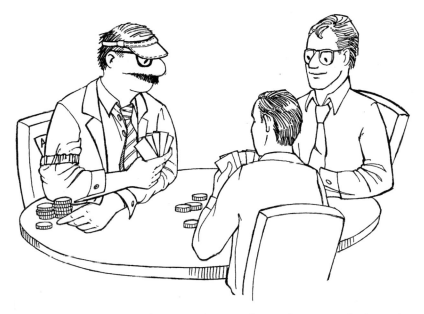

Figure 9-4   Fourier transformation is somewhat analogous to playing poker.

nuclide at a time. Therefore hydrogen signals can be observed completely separate from those signals resulting from any other nuclides. It may appear from the hypothetical spectrum in Figure 9-5 that ^{19}F and ^{1}H are close enough in resonance frequency to cause accidental overlap. The separation is more than 4% (megahertz apart), whereas the chemical shift ranges of each nuclide are measured in parts per million (hertz apart). There is no overlap.

CHEMICAL SHIFT

Within a single nuclear species (for example, ^{1}H), more than one peak may be present in an NMR spectrum. Pragmatically, it became obvious early in the development of NMR that the number of these peaks observed at low resolution was a measure of the number of chemically distinct hydrogen atoms in the molecule. For instance, ethanol has the chemical formula CH_3CH_2OH and exhibits three

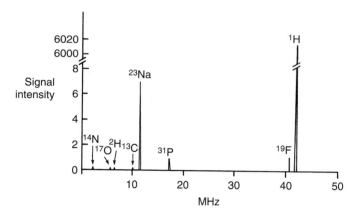

Figure 9-5 The hypothetical nuclear magnetic resonance spectrum of the human body at 1.0 T.

groups of signals in the NMR spectrum (Figure 9-6).

 The pattern of differing Larmor precession frequencies is called **chemical shift.**

The reason for the difference in resonant frequency for a single nuclear species is intimately related to the chemical structure of the molecule in which that particular

nucleus is bound. Each nucleus is surrounded by a cloud of electrons. Because these electrons are moving charged particles, they generate their own magnetic fields that will add to or subtract from the applied external field. These additions and subtractions are noticed by the nuclei, and the exact resonance frequencies are consequently altered slightly.

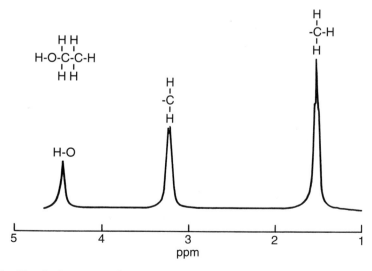

Figure 9-6 The hydrogen nuclear magnetic resonance spectrum of ethanol consists of three peaks corresponding to the three types of hydrogen atoms according to how each is bound in the molecule.

However, electrons are very small, and each one carries only a small charge. Their effects on the nucleus are small compared with the size of the external magnetic field. In general, the effect of these seemingly small electronic effects is sufficient to generate a unique NMR spectrum for every molecule.

A classic example of chemical shift of a single nuclear species is fat and water (Table 9-1). The hydrogen nuclei in fat are effectively shielded by an abundance of electrons and therefore resonate at a 150 Hz lower frequency than hydrogen in water at 1.0 T.

In the molecule shown in Figure 9-6, there are three types of hydrogen atoms, two types of carbon atoms, and one type of oxygen atom. This classification is based on the manner in which the atoms are joined in the detailed chemical structure. There will be three signals in the proton (hydrogen) NMR spectrum, two in the carbon NMR spectrum, and one in the oxygen NMR spectrum.

MAGNETIC FIELD DEPENDENCE

The magnitude of the chemical shift measured in units of frequency varies with the strength of the external magnetic field used to obtain the NMR spectrum. As the strength of the magnet is increased, the frequency difference, and therefore the separation between peaks when measured in units of hertz, increases in a linear fashion (Figure 9-7).

TABLE 9-1	Fat and Water Chemical Shift
Field Strength (T)	**Chemical Shift (Hz)**
0.2	30
0.5	75
1.0	150
1.5	225
3.0	450
4.0	600

THE PPM SCALE

A system was adopted to simplify the reporting of an NMR spectrum. It records the chemical shift in a way that is independent of the strength of the external magnetic field. The system used to express the chemical shift is the *PPM* (parts per million) *scale* in which PPM is the difference in frequency divided by the resonant frequency of one of the peaks, all multiplied by 1 million.

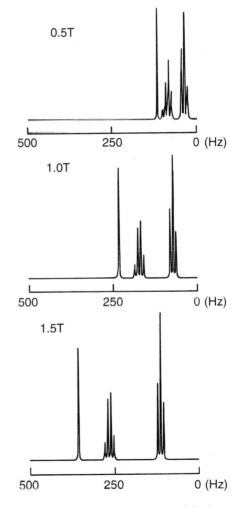

Figure 9-7 The ethanol spectra of hydrogen at three magnetic field strengths show that chemical shifts resulting in peak separation become more obvious at higher field strength. The frequency scale is relative to a standard.

PPM (Parts per Million)	

$$PPM = \frac{f-f_0}{f_0} \times 10^6$$

where f is the resonant frequency under investigation and f_0 is the resonant frequency of a standard.

Two other features facilitate the use of the PPM scale. A reference must be established, and the direction of the scale is reversed. For example, if one peak resonated at 100,000,000 Hz and another at 100,000,500 Hz, they differ by 500 parts in 100 million, or 5 ppm. For ^1H, most resonance peaks occur over a range of 10 ppm, whereas for ^{13}C, resonance signals range over more than 200 ppm.

 The difference in resonant frequency between fat and water protons is 3.5 ppm.

In addition an arbitrary reference standard has been adopted for most nuclides, including ^1H, and it is tetramethylsilane (TMS). Its unique resonance position in each of these NMR ranges is given the value 0. The units of parts per million are dimensionless but are still accorded a frequency scale.

Relative to the reference, the value for the chemical shifts can be positive or negative, depending on whether the resonance is at a higher or lower frequency than the standard TMS. As a matter of experience, as well as choosing of a "good" reference, most values are positive.

One further note is appropriate. The analytical NMR spectrometers that were in use when these conventions were being written were operated at constant frequency, and the strength of the magnetic field was altered to create a spectrum. Thus the plot to the left of the reference (TMS) was called **upfield** and to the right **downfield.** The opposite situation occurred when the frequency-swept machines were put in wide use. The frequency is simply plotted with increasing values to the left to prevent two different displays.

Resonant peaks at higher frequency are downfield; those at lower frequency are upfield.

SIGNAL INTENSITY

NMR spectra are also described by the relative amounts of each type signal in the spectrum. This is the same as the relative number of atoms in chemically shifted unique groups. The amount of signal is given not by the peak height but by the area under the curve that represents the peak.

This relationship is readily made linear in the case of ^1H NMR. The system is a miniature democracy with the creed, "one hydrogen atom, one vote." This situation arises because the excitation and detection of the NMR signal does not normally select for the chemical shift. In the case of ethanol the hydroxyl (OH) group gives one unit of intensity; the methylene (CH_2) group, two units of intensity; and the methyl (CH_3) group, three units of intensity (Figure 9-8).

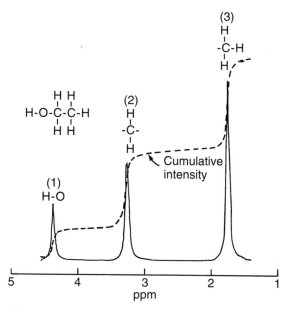

Figure 9-8 The hydrogen nuclear magnetic resonance spectrum of ethanol contains three peaks with sizes that are proportional to the number of nuclei with equal Larmor frequency.

The measurement protocols are more difficult in the study of nuclides other than ^1H, but they can be made sufficiently precise to identify chemical composition and structure. Because of this, NMR spectroscopy has become one of the prevalent methods of both quantitative and qualitative analysis in chemistry and biomedical applications.

J-COUPLING

The concept and observation of J-coupling is another critical aid to NMR. At first, J-coupling was viewed as a nuisance. However, it soon became a well-understood indicator of detailed molecular structure. The J-coupling appears in the spectrum as additional lines appear (splittings) in any particular resonance peak. This creates a finer, more precise spectrum (Figure 9-9).

The origin of J-coupling is in the interaction of spins within the same molecule. In general, those spins close to each other exhibit stronger couplings than those farther away. The magnitude of the J-coupling, expressed in hertz, is independent of field strength. The effect on the spectrum is proportional to the separation in chemical shift between the coupled nuclei. As a result, high field NMR spectra are easier to interpret than those obtained at low field.

The NMR spectroscopist generates a large number of spectral patterns expected from structural subsets. The spectroscopist then identifies structures of molecules as a whole by the interpretation of these couplings. The extra information in the J-coupling is a substantial asset in structure determination.

The figures used here to illustrate the principle of NMR spectroscopy are chosen for ease of understanding, not for completeness of presentation. Organic chemistry and biochemistry have millions of molecules that have been studied by NMR. In most cases, the NMR spectra are considerably more complicated than the ones given here. However, a trained spectroscopist can interpret and explain these spectra in terms of molecular structure and configuration.

Some words of caution: NMR spectroscopy is a daunting, complex, but rewarding intellectual proposition, and the same can be said for MRI. The expectation is that the best features of both can be combined into imaging spectroscopy for medical diagnosis. Such techniques are evolving. Spatially localized MR spectra can be measured with confidence if sufficient time and energy are devoted to the project.

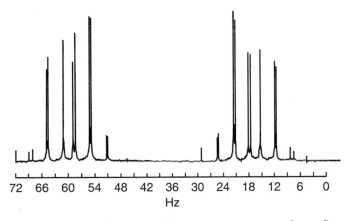

Figure 9-9 This hydrogen nuclear magnetic resonance spectrum shows fine structure as a result of J-coupling.

MEDICALLY IMPORTANT NUCLEI

NMR spectral information has been used to enrich chemistry for the past 40 years; it is just now attracting the interest of the medical community. With the application of in vivo MRS, it is possible to obtain various spectra from patients and therefore gain information about the chemistry of life. Progress toward clinical utility is slow, but the rate of progress is increasing.

Hydrogen

The in vivo MR hydrogen spectrum is dominated by the signal from water. The second most common contributor to the MR signal is the triglycerides found in adipose tissue (fat). Depending on the location of the volume of interest, fat may be the only tissue present, though water is usually evident. The strong (at least in the NMR world) signal from the hydrogen nucleus makes this nuclide the one of choice for MRI.

MRI is relatively easy when the dominant signal is from the hydrogen in water. Image quality is compromised when fat is present. However, the presence of these two signals only causes problems at high magnetic field strength. At low magnetic field strength the difference between the fat signal and water signal is small enough that it is overwhelmed by the gradient magnetic fields used to make the image.

At higher magnetic fields this difference is not overwhelmed by the gradient magnetic fields, and distinct fat and water images that are slightly offset from each other are produced. The resulting image contains a chemical shift artifact (Figure 9-10). The fat and water

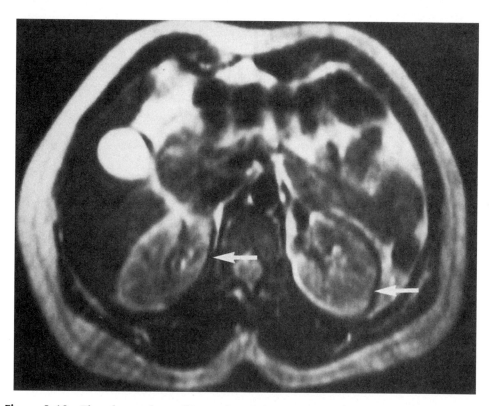

Figure 9-10 The observed curvilinear rim of decreased signal intensity adjacent to the renal cortex is an artifact caused by the chemical shift between hydrogen in fat and hydrogen in water. (Courtesy George Oliver, St. Louis, MO.)

signals are 10,000 times stronger than the signal from other hydrogen-containing metabolites. The use of hydrogen NMR to study these metabolites is thus a strong challenge.

Currently, the use of fat and water suppression (i.e., removing these signals from the MRS region of interest) permits the noninvasive observation of at least 15 different metabolites in the brain. The MRS conditions for convenient measurement select signals from N-acetyl aspartate, creatine, phosphocreatine, choline, and lactate. The lactate is often used as an indicator of a pathologic condition, whereas the other compounds are found in most subjects. The database for ^{1}H MRS is accumulating rapidly. The widespread diffusion of this database will encourage the clinical use of MRS in the future.

Phosphorus

Another nuclide currently receiving attention in MRS is the phosphorus isotope ^{31}P. This nuclide is the only one of phosphorus found in nature. Phosphorus is present in all human tissue and is a reporter of metabolism. It has a spin quantum number of $\frac{1}{2}$ and is similar in its spectral properties to hydrogen. In other words, it is well behaved in its MR spectral properties.

One important phosphorus-containing metabolite is adenosine triphosphate (ATP). Others include adenosine diphosphate (ADP), a byproduct of ATP metabolism, and adenosine monophosphate (AMP), a building block for the formation of ADP and ATP. Creatine phosphate (PCr), a chemical intermediate for the storage of biochemical energy, is also evident in the ^{31}P MR spectrum from some tissues.

All of these metabolites enter into reactions in which phosphoric acid, known to physiologists as *inorganic phosphate* (Pi), is either formed or consumed. One interesting application of ^{31}P MRS is to determine the intracellular pH from the chemical shift of the inorganic phosphate signal. Thus the MR spectrometer is a sophisticated, expensive, but noninvasive pH meter.

An overlay of all these phosphorus signals appears in the MR spectrum of most tissues and provides a window into the energy state of the tissue. A representative ^{31}P spectrum is shown in Figure 9-11.

Phosphorus MR is being used to understand and perhaps diagnose metabolic disorders, assess damage in heart attacks, and monitor the effects of drugs and drug therapy.

Carbon

Almost every chemical compound in living systems contains the carbon atom. Therefore it is anticipated that any method to observe carbon with MR spectroscopy would be advantageous. Nature has conspired to provide carbon in an NMR silent form.

The ordinary nuclide of carbon, ^{12}C, is nonmagnetic because it has paired nucleons and therefore does not generate an NMR spectrum. The magnetic form of carbon, ^{13}C, is present in all tissue to the extent of 1.1%. A number of laboratories are studying this scarce nucleus, though the studies are experimentally demanding.

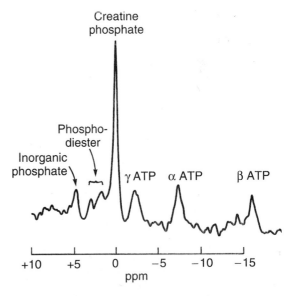

Figure 9-11 A representative ^{31}P nuclear magnetic resonance spectrum. (Courtesy Bud Wendt, Houston, TX.)

The scarcity of ^{13}C permits the tagging of experimental molecules by as much as 100-fold. The tagged molecules can be followed through a number of interesting and intricate metabolic events with MRS. A representative ^{13}C NMR spectrum is shown in Figure 9-12.

Sodium

Sodium is abundant in the body primarily as sodium chloride and other salts. The common isotope of sodium is ^{23}Na; its spin quantum number is ⅔. A spectrum of ^{23}Na is shown in Figure 9-13. There are indications that the MR signal of sodium can be used to probe the intramolecular and intermolecular environments of the molecule and to report them separately.

Fluorine

Fluorine has two advantages for observation in human tissue. Its gyromagnetic ratio is nearly as great as that of hydrogen, and the only nuclear species is ^{19}F, with a spin of ½. Atom for atom, it is as easy to observe as hydrogen. However, it is almost totally absent from the human body. Indeed, high concentrations of fluorine can be toxic.

In the event a safe agent can be identified, which does occur, fluorine becomes a nearly perfect tracer, or indicator, of metabolism. In a

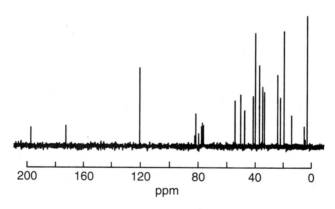

Figure 9-12 A representative ^{13}C nuclear magnetic resonance spectrum. (Courtesy Bud Wendt, Houston, TX.)

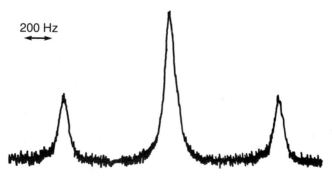

Figure 9-13 A representative ^{23}Na nuclear magnetic resonance spectrum. (Courtesy Bud Wendt, Houston, TX.)

typical measurement there would be no ^{19}F before the measurement, the agent would be introduced, and the arrival of ^{19}F at the volume of interest can be monitored.

In the vocabulary of imaging these are *dark field measurements*. There is no signal at the beginning and then an abundant signal as the ^{19}F arrives at the observation site. Figure 9-14 shows experimental ^{19}F images focused on blood substitute materials and pO_2 imaging.

Forms of materials that carry ^{19}F are the new perfluorocarbon artificial bloods and 5-deoxyfluoroglucose (5-FDG). In addition, chemotherapeutic agents for the treatment of cancer often carry ^{19}F in their chemical structure. Research is being conducted in the use of these agents to monitor blood flow, follow metabolism, and understand the effectiveness of cancer therapy regimens.

Nitrogen

Nitrogen is nearly as common in biology as carbon. All amino acids, peptides, proteins, deoxyribonucleic acids (DNA), and ribonucleic acids (RNA) are rich in nitrogen. Ordinary nitrogen is ^{14}N, with a spin quantum number of 1. The observation of this nuclide is difficult. It has an unfavorable gyromagnetic ratio and is inherently insensitive. In addition the spectral lines are usually extremely broad and hard to detect.

A rare nuclide of nitrogen, ^{15}N, has a spin of ½ and would seem to be suitable for study. However, its gyromagnetic ratio is also

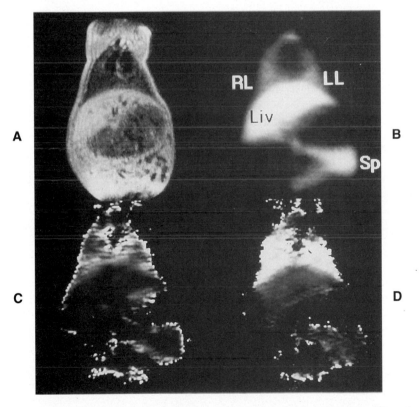

Figure 9-14 Images through the midtorso of a pig. **A,** Sow image. **B,** ^{19}F spin echo image. **C,** Calculated pO_2 T1 weighted (T1W) ^{19}F image during normal breathing. **D,** Calculated pO_2 T1W ^{19}F image during 100% oxygen breathing. (Courtesy Stephen Thomas, Cincinnati, OH.)

unfavorable, and its observation is exceedingly difficult. If nitrogen is to be useful in medicine, it will require expensive ^{15}N-enriched substrates and long observation times.

CHALLENGE QUESTIONS

1. The distribution of frequencies observed in an MR signal is known as what quantity?
2. List at least three other elements that could possibly be used to make a magnetic resonance (MR) image.
3. What happens to the appearance of an NMR spectrum at high magnetic field strength?
4. What is J-coupling?
5. What is chemical shift as it relates to NMR spectroscopy?
6. What is the variation in magnetic field homogeneity expressed in parts per million for a 1 T ± 10 μ T magnet?
7. What is the chemical shift difference in the resonant frequency between fat and water protons?
8. What is the gyromagnetic ratio for hydrogen?
9. What is the frequency difference for proton spins in water versus those in fat at 1.5 T?
10. Along which axis does the chemical shift artifact appear?

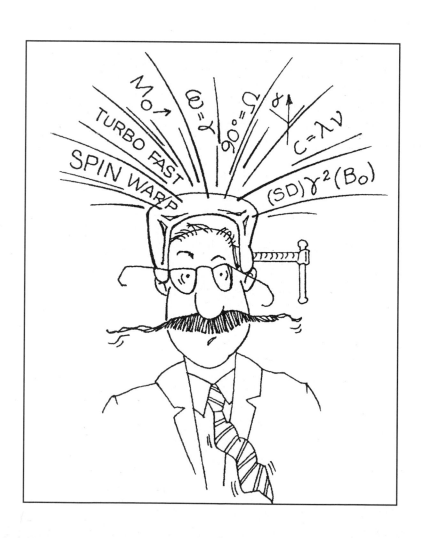

Part II

The Imaging System

Chapter 10

Magnetic Resonance Imaging Hardware

OBJECTIVES

At the completion of this chapter, the student should be able to do the following:

1. Name the three major components of a magnetic resonance imaging (MRI) system and the subassemblies of each.
2. List the three types of MRI systems and describe features of each.
3. Discuss the purpose of shim coils.
4. Identify the principal controls on the MRI operating console.
5. Describe distinguishing features of the MRI computer.

OUTLINE

The basic physics of magnetic resonance imaging (MRI) have been covered in the previous chapters, and the equipment used in the process is discussed in this and the following three chapters.

An MRI system contains three major components, each of which consists of several subsystems. The major components are the gantry, the operating console, and the computer. In this regard, an MRI system is similar to a computed tomography (CT) imaging system. Here, however, most similarities end. These principal components are shown in Figure 10-1.

 Gantry, operating console, and computer are the three principal components of an MRI system.

The gantry contains the main magnet and several other electromagnetic devices essential to MRI. Unlike CT, there are no moving parts in the MRI gantry. The operating console resembles a CT console, and although many of the control designations are similar, they also serve different functions. The MRI computer is powerful and fast such as that used in multislice CT.

Each of the three types of MRI systems—superconducting electromagnet, resistive electromagnet, and permanent magnet—uses similar computers. The operating consoles have similar functional controls that appear the same. However, the gantries are completely different. Each has a distinctive appearance that makes them easily recognizable. Because most MRI systems are superconducting, this discussion focuses on that type.

THE GANTRY

The gantry can be intimidating to a patient, especially after it is placed on the examination couch and moved into the patient aperture. A patient then hears the resounding thump, thump, thump of the gradient coils, suggesting that this is indeed a big and intimidating machine. However, it is not a machine because there are no moving parts. The gantry does have many subsystems and several different electromagnetic coils.

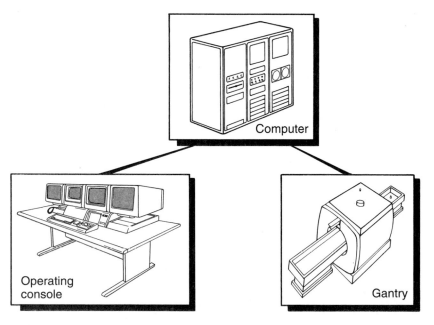

Figure 10-1 The principal components of a magnetic resonance imaging system are the gantry, the operating console, and the computer.

A

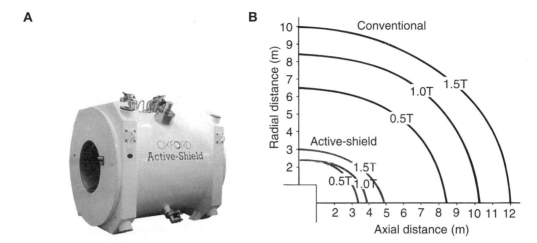

B

Figure 10-2 **A,** This 1.5-T superconducting magnet is actively shielded. **B,** The active shield reduces the magnetic fringe field distance by one third. (Courtesy Oxford Magnet Technology.)

Superconducting Magnetic Resonance Imaging System

Figure 10-2 is a typical superconducting MRI magnet. Superconducting MRI magnets are approximately 3 m across by 3 m high, with a length of 2 m. The massive size is due principally to the requirement of maintaining the primary magnetic coils at a super-cooled temperature or cryogenic state. This cryogenic state is accomplished with multiple insulating chambers.

 Cryogens are liquefied gases that produce supercold temperatures near absolute zero. Liquid nitrogen and liquid helium are used in MRI.

The gantry of a superconducting MRI system can be considered to have three subassemblies: the patient couch, the primary electromagnet assembly, and the various secondary electromagnets (Figure 10-3). Often the secondary electromagnets are at room temperature, unlike the primary electromagnet that is immersed in liquid helium.

The patient couch performs the two functions of support and position. The couch should be able to accept patients who weigh up to 130 kg (286 lb) at near floor level and raise the patient with a power assist to the level of the gantry patient aperture. From this position outside the gantry, the couch should be capable of moving to the imaging position under power assist to within ± 1 mm.

Precise positioning is essential during examination. Once at the imaging position, the patient is not moved during the examination.

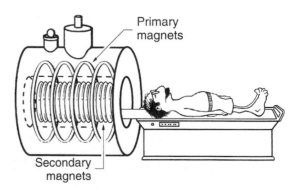

Figure 10-3 The patient couch, the primary electromagnet assembly, and the secondary electromagnets are the three superconducting magnet subassemblies.

This precision is obtained with specialty gears and electronic registers. Each revolution of the smallest drive gear corresponds to a 1-mm movement of the couch. Each revolution also activates an electronic counter so that the couch position can be visually displayed. Table 10-1 lists minimum acceptable specifications for the patient couch.

At installation, the service engineer adjusts the two or three positioning laser lights to intersect at a point on the axis of the MRI gantry (Figure 10-4). Usually, this position is then set at zero on the couch position indicator.

The primary electromagnet assembly is not visible. It is enclosed in a decorative plastic housing. Even with the housing removed, the primary electromagnet assembly cannot be seen because it is deep within the chambers of the cryostat. The innermost chamber of the cryostat houses an aluminum cylinder onto which the superconducting wire is wound (Figure 10-5).

The cryostat is a large, insulating container of many concentric chambers.

Similarly, the secondary magnetic coils are not visible. They are also covered by a decorative protective housing. The relative position of these magnetic coils in the gantry is shown in Figure 10-6.

There are three secondary magnetic coils, and they are independent. Nearest to the patient is the radiofrequency (RF) coil. The RF coil is not an electromagnet in the normal sense. It does produce a magnetic field, an

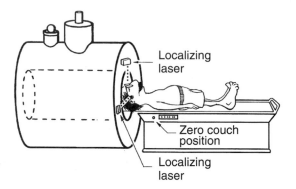

Figure 10-4   Two or three positioning laser lights are adjusted to intersect on the axis of the primary magnetic field of a magnetic resonance imaging system.

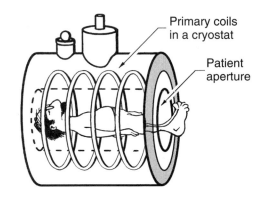

Figure 10-5   Relative position of the primary magnetic coils in the magnet.

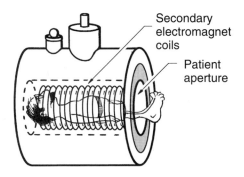

Figure 10-6   Relative position of the secondary magnetic coils in the magnet.

TABLE 10-1	Minimum Specifications for an MRI Patient-Positioning Couch	
Descriptor	**Performance Standard**	
Patient capacity	130 kg	
Lift speed	1 cm/s	
Translation speed	10 cm/s	
Position accuracy	±1 mm	

MRI, Magnetic resonance imaging.

incidental byproduct to its use as an RF antenna. The RF coil is a separate, removable assembly and therefore is not cryogenic but kept at room temperature (Figure 10-7).

The secondary magnetic coils adjacent to the patient aperture are the gradient coils. These coils are large electrical conductors that produce the transient gradient magnetic fields. They are switched on and off rapidly. This current switching results in the conductors' heating and expanding, and these cause the thumping sound. These coils are also usually at room temperature.

Between the gradient coils and the primary electromagnet assembly for earlier systems, shim coils were positioned to make the B_0 field more homogeneous (uniform field intensity). Usually the shim coils were at room temperature, but in advanced MRI systems, they were in the cryostat.

However, shim coils have largely been abandoned because of expense and the bore space they occupied. Now, small pieces of ferromagnetic materials are used along with gradient magnetic field offsets to obtain excellent B_0 homogeneity.

Resistive Electromagnet Imaging System

The patient couch of a resistive electromagnet imaging system appears the same as that of a superconducting MRI system and will have similar performance characteristics. Unlike the superconducting MRI system, the primary magnet can usually be visualized.

Figure 10-8 shows the typical configuration for the primary magnet of the resistive electromagnet imaging system. In this illustration there are three white rings, two large and one small. There is a fourth small ring on the backside of this electromagnet.

These rings each contain a coil of wire conducting a large electrical current, approximately 30 to 50 amperes (A). The two large coils produce the B_0 magnetic field, whereas the two smaller coils on each end help to extend the length of the field and make it uniform.

The secondary electromagnets of a resistive magnet imaging system are often visible. The shim coils and gradient coils are usually con-

tained within the primary magnet. This subassembly defines the patient aperture. The RF probe is a separate operator-interchangeable assembly.

Resistive electromagnet MRI systems have made something of a comeback. Many 0.2-T and 0.5-T magnets are now resistive with an iron core. These magnets look like large C-arms with a vertical B_0 field.

Permanent Magnet Imaging System

The subassemblies of a permanent magnet imaging system are not visible because of a decorative housing. There is no hint of how

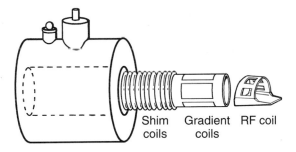

Figure 10-7 Relative position of the shim coils, gradient coils, and radiofrequency *(RF)* coil.

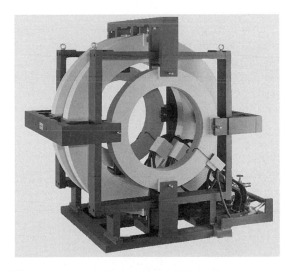

Figure 10-8 A four-coil resistive electromagnet for magnetic resonance imaging. (Courtesy Bruker Instruments.)

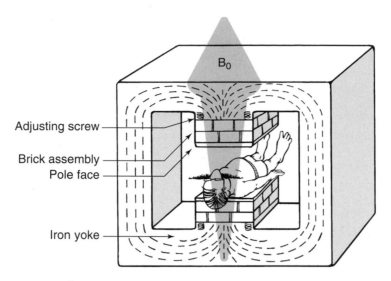

Figure 10-9 A permanent magnet MRI system.

the subassemblies appear except for the RF probe, which is identifiable and operator interchangeable.

The cutaway view of the permanent magnet MRI gantry in Figure 10-9 shows that the primary magnetic field is produced by two assemblies of bricklike magnets. These primary magnets are attached to a massive iron yoke.

The iron yoke plays the same role with the MRI gantry as it does for a transformer and is similar in design. The iron yoke provides a return path for the lines of the primary magnetic field. The result of the yoke's presence is to increase the B_0 magnetic field intensity within the patient aperture.

There are no shim coils in a permanent magnet MRI system. Shimming the primary magnetic field is accomplished by mechanically adjusting the two finely machined pole pieces.

THE OPERATING CONSOLE

The operating console of an MRI system (Figure 10-10) appears similar to that of a CT imaging system, but there are substantial dif-

ferences. In general, two sets of controls are found on the operating console of an MRI system. One set is for image acquisition and the other for image processing.

Some controls are activated by special function keys, but most are under computer command. The operator responds to a video prompt by keying commands through a mouse or trackball interface. As with CT, physicians' viewing consoles are also available as an option on an MRI system.

Many similarities exist between MRI and CT operating consoles. In general, the operating controls associated with start-up and image processing are very similar. The image acquisition controls are different. The principal control functions on the console of an MRI system are as follows:

Start-up

1. Power on/off—This is usually a key switch or push switch that is used to energize the system.
2. Emergency off—This should be used only if the patient is in imminent danger or if continued operation could result in a damage to the imaging system.

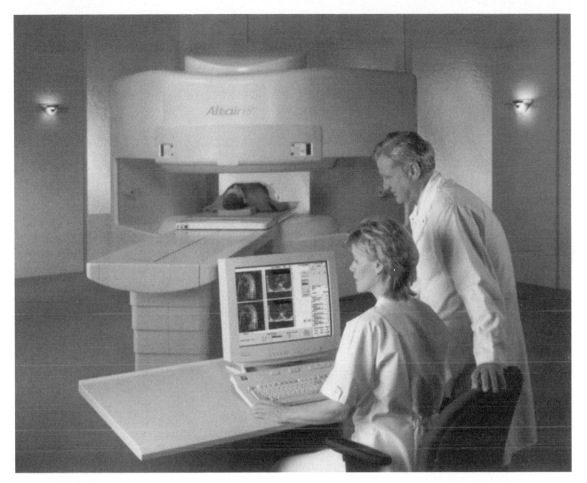

Figure 10-10 A magnetic resonance imaging operating console. (Courtesy Hitachi Medical of America.)

3. Intercom—This device allows communication with the patient.
4. Cathode-ray tube (CRT) flat panel control (LCD)—Several knobs control brightness, contrast, and power to the video monitor.
5. Annotation—Alphanumerical and special function keys input patient and image data for final hardcopy images.

Prescan Calibrations

1. Tune the transmit/receive coils—The size and shape of the patient change the load (electronic impedance) of these coils. The impedance of the coil is tuned to match that of the patient for maximum RF efficiency. Impedance mismatch results in higher noise and therefore reduced contrast. Active tuning of RF coils requires time; therefore some sensitivity has been sacrificed with coils that perform well over a large range of impedances and therefore are not tuned for each patient.
2. Tune the center frequency—Exact tuning establishes slice position and type of protons (fat versus water) for imaging.
3. Calibrate pulse amplitude—The flip angle (α, 90˚, 180˚) is determined by the time the RF is on and the power of the RF (pulse amplitude). Often, just the 90˚ RF pulse is

measured; other flip angles are then scaled to this value.

4. Calibrate receiver gain—This is an amplifier adjustment to ensure the signal is not too low, resulting in noisy images or too high, resulting in data clipping and image distortion.

Image Acquisition

1. Tuning controls—Several keystrokes under computer command are designed to adjust the resonant frequency of the system to accommodate the patient or part being imaged. More often, this is an automatic function.

2. Pulse sequence—The operator usually has a choice of partial saturation, inversion recovery, spin echo, gradient echo, fast spin echo, or echo planar imaging.

3. Repetition time (TR)—This is the time between initial RF pulses. Increasing TR lengthens the scan time. However, with longer TR, more slices per scan are possible with multislice pulse sequence techniques.

4. Inversion time (TI)—This is used with an inversion recovery pulse sequence. TI is the time between the 180° and 90° RF pulse.

5. Echo time (TE)—TE is used with inversion recovery and spin echo pulse sequences. The longer the TE, the more T2 weighted (T2W) the image.

6. Matrix size—The number of pixels is usually 256×256. A larger matrix results in better spatial resolution but requires a longer imaging time.

7. Number of signal acquisitions (NSAs)—This is also represented by number of excitations (NEX) for signal averaging. The more magnetic resonance (MR) signal acquisitions, the better the contrast resolution because the signal-to-noise ratio increases as the square root of the NSAs. Imaging time increases directly as the number of acquisitions increases.

8. Field of view (FOV)—Reducing the FOV increases the spatial resolution but may require more signal acquisitions to maintain an adequate signal-to-noise ratio.

9. Slice thickness—Reducing slice thickness improves the spatial resolution by reducing partial volume effects. More acquisitions may be required to maintain an adequate signal-to-noise ratio.

Image Processing/Display/Manipulation

1. Window width/level—This control is used to set the contrast and shades of gray for the displayed image. The ranges are usually much wider for MRI than for CT.

2. Cursor on/off—This is used to place a cursor on the image and provide for joystick, trackball, or mouse manipulation of the cursor.

3. Region of interest (ROI)—ROI is used for calculation of area of measure and average and standard deviations of pixel values.

4. Zoom—This is used to magnify the image. Some systems provide fixed magnification factors, and others have continuously variable factors. This is an electro-optical zoom. Reconstructive zoom is not possible in MRI as it is in CT.

5. Profile/histogram—This plots the pixel values along an identified axis as either a line graph or a histogram.

6. Highlight—This control selects pixel values within a given range for special attention. They may appear white or black or blink. Special reconstruction algorithms are available for surface rendering and volume rendering.

7. Collage—This provides for the simultaneous display of multiple images or portions of an image on one video screen. It is particularly helpful in MRI because so many images are acquired.

THE MAGNETIC RESONANCE IMAGING COMPUTER

Computers generally come in one of three sizes: microcomputers, minicomputers, and mainframe computers. The explosion in computer technology has erased some of the distinguishing features among these three types of computers.

Minicomputers are used in radiologic imaging, including MRI. An earlier version of a minicomputer required several instrumentation racks. Now, however, minicomputers are found in single, desk-size cabinets.

The basic requirement for a computer in MRI is that it must have high capacity and be fast. The capacity to store data for manipulation must be high because of the nature of the MR signal and the number of signals required for an image. The computer must be fast to handle the high rate of data acquisition and to accommodate the enormous number of calculations required to produce an image. Image processing times of less than 1 second are required. Image processing is essentially simultaneous with MRI.

Storage Capacity

MRI produces quantities of data far in excess of those encountered with other medical imaging modalities. A typical electrocardiogram-gated MR cardiac examination may produce 50 images of 128 × 128 pixels each. If each pixel is 2 bytes deep, this amounts to 1.6 megabytes (MB) of data. A three-dimensional head image may yield spin echo images at TEs of 20 ms for T1 weighted (T1W) or proton density, weighted (PDW) images and 80 ms for T2W images. Each image will cover approximately 350 mm FOV with a 256 × 256 matrix, each pixel 2 bytes.

A typical personal computer has a disk storage capacity of perhaps 10 to 20 gigabytes (GB) and a usable random-access memory (RAM) of at least 128 MB. RAM of 512 MB to 1 GB with a 40 to 80 GB hard disk is currently standard for MRI computers. Such a configuration allows local storage of approximately 100,000 uncompressed 256 × 256 images. Image compression results in approximately five times the number of images.

Computer Speed

Not only must the storage capacity of the computer be large, but the computer must also perform computations quickly. In one common two-dimensional Fourier transformation (2DFT) image reconstruction method, computation of a single 256 × 256 image requires 512 × 256 fast Fourier transforms (FFTs).

Each FFT requires 2048 complex multiplications, and these are the most time-consuming parts of the FFT algorithm. A complex multiplication may be computed with four real multiplications. Therefore the 256 × 256 2DFT image needs approximately 4.2 million multiplications.

For the maximum precision resolution in the data to be preserved, the FFT should be computed with floating-point numbers. A floating-point operation, such as a real multiplication, is referred to as a *flop*. The image will thus require 4.2 million flops. Reconstructing the image in 1 second requires approximately 4,000,000 flops per second.

Only with the assistance of an array processor or digital signal processor (DSP) can such a computational rate be achieved. Typical DSP speeds range from 10 to 40 MFLOPS. Such speed is based on idealized situations; practical performance is slowed by limitations on the rate at which data may be moved on and off the disk and by data bus speed.

High performance MRI systems may incorporate multiple DSPs. Consequently, images appear immediately after data collection.

The Operating System

Image reconstruction is not the only chore to be handled by the computer. The same computer that performs the image reconstruction often organizes data acquisition. The program that controls such a computer is called the *operating system*.

For the computer to perform several tasks at once—such as data acquisition, image reconstruction, and image manipulation—the operating system must be **multitasking**. A multitasking operating system allows the computer hardware to be shared by several programs.

A good operating system minimizes the impact of sharing by knowing when each program does not need to use the computer. An example occurs during the latter part of TR, when the acquisition program is just waiting for the nuclear spin system to recover to equilibrium. Another example is the interval between when the reconstruction requests the raw data of an acquisition from the disk and when those data are delivered.

For a physician to review completed studies on one console while an examination is being performed on another, the operating system must be **multiuser**. This means that the operating system allows several users simultaneous access to the computer.

 A multiuser operating system is inherently a multitasking operation system.

Ideally, each computer user thinks that the full computer is at the user's disposal and does not notice the other users of the system. When the manufacturer does not provide a multiuser operating system, the physician's console often has its own computer, which communicates efficiently with the main console computer.

CHALLENGE QUESTIONS

1. What are the three principal components of an MRI system?
2. For any computer, especially those used for MRI, what type of software program controls the data acquisition and image reconstruction?
3. What are the three types of MRI systems?
4. In computer jargon, what is a flop?
5. The thumping noise generated in the gantry of an MRI system is due to what component?
6. An MR image is reconstructed as a 512×512 matrix, 1 byte deep. How many megabytes are required to store that image?
7. What are cryogenic gases?
8. Which image postprocessing procedure is used to accentuate image contrast?
9. What is the main purpose of the iron yoke in a permanent magnet imaging system?
10. What does the word *shim* refer to for an MRI system?

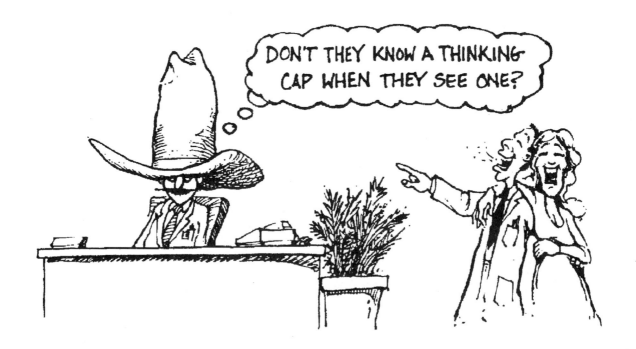

Chapter 11

Primary Magnetic Resonance Imaging Magnets

OBJECTIVES

At the completion of this chapter, the student should be able to do the following:

1. Identify the properties of various types of magnets used for magnetic resonance imaging (MRI).
2. Describe superconductivity and its application to MRI.
3. Discuss the terms *cryogen, cryogenic gas,* and *cryostat.*
4. Convert temperature from one scale to another.
5. Identify differences in imaging between high field and low field.

OUTLINE

PERMANENT MAGNETS
ELECTROMAGNETS
  Resistive Electromagnets
  Superconducting Electromagnets
  Superconductivity
  Superconductor Operation

The equipment necessary to perform magnetic resonance imaging (MRI) is complex and sophisticated. A systematic walk through the major components of the MRI system makes the operation of that system clearer.

A schematic block diagram of a typical MRI system is shown in Figure 11-1. The major components of the gantry of an MRI system can be identified as either the primary magnets or the secondary magnets.

The primary MRI magnet produces the static magnetic field (B_0). Secondary magnets are used to shim the B_0 field and produce gradient magnetic fields (B_X, B_Y, B_Z). These fields are sometimes designated as G_X, G_Y, and G_Z. Finally, the radiofrequency (RF) system can also be considered as a secondary magnet. It includes transmit and receive coils. The shim/gradient coils and RF system are discussed in later chapters.

The primary magnet is the heart of the MRI system. The function of the primary magnet is to provide a sustained B_0 during the MRI examination. The maintenance of a homogeneous B_0 is required because B_0 homogeneity affects image resolution, uniformity, and distortion.

At least two criteria in the selection of an MRI system are driven by the type of primary magnet: the desired field strength and siting limitations. Field strength and siting limitations are interrelated because for a given magnet design, increasing field strength increases the size of the associated fringe magnetic field. Fringe magnetic fields are the component of B_0 that extend outside the magnet and its housing (see Chapter 13).

Basically, two types of magnets are used to generate B_0: permanent magnets and electromagnets. Electromagnets can be further classified as resistive electromagnets and superconducting electromagnets (Box 11-1). Each magnet type has advantages and disadvantages with respect to these two important, often overriding, criteria: field strength and siting limitations. Although the following discussion considers each type of magnet, the main focus is on superconducting electromagnets, the type used in more than 95% of installed

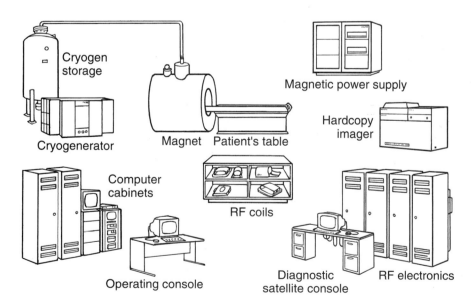

Figure 11-1 Schematic diagram of the principal components of an magnetic resonance imaging system.

MRI systems. A brief comparison of these systems is given in Table 11-1.

PERMANENT MAGNETS

The permanent magnet is the most familiar type of magnet. This is the type of magnet used to demonstrate magnetic fields in science classes and to fix paper to refrigerators. Permanent magnets are components of compasses, motors, and audio speakers. They are inexpensive and widely used for simple applications.

 Permanent magnets occur naturally, or they can be synthesized.

The earliest commercial magnets were made of iron and called *ferrite magnets.* In the 1930s, an alloy called *alnico* (**al**uminum, **ni**ckel, and **co**balt) was developed with a slightly higher magnetic field than ferrite magnets. Alnico magnets have been made with ever-increasing magnetic field intensities. More recently, rare earth magnets have been introduced, which have even higher magnetic field intensity (Figure 11-2).

Although magnetic field strengths of up to approximately 1.2 T can theoretically be achieved with permanent magnets, field strengths of only about 0.3 T are practical for whole-body MRI systems. Figure 11-3 shows a typical permanent magnet MRI system.

This design is often called an *open* MRI system because it enables parents to remain with their child during imaging. Open permanent magnet systems also make claustrophobic or anxious patients more comfortable. The magnetic field is typically produced by individual brick-size ferromagnetic ceramic materials that are rendered magnetic by charging them in the field of an electromagnet (Figure 11-4).

Once magnetized, these bricks are then carefully oriented into an array, up to 1 m on a side, containing two to five layers. The fabrication of such a large magnet made from smaller magnets is not a trivial task. The forces exerted are enormous, and if one brick is positioned incorrectly, contrary magnetic fields can result and cause the whole assembly to fragment violently.

A variety of magnetic bricks are shown in Figure 11-5. Two assemblies are positioned opposite one another at a distance appropriate for head (50 cm) or whole-body (100 cm) imaging. A typical permanent magnet design is shown in Figure 11-6. In such a design the four corner posts are iron and provide a return path for the magnetic field.

A pole face is positioned on each magnet assembly (Figure 11-7). These pole faces are

---

Box 11-1 | *Types of Magnets Used to Generate B_0*

MRI B_0 MAGNETS

Permanent   Electromagnets

                Resistive   Superconducting

MRI, Magnetic resonance imaging.

TABLE 11-1	Characteristic Features of Magnetic Resonance Imaging Systems		
	Permanent Magnet	**Resistive Electromagnet**	**Superconducting Electromagnet**
B_0 field intensity	0.1-0.3 T	0.2 T	0.5-4 T
Power requirements	Low	Very high	Low
Cooling requirements	None	Water	Cryogenic
Magnetic fringe field	None	Modest	Strong

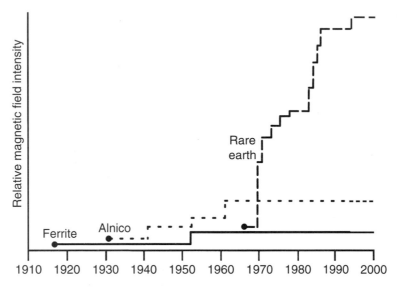

Figure 11-2   Developments in permanent magnet design have caused magnetic field intensity to increase over the years.

carefully machined iron slabs designed to help orient and shape the B_0 field and to increase its homogeneity within the imaging volume. Often there are adjusting screws or other mechanical shimming devices to further refine the homogeneity of the magnetic field after the imaging system is installed in a prepared site.

 Permanent magnets are shimmed with a pole face.

An iron yoke is in physical contact with each permanent magnet, and this contact serves

three purposes. First, it provides a mechanical frame for assembly and stability. Second, it confines the fringe magnetic field by concen-

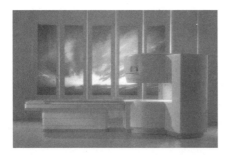

Figure 11-3   A permanent magnet magnetic resonance imaging system featuring an open design provides easy access and comfort for claustrophobic patients. (Courtesy Hitachi Medical Corp.)

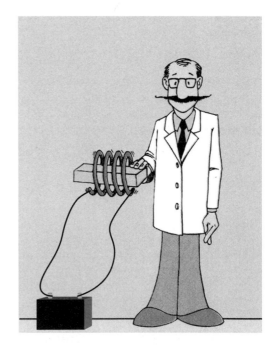

Figure 11-4   A method for rendering ceramic bricks magnetic with an electromagnet.

trating the lines of the magnetic field in this iron yoke. Finally, by containing the fringe magnetic field, the yoke also intensifies B_0 in the imaging aperture. Without an iron yoke, B_0 strength of such an assembly would be much less (Figure 11-8). The yoke is usually made of soft iron laminated and bolted together like a transformer core.

Table 11-2 presents the principal characteristics of a permanent magnet MRI system. The principal advantage of a permanent magnet MRI system is the insignificant fringe magnetic field, which for any MRI system must be no greater than 0.5 mT in any controlled area. This level is chosen out of consideration for patients with cardiac pacemakers; it is not hazardous to others.

The 0.5-mT field is within a few centimeters of the permanent magnet gantry because of the mass and design of the iron yoke. Other advantages of a permanent magnet MRI system include low electric power consumption and the absence of a cooling system.

The principal disadvantage of a permanent magnet MRI system is the limited B_0 intensity. This places some restrictions on the type and

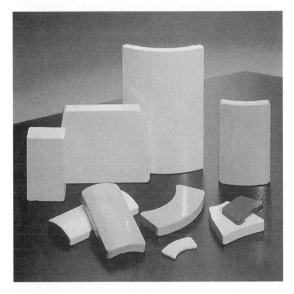

Figure 11-5 Individual magnets of varying sizes and shapes are assembled to produce the strong magnetic field of a permanent magnet magnetic resonance imaging system. (Courtesy Sumitomo Special Metals.)

complexity of imaging allowed. Other disadvantages include the relatively poor magnetic field homogeneity, usually about 20 parts per

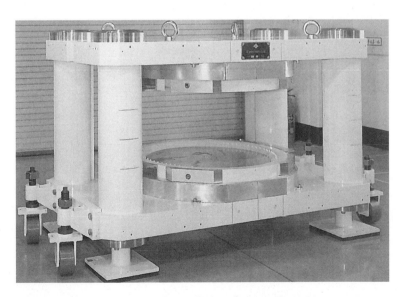

Figure 11-6 Typical permanent magnet design for imaging. (Courtesy Sumitomo Special Metals.)

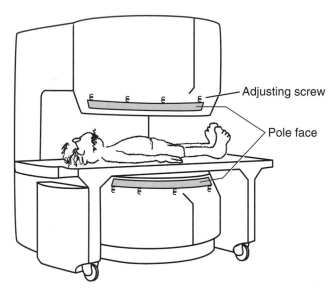

Figure 11-7 Permanent magnets are shimmed by positioning precisely machined pole faces.

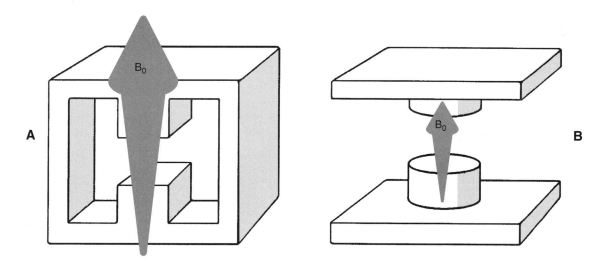

Figure 11-8 The presence of an iron yoke (**A**) with a permanent magnet imaging system intensifies the B_0 field in comparison to one without (**B**). The yoke provides a return path for the lines of the magnetic field.

million (ppm), and the excessive weight. Poor magnetic field homogeneity results in reduced spatial and contrast resolution. The weight of a permanent magnet MRI system limits its use to fixed sites.

Permanent magnets are attractive for low magnetic field imaging applications because of their minimal fringe magnetic fields, low power requirement, and open architecture. However, the use of permanent magnets in

TABLE 11-2 Characteristics of a Permanent Magnet Magnetic Resonance Imaging System	
Feature	Value
Magnetic field (B_0)	Up to 0.3 T
Magnetic field homogeneity	10-50 ppm
Weight	90,000 kg
Cooling	None
Power consumption	20 kW
Distance to 0.5-mT fringe field	<1 m

clinical MRI is limited. This is because the maximum B_0 intensity is low. Permanent MRI systems compromise the ability for some clinical applications, such as echo planar imaging.

Although the fringe magnetic fields tend to be small, the weight of a well-designed permanent magnet MRI system can approach 90,000 kg (approximately 100 tons). This imposes significant mechanical considerations on the chosen location and usually excludes all but ground floor siting.

There is a fundamental difference between a permanent magnet MRI system and one of

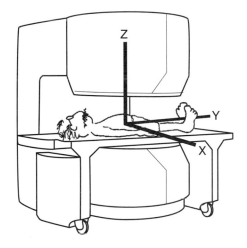

Figure 11-9 The long axis of the patient is the Y-axis in a permanent magnet magnetic resonance imaging system corresponding to the axis identification of vector diagrams.

electromagnet design. The B_0 field of a permanent magnet imaging system is vertical (Figure 11-9). Therefore the Z-axis is vertical rather than horizontal as in most superconducting electromagnet imaging systems. The long axis of the patient in a permanent magnet imaging system is the X-axis, and the lateral direction is the Y-axis. This corresponds to the axis identification in vector diagrams.

ELECTROMAGNETS

Electromagnets make up the second type of primary magnet system for imaging. It is useful to discuss resistive electromagnets and superconducting electromagnets separately because they have significantly different operating characteristics. However, the physics of image production is exactly the same regardless of magnet type, especially when comparing equal B_0. Neither the patient nor the secondary magnets can identify the origin of the B_0. There are no characteristic image distinctions.

Resistive Electromagnets

Resistive electromagnets are making something of a comeback, having nearly disappeared from the commercial MRI scene. The B_0 in a resistive electromagnet imaging system is produced by a large, classical electromagnet. All of the early MRI investigations were conducted with such resistive air-core electromagnets. The two outside coils of the classical four-coil design are smaller in diameter, rendering the B_0 more uniform in the imaging volume between the two large inside coils (Figure 11-10).

One variation of a resistive electromagnet MRI incorporates the design shown in Figure 11-11. This arrangement results in a vertical B_0 field, which can be intensified by coupling to a permanent magnet.

The most common design of solenoid resistive electromagnets uses aluminum strips wound spirally around a tube in several thousand layers. The advantage in cost and weight

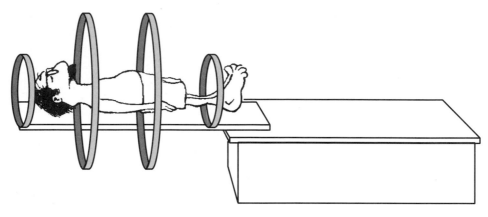

Figure 11-10 A resistive electromagnet usually has four separate coils to intensify B_0 and make it uniform.

dictates aluminum as the preferred resistive electromagnet material. The mass density of aluminum is approximately one third that of copper; however, it has only about 60% the conductivity of copper. Table 11-3 gives the principal characteristics of a resistive electromagnet MRI system.

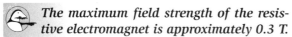 *The maximum field strength of the resistive electromagnet is approximately 0.3 T.*

Resistive electromagnet imaging systems have some advantages. They are less expensive than superconducting electromagnet imaging systems because they operate at lower field strengths and they do not require the precision and homogeneity of a superconducting imaging system. Magnetic field homogeneity of 10 to 50 ppm exists for most resistive MRI sys-

tems. Shimming this type of magnet is somewhat less difficult than shimming a superconducting system.

Because such a resistive electromagnet is readily brought up to designed magnetic field strength, it is just as easily turned off. This removes the hazard of ferromagnetic projectiles during nonimaging time. It is a simple matter to remove metallic objects that become attracted to and stuck in the magnet.

Siting the resistive electromagnet imaging system is easier than siting a superconducting electromagnet in terms of fringe magnetic fields. A resistive electromagnetic imaging sys-

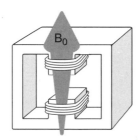

Figure 11-11 This resistive electromagnet configuration produces a vertical B_0 field.

TABLE 11-3	Characteristics of a Resistive Electromagnet Magnetic Resonance Imaging System
Feature	**Value**
Magnetic field (B_0)	Up to 0.3 T
Magnetic field homogeneity	10-50 ppm
Weight	4000 kg
Cooling	Water, heat exchanger
Power consumption	80 kW
Distance to 0.5-mT fringe field	2 m

tem also weighs less than permanent magnet imaging systems (4000 kg versus 90,000 kg). For these reasons, siting the resistive electromagnet imaging system is often the simplest.

The principal disadvantage of this type of imaging system is electric power consumption. A resistive electromagnet imaging system is the most power hungry of the three. A 0.2-T imaging system may require 60 to 80 kW, and this is a continuous power drain when the magnet is on. In addition, requirements for cooling the magnet must be met. Resistive electromagnets are water cooled, with a closed primary loop communicating with a secondary single pass system through a heat exchanger.

Superconducting Electromagnets

Electromagnets are created by conducting electric current through coiled wire. MRI systems based on superconducting electromagnet technology have the principal characteristic of high B_0 magnetic field strength.

Most superconducting clinical imaging systems operate at 0.5 T, 1.0 T, or 1.5 T. Superconducting imaging systems at 3 T and 4 T are in clinical operation at many sites, but these are specialty systems. Superconducting electromagnets used for analytical spectroscopy and high-energy physics now exceed 14 T. These systems can achieve such high fields because of their high electric current and small bore size.

High field superconducting magnets have relative advantages and disadvantages when compared with low field systems. Higher B_0 requires more intense gradient magnetic fields, resulting in broader RF bandwidth.

Longitudinal relaxation time (T1) increases with increasing B_0 and requires relatively longer repetition time (TR) for the same T1 weighting (T1W). B_0 has no effect on transverse relaxation time, T2, at field strengths below approximately 2 T. At higher B_0, T2 decreases slightly.

The precessional frequencies of fat and water protons are separated by approximately 3.5 ppm. At 0.3 T this amounts to only 45 Hz and is not noticeable. At 3 T the chemical shift

is 450 Hz and results in a distinct artifact. Artifacts caused by magnetic susceptibility, blood flow, and patient motion are more severe at high B_0.

The most common magnets today use superconducting technology to achieve intense, highly homogenous magnetic fields. Table 11-4 presents the principal characteristics of a clinical superconducting electromagnet MRI system.

Superconductivity

At room temperature, all materials resist the flow of electric current. Superconductivity is the property of some materials that allow them to conduct electricity with no resistance. Such materials reach superconductivity as temperature is lowered to a critical temperature (T_c). This critical temperature varies with each superconducting material.

 Superconductivity means that once the electric current begins to flow, it will flow indefinitely.

All clinical superconducting electromagnets use niobium-titanium (NbTi) alloys that have a critical temperature of approximately 9 Kelvin (K). The way to achieve such a low temperature is to immerse the conductor in liquid helium.

TABLE 11-4	Characteristics of a Clinical Superconducting Electronmagnet Magnetic Resonance Imaging System
Feature	**Value**
Magnetic field (B_0)	0.5 T to 4 T
Magnetic field homogeneity	0.1-5 ppm
Weight	10,000 kg
Cooling	Cryogenic
Power consumption	20 kW
Distance to 0.5-mT fringe field	10 m

Liquid helium vaporizes at 4 K and therefore easily maintains the NbTi conductor below its critical temperature. Liquid nitrogen, which vaporizes at 77 K, was used to insulate the liquid helium. Liquid nitrogen is seldom used in current cryostats. Liquified gases that are used to keep the conductors cold, such as liquid helium and liquid nitrogen, are called **cryogens.**

 The container housing the superconducting wire and the cryogens is a cryostat.

Superconductivity is one of the four electrical states of matter (Box 11-2). In this state, electrons flow in a conductor and experience no resistance. As the temperature of a conventional electrical conductor such as copper is lowered, its resistance decreases (Figure 11-12). Theoretically the decrease is linear to the origin, so its value is 0 at 0 K.

A superconductor such as NbTi has higher resistance at room temperature than copper and is therefore a poor conductor at room temperature. Its resistance decreases linearly with temperature just as copper. However, when it reaches its T_c, its resistance immediately drops to zero.

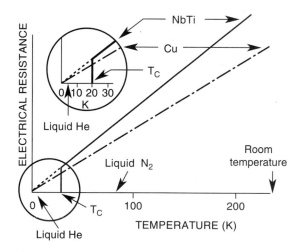

Figure 11-12 The electrical resistance of a conductor (Cu) and a superconductor (NbTi) as a function of temperature. T_c, Critical temperature.

There is much scientific investigation of superconductivity at this time that may profoundly affect the future of MRI. In 1987 Bednorz and Müller won the Nobel Prize in physics for their work on high temperature superconductivity in a new class of materials. They showed that the state of superconductivity could be made to exist in some exotic materials at temperatures above 20 K. The materials showing the most promise are compounds of lanthanum, barium, copper, and oxygen.

Since then, other investigators have demonstrated the state of superconductivity at even higher temperatures (Figure 11-13). If this research results in superconducting wire above the boiling point of nitrogen, 77 K, the cost of MRI systems will be greatly reduced. The design and production of the cryostat would be greatly simplified to accommodate the cheap and readily available liquid nitrogen.

There are several advantages to superconducting MRI magnets. The high magnetic field intensity is essential if spectroscopy is planned; however, the tolerances on field homogeneity are more restrictive at such high B_0 intensities.

Higher B_0 intensity is desirable because the increased magnetic resonance (MR) signal from such imaging systems results in higher signal-to-noise ratio (SNR), allowing shorter examination times and fewer motion artifacts. In addition, because of the increased SNR, higher spatial and contrast resolution images are obtained with these systems.

The field of the superconducting electromagnet can also be homogenized or shimmed to a degree not achievable with the other magnet systems. The solenoidal design of super-

Box 11-2	*The Four Electrical States of Matter*

1. Insulator
2. Semiconductor
3. Conductor
4. Superconductor

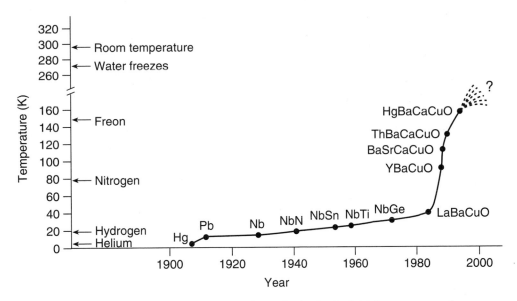

Figure 11-13   Recent years have shown a dramatic rise in the initial temperature for super-conducting materials.

conducting magnets makes them inherently homogeneous. Shimming is important for small field of view (FOV) imaging, optimal fat suppression, fast imaging, and spectroscopy.

Homogeneity of less than 1 ppm over a 40 cm FOV is obtainable with superconductive shimming. At 1 ppm, a 1-T imaging system has a B_0 of 1 T $\pm$ 1 μT (see Chapter 12).

The principal disadvantage of these systems is their intense fringe magnetic field, which can compromise site selection. At a magnetic field strength of 1 T, the 0.5 mT (5 gauss) fringe magnetic field associated with pacemaker exclusion extends some 10 m in all directions.

The extent of the fringe magnetic field may be reduced by passive or active shielding. Passive shielding consists of placing ferromagnetic material in the walls of the examination room or around the magnet (Figure 11-14). With a 2-cm ferromagnetic shield, the 0.5-mT isomagnetic line of a 1-T imaging system can be reduced to a distance of perhaps 5 m from 10 m. However, this passive shielding is heavy (as much as 9000 kg) and expensive but quite standard for current magnets.

Active shielding uses a second set of superconducting coils positioned outside the primary coils but still inside the cryostat with electric current of opposite direction of the primary current. This produces a magnetic field that counteracts the primary magnetic field, resulting in reduced fringe magnetic field outside the magnet. Although active shielding is expensive and may not appreciably change the weight of the system, it is generally standard now.

The effect of other magnetic fields and ferromagnetic objects on the fringe magnetic field of actively shielded magnets is poorly understood and unpredictable. Figure 11-15 shows the approximate distance to the 0.5-mT exclusion line for a 0.5 T, 1 T, 1.5 T, and 2 T unshielded magnet and for a magnet passively or actively shielded.

A new clan of superconducting electromagnets has been developed to compete with the "open architecture" of permanent magnet imaging systems. Such imaging systems are designed around two magnets stacked so that the B_0 field may be 1.0 T with an imaging

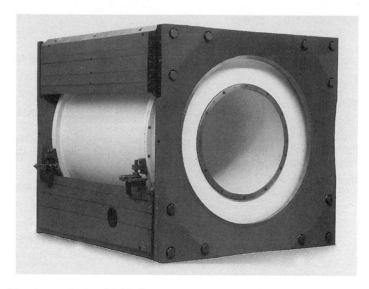

Figure 11-14 A passively shielded superconducting imaging system. (Courtesy Seimens Medical Systems.)

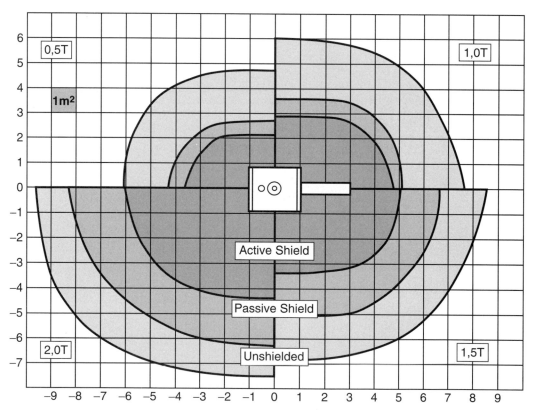

Figure 11-15 Distance to the 0.5-mT fringe magnetic field line for several imaging field strengths, both unshielded and shielded.

aperture of 50 cm. If actively shielded, the 0.5-mT fringe magnetic field is restricted to a 4-m distance.

Another disadvantage of the superconducting magnet is the need for cryogenic gases. Maintenance of the NbTi superconducting wire in a superconducting state requires an environment below its critical temperature of 9 K. The NbTi wire is wound on aluminum formers that are immersed in liquid helium, which vaporizes at 4 K.

External forces, principally in the form of thermal radiation, will cause the liquid helium to heat and vaporize over time. Because liquid helium is expensive, its vaporization is reduced by surrounding the helium compartment with concentric insulating compartments (Table 11–5).

In some magnets, the compartment containing the coils and liquid helium is separated from an outer vessel containing liquid nitrogen by a vacuum shield. Liquid nitrogen, which vaporizes at 77 K, is used instead of liquid hydrogen (20 K) or liquid neon (27 K) because it is less expensive. Furthermore, because of its high boiling point, liquid nitrogen also vaporizes more slowly.

Temperature Scales
$T_C = 5/9 (T_F - 32)$ $T_F = 9/5 T_C + 32$ $T_K = T_C + 273$ where the subscripts C, F, and K refer to Celsius, Fahrenheit, and Kelvin, respectively.

The liquid nitrogen is also protected by a vacuum shield from the environment. This arrangement of multiple thermal compartments is shown in Figure 11-16. The whole assembly is approximately 3.0 m in diameter, but because of the multiple thermal layers, the bore of the assembly is only approximately 1 m. Advanced magnet design eliminates the nitrogen compartment in favor of superior vacuum

compartments with liquid helium–replenishing devices called **cryogenerators.** Figure 11-17 shows an actively shielded 1.5-T imaging system with a cryogenerator.

These several thermal shields are designed to maintain the superconducting condition of the electromagnet. Despite rather rigorous designs, both liquids tend to vaporize, the nitrogen more readily than the helium. Vaporization rates of approximately 1.0 l/hr for nitrogen and 1.0 l/day for helium are experienced in some imaging systems. However, advanced cryostats of actively shielded magnets can go 3 years without helium refill.

Nitrogen costs about as much as milk, whereas helium costs as much as fine wine. At $10 per liter for helium and $0.50 per liter for nitrogen, the annual cost for supplying such cryogens can exceed $30,000.

Superconductor Operation

Once the superconducting electromagnet is energized or "brought up to field," it no longer requires external electrical power to maintain the B_0. This dramatically reduces the power requirements of the site relative to resistive electromagnets.

However, the disadvantage of the superconducting system is that the coil windings must be maintained at cryogenic temperature, which

TABLE 11-5	Notable Temperatures and Characteristic Effects

Temperature (K)	Characteristic Effect
0	Absolute zero; all motion stops.
4	Helium vaporizes.
9	NbTi superconducts.
77	Hydrogen vaporizes.
273	Ice melts.
293	Room temperature is achieved.
373	Water boils.

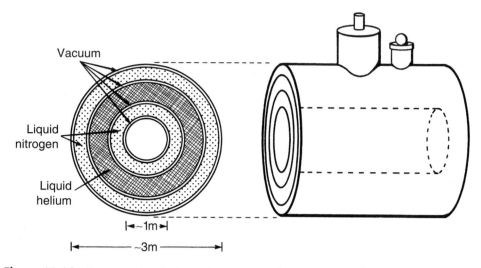

Figure 11-16 Cross-sectional view of a superconducting magnet for magnetic resonance imaging.

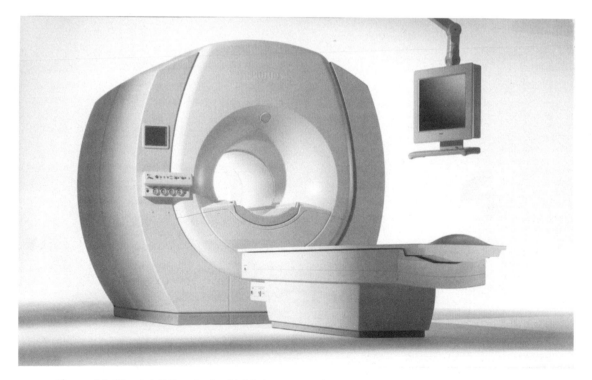

Figure 11-17 A 1.5-T actively shielded superconducting magnet designed with an integral cryogenerator. (Courtesy Philips Medical Systems.)

requires the occasional replenishing of liquid helium and/or liquid nitrogen. This replenishing must be performed by trained service personnel.

 Advances in magnet design have reduced helium boil-off and eliminated liquid nitrogen.

How then is the MRI system connected to a power source that is resistive in nature and the magnet brought up to designed magnetic field strength in the superconductive state? A direct current (DC) is supplied to the magnet through a resistive power supply. The primary coil has a shunt across it, but there is a heater on the shunt, causing it to behave as a resistive conductor (Figure 11-18, *A*).

Electron flow is from the resistive power supply and through the primary coil. As this electric current exits the primary coil to complete the circuit, it senses the high resistance of the shunt (Figure 11-18, *B*).

When the electric current designed to produce a given B_0 is attained, the shunt heater is turned off and the shunt becomes superconducting (Figure 11-18, *C*). Now the electric current must choose between the resistive power supply and the superconducting shunt. The shunt wins, and the power supply is unplugged.

If the superconductor becomes resistive, it heats up. As it heats, it becomes more resistive. The result of such a situation is a **quench.** Quenches may be controlled, as when a magnet is "ramped down." On the other hand, quenches may occur as a result of a lack of liquid helium or mechanical trauma to the cryostat that causes the conductor to come in contact with a warmer component of the cryostat. If this contact happens, an uncontrolled quench occurs, and the energy stored in the magnet is converted to heat.

Much of this heat boils off the cryogens. However, some of this heat may raise the temperature of the cryostat and damage the superconductive windings. Such a violent quench can destroy a magnet.

 A quench occurs when a superconducting magnet warms and the electromagnetic coil becomes resistive.

In the event of an unplanned quench, one may first hear a hissing noise caused by the release of helium, nitrogen, or both. Everyone should be immediately evacuated because both gases can displace oxygen and cause asphyxiation. Then, as you are dying, your voice will sound like that of Donald Duck.

The cryogenic gases are supplied to the MRI facility in large, thermoslike vessels called **dewars.** The dewars require special handling and storage. Only specially trained service personnel should replenish cryogens because of the potential hazards to skin, which can be burned severely by contact with a cryogen.

CHALLENGE QUESTIONS

1. What is the difference between an electromagnet and permanent magnet?
2. What happens when a superconducting magnet quenches?
3. What level of magnetic field intensity (B_0) can be obtained with a permanent magnet, resistive electromagnet, and superconducting electromagnet?
4. State the critical temperatures for NbTi superconducting wire, liquid helium, liquid nitrogen, and water.
5. A comfortable room temperature is considered to be 70° F. What is that temperature expressed in degrees Celsius and Kelvin?
6. Superconducting MRI magnets are made more homogeneous with electromagnetic shim coils. How is this accomplished with a permanent magnet imaging system?
7. What is so special about absolute zero?
8. List some advantages to the use of a resistive electromagnet for MRI.
9. Describe the four electrical states of matter.
10. Define *superconductivity*.

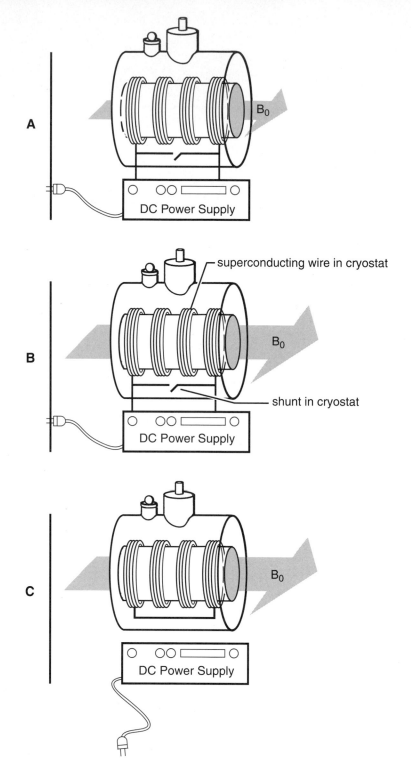

Figure 11-18 Achieving superconductivity with a resistive power source. **A,** Heater on the shunt causes it to behave as a resistive conductor. **B,** As the electric current exits the primary coil, it senses the high resistance of the shunt. **C,** The shunt becomes superconducting when the shunt heater is turned off.

Chapter 12

Secondary Magnetic Resonance Imaging Magnets

OBJECTIVES

1. At the completion of this chapter, the student should be able to do the following:

1. Identify shim coils and their purpose.
2. Understand the shape and positioning of the three sets of gradient coils.
3. Describe quadrature detection and its relevance to magnetic resonance (MR) signal detection.
4. Discuss the difference between homogeneous and inhomogeneous radiofrequency (RF) probes.
5. List the advantages and disadvantages of surface coil imaging.

OUTLINE

On one hand, magnetic resonance imaging (MRI) requires a uniform static magnetic field (B_0) to produce a free induction decay (FID), a spin echo (SE), or a gradient echo (GRE) and on the other hand, precisely fashioned gradient magnetic fields to provide spatial location. The gradient magnetic fields are produced by secondary electromagnetic coils that are usually the resistive type but can be superconducting.

In addition to the gradient coils that produce the gradient magnetic fields, there are shim coils and the radiofrequency (RF) probe. These secondary coils are positioned inside the bore of the cylinder of the gantry.

Indeed, the gradient coils and shim coils are designed to produce precise magnetic fields to superimpose on the primary static magnetic field. The RF probe is used to transmit RF into the patient and receive the induced signal from the patient.

SHIM COILS

Shimming is the process of making the B_0 field uniform throughout the imaging volume. The shimmed volume will determine the volume of the static magnetic field suitable for imaging. Figure 12-1 shows a cylinder about 1 m in diameter with 13 separate coils wound around the cylinder, each attached to its own power supply. These are the shim coils.

 Magnetic field uniformity is termed homogeneity.

The Parts per Million Scale

The specification of magnetic field homogeneity as parts per million (ppm) is borrowed from nuclear magnetic resonance (NMR) spectroscopy. This allows field homogeneity to be expressed independent of field strength. If a 1.0-T magnet were perfectly homogeneous throughout the imaging volume, it would be stated as $\pm$ 0 ppm. A homogeneity of $\pm$ 1 ppm is a variation of $\pm$ 1 μT throughout the imaging volume of a 1.0-T magnet (1 T = 10^6 μT). A homogeneity of $\pm$ 5 ppm in a 1.5-T magnet would be $\pm$ 7.5 μT.

 Magnetic field homogeneity is approximately 20 ppm with permanent magnets, 1 ppm with superconducting magnets.

For a 1.5-T field, the proton Larmor frequency is 63 MHz. If field homogeneity of 10 ppm is achieved, the resonance frequency in the shimmed volume will be 63 MHz $\pm$ 630 Hz. For a 0.5-T system operating the same way, 10 ppm homogeneity means the proton Larmor frequency is 21 MHz $\pm$ 210 Hz.

Shimming the Magnet

The imaging volume in an MRI system generally consists of a cylinder with a diameter of approximately 60 cm and a length along the Z-axis of 50 to 70 cm. A conventional six-coil superconducting magnet will normally produce a magnetic field with homogeneity of approximately $\pm$ 5 ppm.

Previously, the common practice was that once a magnet was properly shimmed, the procedure was not repeated unless operating techniques or site environment changed greatly. With higher resolution imaging techniques and chemical shift-sensitive fat suppression, better B_0 homogeneity is required.

Current superconducting magnets are designed and manufactured according to good specifications. Gross shimming is performed at the factory with the installation engineer only completing minor corrections. What used to take up to 2 weeks now takes just hours.

 Shimming is the process of making the B_0 field homogeneous.

An actively shielded magnet incorporates superconducting shim coils in the cryostat

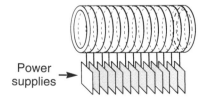

Power supplies →

Figure 12-1 Shim coils are spaced on a cylinder with a precise electric current and polarity to make the magnetic field homogeneous within the imaging volume.

with the primary magnet. This seems to be the most effective shim design of all. Field homogeneity of less than $\pm$ 1 ppm is attainable with superconducting shim coils.

During installation of an MRI system the magnet is brought up to field, and the homogeneity of the B_0 field is optimized with the bore clear of gradients or RF coils. For superconducting electromagnets, this homogeneity may be accomplished with the aid of superconducting coils within the cryostat itself.

An alternative method, passive shimming, consists of the positioning of ferromagnetic strips in precise locations on the magnet to alter the static magnetic field. The gradient coils are then inserted into the magnet bore, and room temperature shimming is performed.

Room temperature or resistive shim coils are configured to alter the magnetic field on the basis of spherical coordinates. The "first order" terms are the familiar x, y, and z directions. Second order terms include x^2, y^2, z^2, xy, yz, and so on. These "higher order" terms are only required for extremely high homogeneity applications, such as spectroscopy.

The most common method for shimming conventional MRI systems is to offset the baseline currents of the X, Y, and Z gradient coils. This method can usually achieve the desired degree of field homogeneity with additional hardware. The ability to use only the three first order shims is partly the result of the superior homogeneity of modern superconducting magnets. However, for systems used for spectroscopy in which a higher degree of homogeneity is required, an independent set of coils may be necessary.

During prescan calibration, additional shimming may be required because of patient size, shape, and magnetic susceptibility. The patient reduces the field homogeneity. For SE imaging, such prescan shimming is not required. However, at high B_0 with fast imaging and especially for magnetic resonance (MR) spectroscopy, prescan shimming may be necessary. Such prescan shimming is computer controlled and requires little technologist time.

GRADIENT COILS

If room temperature shim coils are used, another cylinder is positioned inside the cylinder on which the shim coils are wound. The gradient coils are positioned on this second cylinder. If room temperature shims are not used, the gradient coils are just inside the primary magnet housing.

There are three sets of gradient coils, one each for the X, Y, and Z directions. Figure 12-2 shows the configuration of such coils. Gradient coils are not coils of wire in the normal sense. Instead, they are broad, thick copper-conducting bands (Figure 12-3).

These bands are referred to as *conductors* and typically measure 10 mm wide and 4 mm thick. The large size is necessary to reduce resistance and carry the intense electric current (up to 30 A) required to generate the gradient magnetic fields (up to 40 mT/m). Gradient magnetic fields are measured in millitesla per meter, and when fast imaging is required, bigger is better.

These coils must be able to switch on and off rapidly. Switching times of less than 500 μs are necessary for many MRI applications. Advanced gradient coils, such as those used for echo planar imaging, can produce gradient fields of up to 40 mT/m, with switching times of as little as 50 μs.

 The rate of rise to maximum gradient amplitude is the slew rate. The time required to switch gradient coils on or off is rise time.

A typical slew rate curve is shown in Figure 12-4. This representation shows that the maximum gradient field, 40 mT/m, is obtained in a rise time of 250 μs. Therefore the slew rate is 160 T/m/s.

Slew Rate
40 mT/m in 250 μs
40 mT/m/250 μs
4×10^{-2} T/m/2.5×10^{-3} s
160 T/m/s

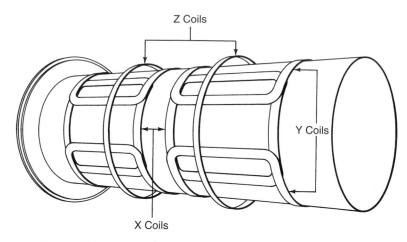

Figure 12-2 The positioning of the three sets of gradient coils.

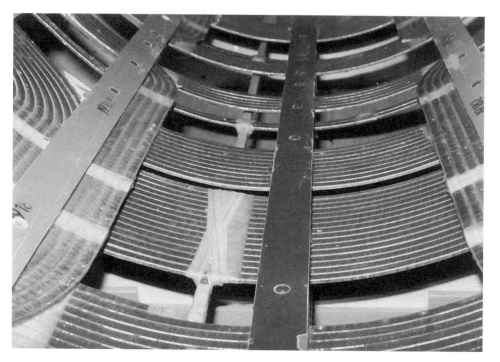

Figure 12-3 Gradient coils consist of large, band-type conductors.

Because the gradient coils are not brought to design amplitude instantaneously, they are generally represented as a trapezoid, as in Figure 12-5.

For routine SE imaging, slew rate is important because it limits the minimum time-to-echo (TE) that is available. For fast imaging, slew rate is exceptionally important because it is the limiting specification for short repetition time (TR), short TE, and total imaging time.

The switching of the gradient coils produces the "thump, thump, thump" in the imaging

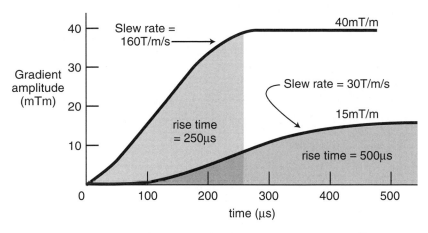

Figure 12-4 The slew rate is the time required to energize or switch off a gradient coil.

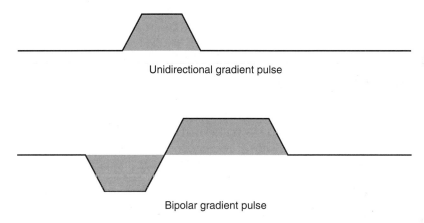

Figure 12-5 The representation of gradient pulses in a pulse sequence diagram.

aperture that is heard by the patient. When a gradient coil is switched on, the electric current causes the conductor to expand as a result of resistive heating. When the gradient is switched off, the conductor cools and contracts. The alternate expansion and contraction simulates an audio speaker cone, and a thumping sound is the result.

Because the gradient coils are generating magnetic fields, they also tend to torque or twist. If this happens without constraints, the coils change shape, and the resulting magnetic field is altered.

MRI systems incorporating high slew rate gradient coils induce **eddy currents** more efficiently. The rapidly changing gradient magnetic field can induce eddy currents in anything nearby (patient, coils, probes), but most important, in the conductive structures of the interior of the annulus of the cryostat, and can create image artifacts and loss of spatial and contrast resolution.

The principal method for controlling eddy currents is the use of shielded gradients. The gradient magnetic fields are effectively shielded from producing eddy currents at the surface of the cryostat.

For the prevention of physical distortion, the gradient coils are imbedded in a strong epoxy resin casing. This casing prevents the coils from moving when they are energized and dissipates the heat generated by the gradients. The casing is also designed to muffle the sound of the gradient switching for patient comfort.

Because gradient coils are designed to have low resistance, heating does not really become a problem until echo planar imaging (EPI) speeds are approached. Sometimes water-cooling is used.

Z Gradient Coils (G_Z, G_{SS})

The Z gradient coils are usually a pair of circular coils, each of which is wound on the cylinder at opposite ends of the imaging volume (Figure 12-6). If a direct current with opposite polarity is passed through the two coils, a small change in the magnetic field along the Z-axis of the gantry is produced. The currents used for SE imaging are approximately 20 A, producing a linear change in main magnetic field strength of 10 to 40 mT/m.

This change in magnet field strength allows for selection of a slice along the axis of the gantry. When transverse slices are required, the Z gradient is the **slice selection gradient**. The stronger the Z gradient electric current is, the stronger will be the Z gradient magnetization, and this will result in thinner slices.

 The Z gradient magnetic field is symbolized by B_Z or B_{SS}, for slice selection.

The B_Z coils are much more efficient than the B_X and B_Y coils because all segments of the coils contribute to the gradient magnetic field. There is a larger gradient per ampere-turn.

X Gradient Coils (G_X, G_R)

As shown in Chapter 2, the magnetic field lines of a circular coil of wire are along the axis of that coil. As a result, the X and Y gradient coils are more difficult to fabricate and position on the cylinder because they cannot be made as circles. Figure 12-7 shows the way the X gradient magnetic field is induced by a pair of coils—actually four saddle-shaped coils in sets of two—positioned on either side of the cylinder.

By convention, these coils are positioned so that the gradient magnetic field is across the patient laterally. The axis is therefore the horizontal axis across the patient from side to side.

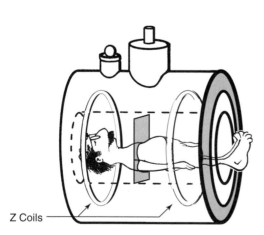

Figure 12-6 Z gradient coils change the gradient magnetic field along the Z-axis. This field, B_{SS}, is often used to select a transverse section of the patient for imaging.

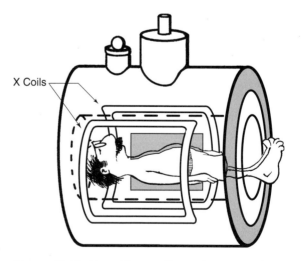

Figure 12-7 X gradient coils produce a gradient magnetic field across the patient. For transverse imaging, this field is frequency encoded and called the *read gradient magnetic field* (B_R).

These coils behave in precisely the same way as the B_Z coils. Direct current of opposite polarity is applied to produce a gradient magnetic field. The X gradient current and induced gradient magnetic field are similar in magnitude to the Z gradients.

The X gradient magnetic fields provide spatial localization along the X-axis, side-to-side across the patient, and can also be used for slice selection (sagittal images), phase encoding, or frequency encoding.

 For transverse images, the X gradient magnetic field is usually frequency encoded and symbolized as B_X or B_R, for the read gradient.

Y Gradient Coils (G_Y, G_Φ)

A gradient magnetic field along the Y-axis of the patient is produced by a set of coils that look and operate exactly like the X gradient coils (Figure 12-8). By convention, the Y-axis is the vertical axis through the patient in the anterior-posterior direction.

The Y gradient is normally, though not necessarily, used for phase encoding the MR signal during transverse imaging and is symbolized as B_Y or B_Φ. It can also serve to perform slice selection (coronal images) and to frequency encode. Together, the Y and X gradient allows precise determination of where the contribution to the MR signal from each voxel originated within the transverse imaging section.

 For transverse images, the Y gradient magnetic field is usually phase-encoded and symbolized as B_Y or B_Φ.

The previous discussion is an instructional convenience that correctly applies to images of the chest and abdomen. Transverse images of the head are usually acquired with the phase-encoded gradient running from left to right. With this technique, the number of phase-encoding steps can be reduced to produce a rectangular field of view that better conforms to the elliptical shape of the head.

Combined Gradients

Magnetic fields add vectorially. When energized simultaneously, the currents in the three pairs of gradient coils do not produce three separate magnetic fields but rather a single composite magnetic field.

All three gradients are energized simultaneously to obtain an oblique image (Figure 12-9). If the current through each pair of gradient coils is precisely controlled, the plane for imaging can be precisely specified.

The gradient coils are under coordinated electronic control during the MRI examination by the pulse programmer to achieve the desired gradient magnetic fields. Oblique sections can also be imaged with three-dimensional Fourier transformation (3DFT) techniques.

THE RADIOFREQUENCY PROBE

The RF probe is essentially a coil of wire not unlike the gradient, shim, and primary coils of the MRI system. It differs, however, in that it must accommodate a high-frequency alternating current of 10 to 200 MHz, depending on B_0

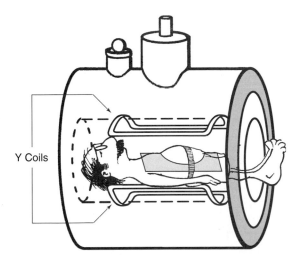

Figure 12-8 Y gradient coils produce a gradient magnetic field through the patient from front to back. For transverse imaging, this field is usually the phase-encoding gradient magnetic field, B_Φ.

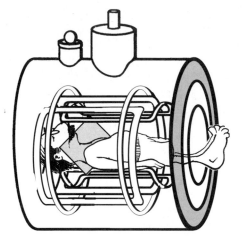

Figure 12-9 When all three gradients are energized at the same time, an oblique plane is imaged.

intensity, so that it can produce a radio signal at the Larmor frequency.

Furthermore, the RF probe must usually be precisely designed to behave as both a transmitter and receiver of RF. The design of the RF probe is one of the more critical engineering

features of an MRI system. Such design has developed into a very exact science.

The signal generated for the RF probe comes from a device called a *frequency synthesizer*. This is the master frequency source for the MRI system. It provides a tunable frequency band from which the Larmor frequency can be accurately determined for each individual examination. This small but precise signal is then amplified by a transmitter that feeds RF energy into the coil.

The simplest RF probe is a coil of wire wrapped around a patient or placed on the body but separated by a covering. The intensity of the emitted RF signal and the sensitivity to the signal received from the patient are maximum in a volume approximately equal to the diameter of the coil.

Outside of this coil diameter, signal intensity and sensitivity decrease rapidly. Such a simple type of coil is easily adaptable to a permanent magnet imaging system (Figure 12-10). This arrangement adds to the simplicity of a permanent magnet imaging system and improves sig-

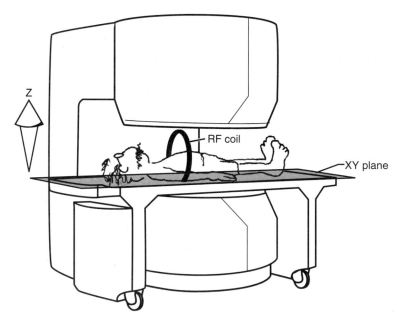

Figure 12-10 A simple, circular radiofrequency *(RF)* coil can be used with a vertical field permanent magnet imaging system because the coil axis is in the XY plane.

nal-to-noise ratio (SNR) at a given magnetic field strength.

For most superconducting electromagnetic imaging systems, the primary static magnetic field is along the axis of the patient. To be used, the simple circular coil has to penetrate through the patient either laterally or anteroposteriorly (Figure 12-11). Because patients object to such treatment, other coil designs and shapes had to be devised.

Initially, the most widely used design for the RF probe was a saddle coil (Figure 12-12, *A*).

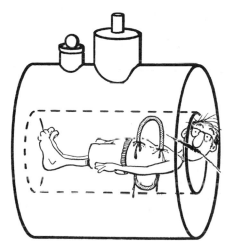

Figure 12-11 Radiofrequency probes for electromagnetic imaging systems are complicated because a simple circular coil would have to pass through the patient for its axis to be in the XY plane.

In such a coil, the intensity of emitted RF and the sensitivity of the received signal are nearly uniform within the confines of the coil. The degree of such uniformity predominantly results in great measure from the precise spacing of the loops of the saddle. However, this type of coil has low signal sensitivity.

Quadrature Coils

Quadrature coil design improves SNR by detecting the MR signal from multiple directions, as shown in Figure 12-13. They view the signal as though they were a pair of stereo lenses. The result is better sensitivity to the MR signal relative to linear coils.

Quadrature coils are also constructed to be more homogeneous for RF transmission and reception. For this reason, quadrature coils have replaced the saddle design for virtually all homogeneous applications (e.g., head, body, knee). There are several types of quadrature coils, which are all much more complicated than the saddle coil. One version, the "birdcage" resonator, is widely used (Figure 12-12, *B*)

There are basically two types of RF probes. Homogeneous volume coils are typically used both to transmit RF and to receive the MR signal. These include the head and body coils and other special application coils, such as an upper extremity/shoulder coil shown in Figure 12-14.

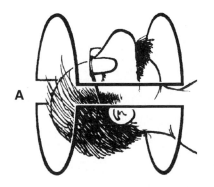 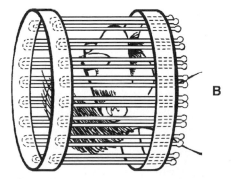

Figure 12-12 **A,** The saddle coil. **B,** The "birdcage" resonator type of quadrature coil.

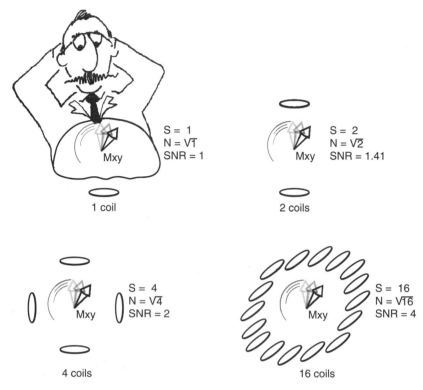

Figure 12-13 Quadrature detection improves signal-to-noise ratio *(SNR)* with multiple pairs of coils.

 Head, body, or extremity coils are known as homogeneous coils; surface coils are referred to as **inhomogeneous coils.**

Most inhomogeneous coils are surface coils, and the word *inhomogeneous* is used because these coils do not transmit RF in a homogeneous fashion. For this reason, they usually receive only. When these coils are used, the RF is transmitted by the head or body coil. The transmitting coil is then electrically silenced or **decoupled** while the surface coil receives the signal.

The MR signal detected from a patient consists of two components: signal and random noise. The signal comes from only the slice of tissue being excited.

The noise detected by the RF coil comes from all the tissue within the sensitive volume of the coil. For example, with the body coil, the

MRI technologist may excite and subsequently detect an MR signal from a slice through the liver, but the noise detected by the body coil comes from the liver, chest, and abdomen within the body coil. This reduces the SNR because of the higher level of noise.

All coils except the body coil improve SNR by reducing the detected noise. Tissue not being examined is eliminated from the coil's sensitive volume. For example, the head coil does not detect noise from the liver because the liver is far from the coil (i.e., outside its sensitive volume). The other coils also improve SNR through increased signal detection by having the signal better "fill" the coil volume.

Body Coils

The most robust RF probe is the body coil. This statement is justified because the body coil can

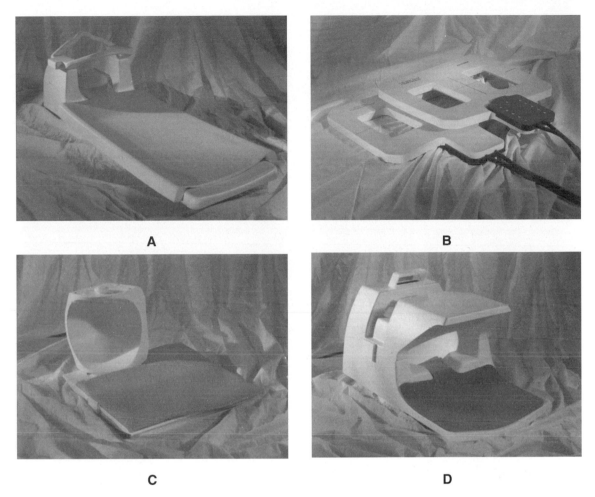

A

B

C

D

Figure 12-14 A basic set of radiofrequency coils would include coils to image the head, body, extremities, and spine. These coils are for **A,** spine and soft tissue neck studies; **B,** chest, abdomen, and pelvis imaging; **C,** imaging across the glenohumeral joint; and **D,** soft tissue, skullbase, neck, and brain imaging. (Courtesy GE Medical Systems.)

image any part of the human anatomy. The body coil is wound on a former and is just inside the gradient coils. The body coil is always a transmit/receive device (Figure 12-15). However, it is often possible to design coils for imaging specific anatomy with better SNR and thereby produce better images than those produced with a single body coil alone.

Head/Extremity Coils

A common alternative to the body coil for imaging cranial anatomy is the head coil. An extrem-

ity coil is available to obtain high-resolution images from the lower extremity. A typical quadrature birdcage head coil (Figure 12-16) can be attached to a neck coil and a thoracic/lumbar surface spine coil to produce images of the total spine.

Surface Coils

For most imaging systems, the RF probe serves as both the transmitter of the RF and the receiver of the MR signal. One notable exception is the surface coil.

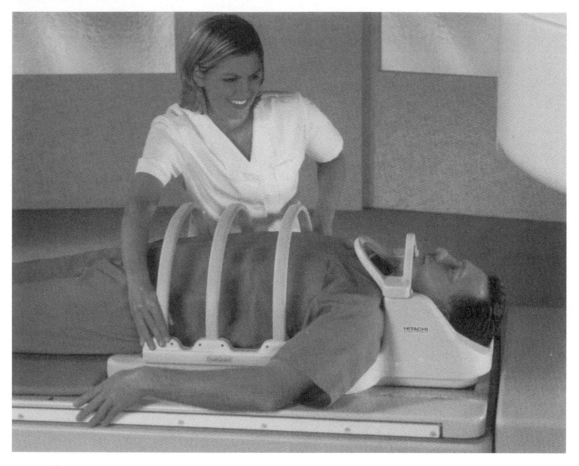

Figure 12-15 A body probe of a quadrature detection phased-array design to image the cervical, thoracic, and lumbar spine simultaneously. (Courtesy Hitachi Medical Systems America.)

A surface coil is a specially designed coil that is usually flat but can also be other shapes and is used to obtain high SNR images of anatomy close to the surface. The disadvantage of its use is reduced field of view (FOV). The surface coil may be encased in a rubberized or plastic matrix to make it somewhat pliable or in a hardened composite material for increased stability. The coil is placed on the surface of the patient at the anatomical region under investigation.

Surface coils come in many different sizes and shapes and are usually fabricated for specific anatomy. A minimal complement of surface coils consists of several flat, circular devices of varying diameters and a "license plate" coil for spine imaging.

Other surface coils include individual probes designed specifically for extremities, joints, or orbit (Figure 12-17). Special coil designs now include breast (Figure 12-18), prostate (Figure 12-19), and almost any other organ of interest. A high-resolution prostate image is shown in Figure 12-20.

When in use, the surface coil is positioned inside the head or body RF probe on the patient but is insulated from the skin. These devices are normally used only as MR signal

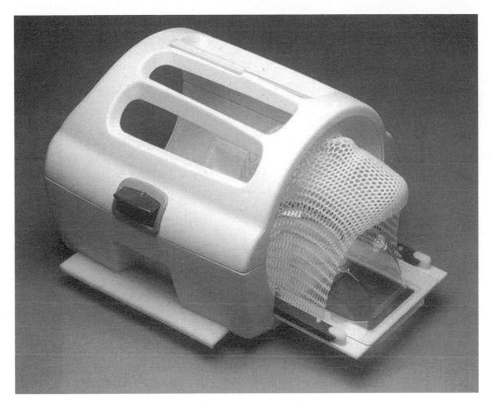

Figure 12-16 Quadrature design, birdcage, head coil shown with oncology mask. (Courtesy Midwest RF.)

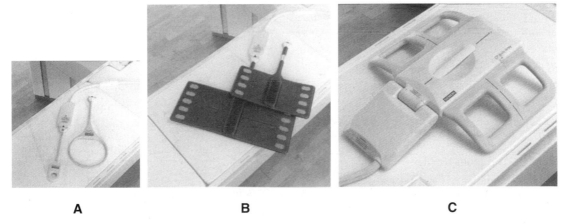

A   **B**   **C**

Figure 12-17 Typical surface coils from small circular **(A)** to rectangular coils for spine **(B)** to large rectangular **(C)** available for magnetic resonance imaging. (Courtesy Siemens Medical Systems.)

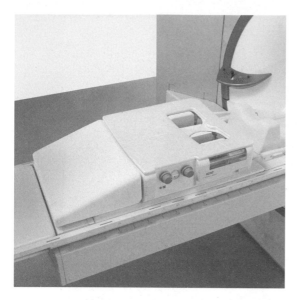

Figure 12-18 Bilateral breast coil for magnetic resonance mammography. (Courtesy Siemens Medical Systems.)

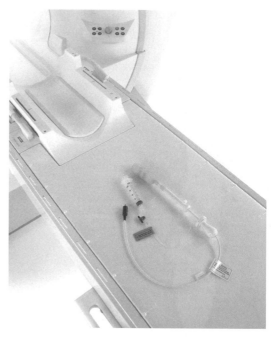

Figure 12-19 Endorectal coils for prostate imaging. (Courtesy Siemens Medical Systems.)

receivers and rely on the head or body coil to transmit the RF. This type of use requires that the two coils be decoupled from one another so that they do not interfere with sensing the weak MR signal or that one does not "intercept" the RF transmission of the other.

Lack of decoupling can cause the receiving coil to heat up, possibly destroy the surface coil electronics, and potentially burn the patient. Special hardware is often used to actively decouple the two coils by detuning one of the coils while the other is operating.

 Surface coils provide better contrast resolution and better spatial resolution.

A surface coil has improved contrast resolution because of higher SNR. A surface coil has improved spatial resolution because of smaller FOV. A surface coil image of the cervical spine, for instance, has a pixel size of 0.4 × 0.4 mm for a 10-cm FOV and a 256 matrix (Figure 12-21). Because a smaller volume of tissue is being imaged, the pixel size for a given matrix with a

surface coil is always less than that for a whole-body RF probe.

Spatial Resolution/Pixel Size
FOV = 10 cm = 100 mm
Matrix size = 256 × 256
Pixel size $= \dfrac{100\ \text{mm}}{256} = 0.39$ mm
2 pixels per line = 0.78 mm/lp
Hence: spatial resolution
$\quad = (0.78\ \text{mm/lp})^{-1}$
$\quad = 1.28$ lp/mm
$\quad = 12.8$ lp/cm

Disadvantages of surface coil imaging include limited FOV and positioning. Because the surface coil is smaller than the head or body probe, it has a smaller sensitive volume, which results in a restricted FOV. This is

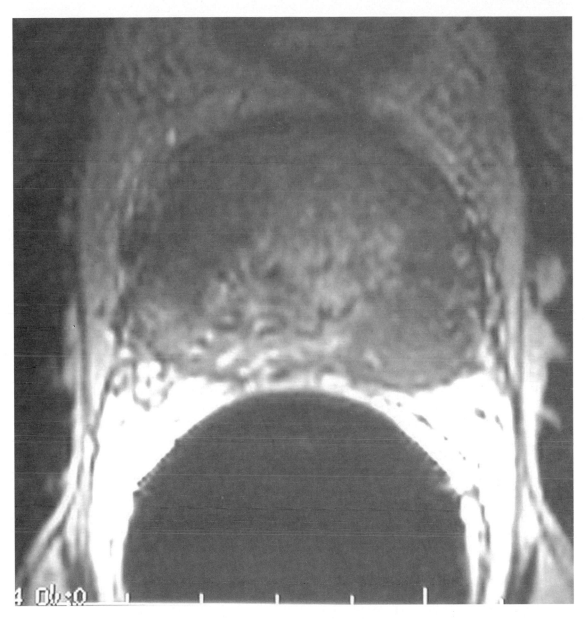

Figure 12-20 High-resolution, T2 weighted, three-dimensional fast spin echo (FSE) image of the prostate acquired with an endorectal coil and pelvic phased-array showing carcinoma (low intensity) on the left. (Courtesy William Bradley, San Diego, CA.)

acceptable if only a small region of anatomy is to be imaged.

However, positioning the surface coil requires more time. To maximize the signal from the small volume, the MRI technologist must pay closer attention to patient setup. The surface coil must be as orthogonal or perpendicular to the XY plane as possible for maximum sensitivity. Just a slight tilt in the coil can result in significant loss of signal. With

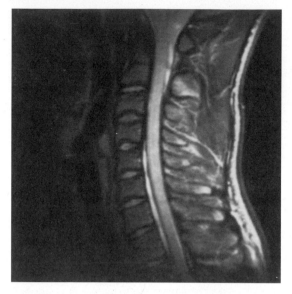

Figure 12-21 A high-resolution image of the cervical spine. (Courtesy Larry Rothenberg, New York, NY.)

experience, MRI technologists learn to position surface coils easily and quickly.

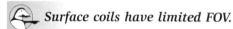

Surface coils have limited FOV.

The principal objection in the use of surface coils is the limited FOV. This deficiency has

been overcome with the development of phased-array or multicoil systems. If several surface coils are connected and positioned so that they have minimal coupling, a single large image can be the result. Each coil must have its own receiver channel for processing that single image of the cumulative sensitive volumes of all the coils (Figure 12-22).

In this situation, the SNR and spatial resolution of each individual surface coil is maintained in the composite image. For example, if four surface coils are used to image the thoracic and lumbar spine, each having a 10-cm FOV acquired at a matrix size of 256×256, the composite image could have up to a 40-cm FOV with a 256×1024 matrix (pixels are added only along the coils). Current routine applications of this technology include imaging of the spine (Figure 12-23), pelvis, and breast.

CHALLENGE QUESTIONS

1. What is the purpose of shim coils in a superconducting MRI system?
2. Surface coil imaging results in better SNR and better spatial resolution. What are its principal limitations?

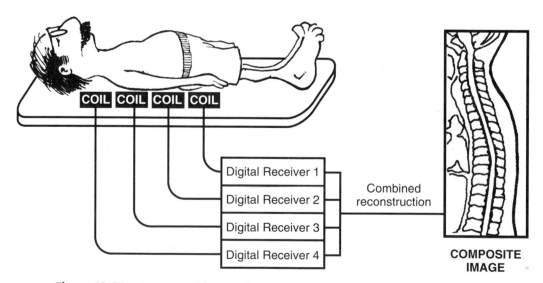

Figure 12-22 An array of four surface coils positioned to image the entire spine.

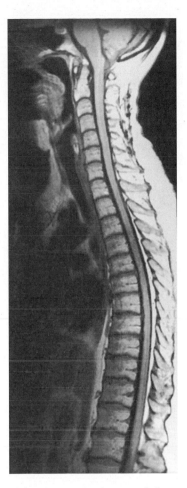

Figure 12-23 Composite image of the entire thoracic and lumbar spine acquired with multiple surface coils. (Courtesy GE Medical Systems.)

3. A superconducting MRI system operating at 3 T is said to have a field homogeneity of ± 1 ppm. How should that be expressed in millitesla?

4. A surface coil with an 8-cm FOV is used to image the orbit with a 512 × 512 reconstruction matrix. What is the limiting spatial resolution for this examination?

5. A gradient magnetic field has a maximum amplitude of 25 mT/m, with a rise time of 100 ms. What is the slew rate?

6. What can be done to improve the spatial resolution of an MRI system?

7. For sagittal plane imaging, which gradient coil must be energized (G_X, G_Y, G_Z)?

8. Surface coils are said to result in better contrast resolution. Why?

9. For a transverse image, is the read gradient magnetic field (B_R) frequency encoded or phase encoded?

10. What is a homogenous RF coil?

Chapter 13

The Purchase Decision and Site Selection

OBJECTIVES

At the completion of this chapter, the student should be able to do the following:

1. List the advantages and disadvantages of both permanent magnets and superconducting electromagnets.
2. Identify the characteristics of the B_0 magnetic field that influence site selection.
3. Name equipment that can be caused to malfunction because of the fringe magnetic field.
4. Describe why the magnetic resonance imaging (MRI) suite must be radiofrequency (RF) shielded.
5. Discuss construction features particularly appropriate for an MRI suite.

OUTLINE

Placing a magnetic resonance imaging (MRI) system in a hospital is not at all like adding an x-ray imaging suite, and this has generated much discussion and publicity. Indeed, more rigorous constraints govern where and how the MRI system can be located.

The first consideration is not where the MRI system will be placed but rather what type and what field strength system will be purchased. Only after the type of imaging system has been decided should the site selection be analyzed. The third phase in this process concerns the actual construction details, which obviously must wait until the site is selected.

SELECTING THE IMAGING SYSTEM

MRI systems not only are used for imaging but also may be configured for magnetic resonance spectroscopy (MRS) as a potential aid to diagnosis. In deciding on an imaging system, the buyer must first decide whether MRS is to be a possible application. Furthermore, if high-resolution, fast imaging is planned, a high field strength imaging system will be required.

Application of MRS has been used to advantage on biological specimens in the laboratory, but its application in the clinic in vivo is being implemented slowly. For those institutions where MRS is of interest, the decision as to the type of imaging system is automatic; a superconducting MRI system of high magnetic field strength is required. Today, that would suggest a 1.5- to 3-T imaging system. However, for such an application, a new facility may be required because of unsuitable existing structures.

Type of Magnet

If spectroscopy is not intended, an imaging system based on permanent or superconducting magnet technology may be considered. Table 13-1 summarizes some characteristics, including field strength, associated with three types of MRI systems. Each type of MRI system has certain advantages and disadvantages (Table 13-2).

Good clinical images can be produced by each of the imaging systems, but currently, superconducting magnets prevail. However, resistive electromagnet MRI systems are increasing market share.

In some respects the development of MRI parallels that of computed tomography (CT). Although third-generation CT imaging systems have considerable market share over fourth-generation CT imaging systems, there is no intrinsic basis to consider one superior to the other. Similarly, the way the magnetic field is generated carries no advantage to the physics of producing a magnetic resonance (MR) image.

The sometimes emotional debate regarding optimum magnet field strength is not easily resolved. It is unclear whether an optimum magnetic field strength exists for MRI; exquisite images can be made with either of the two types of magnets and with B_0 field strength ranging from 0.1 T to 4 T.

TABLE 13-1	Characteristics of Magnetic Resonance Imaging Systems		
Characteristics	**Permanent Magnet**	**Resistive Magnet**	**Superconducting Magnet**
Field strength (T)	0.1-0.3	0.15-0.4	0.5-4.0
Cost ($\$ \times 10^6$)	0.5-1.0	0.8-1.2	1.0-2.5
Approximate size (m)	1.5×2.0	2.1×2.3	2.3×3.0
Weight (kg $\times$ 1000)	3.0-4.5	5.5-9.0	4.5-8.1
Power requirements (kW)	20	80	25
Distance to 0.5-mT fringe field (m)	<1	0.5-2	3-10

TABLE 13-2	Advantages and Disadvantages of Magnetic Resonance Imaging Systems

Advantages	Disadvantages
Permanent	
Low capital cost	Limited field strength
Low operating cost	Fixed field strength
Negligible fringe field	Very heavy
Resistive Iron Core	
Low capital cost	High power consumption
Easy coil maintenance	Water cooling necessary
Negligible fringe field	Potential field instability
Resistive Air Core	
Low capital cost	High power consumption
Lightweight	Water cooling necessary
Easy coil maintenance	Significant fringe field
Superconductive	
High field strength	High capital cost
High field homogeneity	High cryogen cost
Low power consumption	Intense fringe field

The rapidly developing surface coil technology and software advances will probably result in more improvements to image quality and further obscure the debate over B_0 field strength. Therefore the purchase decision will be based on other considerations, some of which, such as service support, ability to upgrade, and corporate commitment, are not discussed here.

Permanent Magnet. The principal advantages of a permanent magnet MRI system are the lack of a significant fringe magnetic field and the open gantry. The 0.5-mT fringe magnetic field will certainly not extend more than 1 m in any direction from the magnet, and protective measures for adjacent areas are therefore unnecessary. This absence of a fringe field allows great flexibility in siting such a system.

 There is essentially no fringe magnetic field with a permanent magnet MRI system.

The principal disadvantage of a permanent magnet MRI system is its weight, which ranges from approximately 5000 kg for a head or extremity imaging system to 40,000 kg for a whole-body imaging system. The heavier systems may be restricted to location on the ground floor because of inadequate load design of upper floors. Certainly the heavier systems are not adaptable to mobile units because of various problems (Figure 13-1).

Superconducting Magnet. The reason superconducting magnets are the most widely used is field strength. A permanent magnet imaging system cannot produce magnetic fields in excess of approximately 0.3 T. Current superconducting magnets provide imaging fields up to 4 T.

 High B_0 field intensity is the principal advantage to a superconducting MRI system.

There are several disadvantages to a superconducting imaging system. The initial cost is very high, sometimes exceeding $2 million. The intensity of the fringe magnetic field can place limits on where the imaging system can be located. Site preparation costs are often excessive for existing buildings. Such costs may require that the imaging system be located in a new, relatively isolated location.

A superconducting MRI system has many advantages. Better image quality is strongly suggested by some. The high B_0 magnetic field is associated with high field homogeneity with most imaging systems. The superconducting MRI magnet consumes no electric power, but this advantage is offset by the requirement for cryogenic gases.

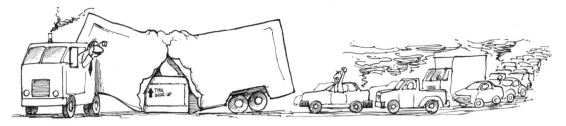

Figure 13-1 Possible fate of a mobile magnetic resonance imaging system with a permanent magnet.

Performance Evaluation

The medical physics community has developed some rather precise methods and test tools for evaluating image quality in MRI. With the large selection of MRI systems available, few purchasers buy a particular system without the assistance of a medical physicist.

Purchasers should not rely on the specifications published by manufacturers for performance characteristics of such imaging systems without independent confirmation. Imaging characteristics such as spatial resolution, contrast resolution, slice thickness, linearity, uniformity, artifact generation, and reconstruction time should be evaluated routinely for MRI.

More important, acceptance testing of MRI systems is essential. Both the American Association of Physicists in Medicine (AAPM) and the American College of Medical Physics (ACMP) have developed protocols for acceptance testing and routine evaluation of MRI systems. Specific test tools are also prescribed (see Chapter 30).

The American College of Radiology (ACR) has developed an accreditation program for MRI facilities that incorporates rigorous routine performance evaluations.

LOCATING THE MAGNETIC RESONANCE IMAGING SYSTEM

Once the imaging system is selected and arrangements have been made for its acceptance testing, its location can be determined. There are four options (Table 13-3).

If the imaging system is located in a new building such as an imaging center, the siting requirements may not be so rigorous. Most new construction will be designed so that only considerations of adjacent imaging appa-

TABLE 13-3	Considerations for Locating a Magnetic Resonance Imaging System
Advantages	**Disadvantages**
New Construction	
Easier to plan for fringe magnetic field	Cost
	Possibly remote
Custom design	
Existing Building	
Proximity to other services	Accommodation of fringe field
Use of existing facilities	Higher renovation cost
Temporary Building	
Short time to operation	Possible compromised patient access
Easier to plan for fringe magnetic field	Unsightly addition
Mobile	
Cost-effective for low workload	Scheduling
	Time required for setup
Learning period for all	

ratus may be necessary. New construction can generally be designed so that shielding of the fringe magnetic field is unnecessary. Exclusion areas may be easy to identify and control.

The decision to locate an MRI system in an existing building, usually a hospital, places considerable demands on the precise site location and its preparation. This may preclude the purchase of a superconductive magnet system of high field strength.

On the other hand, except for possible weight constraints, permanent magnet systems may be sited nearly anywhere in existing buildings. There are essentially no fringe fields with a permanent magnet.

Placing the imaging system in a temporary, but fixed location adjacent to the hospital has many attractions. Site preparation costs are low. The time required to prepare the site is short, allowing for placing a system into operation quickly. Patient and visitor access can be closely controlled.

This approach is appealing because minimum time and expense are involved, and considerable experience can be gained early. This experience can be used to advantage if it is subsequently decided to place an MRI system in a permanent location such as a hospital.

Mobile MRI is most attractive to facilities that cannot justify full-time operation because of low patient load. Mobile operation suffers from the time required to shim the magnet and tune the electronics after each move. This is especially true with superconducting MRI systems. A particular advantage to a mobile system is the lack of long-term commitment on the part of the imaging facility. The experience gained with a mobile system educates all involved (administrator, radiologist, and imaging technologist) for subsequent selection of a stationary facility.

There are two principal concerns regarding site selection for the magnet. First, what will be its effect on equipment and operations in adjacent areas? Second, what characteristics of

these adjacent areas could adversely affect the operation of the MRI system?

Effect of the Magnet on the Environment

Perhaps the first consideration in selecting a site for an MRI system is the influence that the fringe magnetic field might have on equipment and activities in surrounding areas. Any electronic device that operates on the basis of moving electric charges in a vacuum can be influenced by the fringe magnetic field of the MRI system. Devices such as cathode-ray tubes, image intensifier tubes, electron microscopes, and gamma cameras are all susceptible to MRI fringe magnetic fields.

A stationary electron has an associated electric field. In motion, the electron also has a magnetic field. In the presence of a fringe magnetic field, the magnetic field of the moving electron will interact with the fringe magnetic field, causing the electron to stray from its intended

TABLE 13-4	Exclusion of Various Types of Equipment According to the Intensity of the Fringe Magnetic Field
Strength of the Fringe Magnetic Field (mT)	**Devices to Be Excluded**
10	Analog watches, credit cards
5	Operator's console, magnetic tapes and diskettes, electric motors, computers
1	Video cameras and monitors, multiformat cameras, dewars, CRTs
0.5	Cardiac pacemakers, hearing aids, image intensifiers, metal detectors
0.1	Gamma cameras, electron microscopes, CT scanners, PET scanners

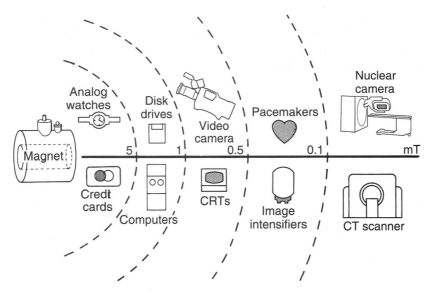

Figure 13-2 The types of objects that should be excluded at several isomagnetic fringe fields.

course. As a part of sensitive electronic equipment, an electron beam will therefore experience a change in direction, which can severely compromise the operation of such equipment.

Table 13-4 presents some general rules for determining exclusion limits of sensitive electronic equipment from an MRI magnet. This requirement is shown in Figure 13-2. It must be recognized that the fringe magnetic field is three-dimensional. It extends to not only the space on the same floor but also the space above and below (Figure 13-3).

This effect of the magnet on the environment is particularly important for superconducting MRI systems. The fringe field of a permanent magnet imaging system will rarely require such consideration.

The intensity of the fringe magnetic field of a superconducting MRI system is related to the strength of the B_0 field. For example, a 0.5-T imaging system has its 0.5-mT fringe magnetic field at a distance of approximately 8 m. For a 2-T magnet, the same fringe magnetic field extends to a distance of approximately 14 m.

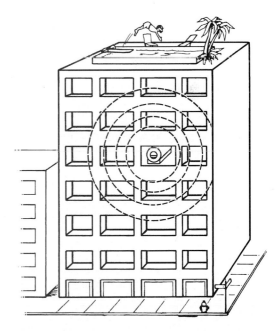

Figure 13-3 The fringe magnetic field is three-dimensional. This characteristic influences the potential locations for such a magnetic resonance imaging system.

Shown in Figure 13-4 are the isomagnetic lines in a frontal plane and side projection. Table 13-5 presents the distance from the center of a magnet to various fringe magnetic field intensities along the axis and transverse for imaging systems of various field strengths.

Manufacturers have devised ways of shrinking the fringe magnetic field, but the cost can be substantial. These methods are either passive or active (Table 13-6).

If a passive shield is used by lining the walls of the room with iron (Figure 13-5), the fringe magnetic field intensity is reduced and the isomagnetic lines pulled closer to the magnet. As a general rule, 10 mm of iron reduces the intensity of the fringe magnetic field by approximately 50%. This rule of thumb is not absolute but varies with the permeability of the iron and the strength of the fringe magnetic field.

Iron is an effective magnetic shield because it has high magnetic permeability and readily attracts the lines of a fringe magnetic field. The principle is the same as that associated with the yoke of a permanent magnet imaging system or the core of a transformer.

The closer the iron can be positioned to the magnet, the less iron is required for the same degree of magnetic field shielding. Figure 13-6 shows some manufacturers' innovative passive self-shielding approaches to

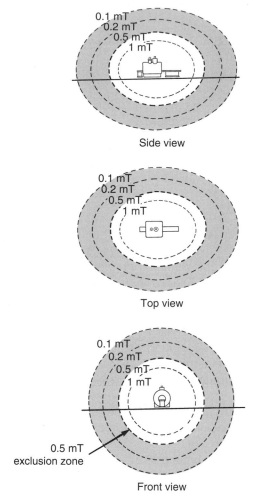

Figure 13-4 The axial fringe magnetic field is elliptical. The transverse field is circular.

TABLE 13-5	**Axial and Transverse Distances to Various Fringe Magnetic Fields for Several Magnet Strengths, Unshielded**			
Fringe Magnetic Field (mT)	**Magnet Strength**			
	0.5 T axial/ transverse (m)	**1.0 T axial/ transverse (m)**	**1.5 T axial/ transverse (m)**	**4.0 T axial/ transverse (m)**
1.0	7.0/5.0	8.5/6.7	10/7.0	13/11
0.5	8.5/6.7	11/8.5	13/9.7	16/13
0.3	11/8.3	13/10	15/12	20/16
0.1	15/12	19/15	21/17	25/20

TABLE 13-6	Methods to Reduce the Fringe Magnetic Field
Passive Shielding	**Active Shielding**
Iron in the wall	Resistive shim coils
Iron at the magnet	Superconducting shim coils

shrinking the fringe magnetic field. In Figure 13-6, *A,* four large triangular iron rods are mounted the length of the magnet at the four corners. In Figure 13-6, *B,* an iron cage is constructed around the magnet. Individual slabs of iron of varying thicknesses are fastened to the cage.

Magnets can be actively shielded by the use of coils wound outside the primary magnet windings. These coils can operate in the resistive state, in which case they would be outside the cryostat. More frequently, they are wound in the cryostat, just around the primary magnet windings and

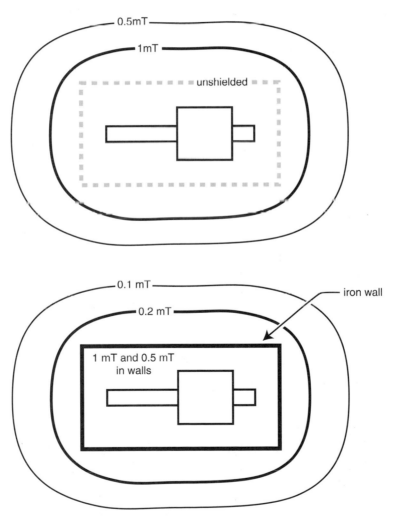

Figure 13-5 The use of iron shielding pulls the fringe magnetic field closer to the magnet.

therefore operate in the superconducting state.

 Superconducting shim coils reduce fringe magnetic field distance and improve B_0 field homogeneity at the same time.

The polarity of the direct current of the active shield windings is opposite that of the primary magnet current, and therefore an opposing magnetic field is produced. This opposing magnetic field cancels much of the fringe magnetic field with little effect on the intensity of the B_0 field.

Effect of the Environment on the Magnetic Resonance Imaging System

A very uniform B_0 magnetic field must first exist in the imaging volume to produce an image. Gradient magnetic fields are introduced

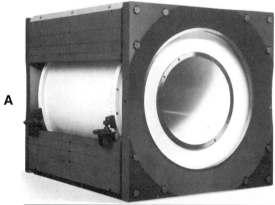

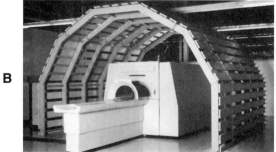

Figure 13-6 The approach of two manufacturers using self-shielding magnets to shrink the fringe magnetic field. (Courtesy **A,** Siemens Medical Systems, and **B,** Philips Medical Systems.)

to shape the B_0 magnetic field precisely for spatial localization.

This shaped magnetic field can be disturbed by large, stationary ferromagnetic objects that interact with the fringe magnetic field of the MRI system. Smaller ferromagnetic objects in motion can be even more bothersome.

Ferromagnetic Interference.   When a mass of ferromagnetic material is positioned external to the magnet, the fringe magnetic field will be deviated into that material (Figure 13-7). This is the basis for the use of iron as a magnetic shield to protect the environment.

What also occurs, however, is a compensating distortion of the B_0 magnetic field in the imaging volume. Such distortion can result in image degradation.

Stationary iron objects external to the MRI suite can usually be compensated for by shimming the magnet with smaller pieces of iron positioned strategically on the external surface of the magnet. Additional shimming can be done with shim coils (see Chapter 12).

Generally, more rigorous site selection in a nonferrous environment is required for magnets of higher field strength because of the requirement for higher B_0 magnetic field homogeneity. If substantial iron or steel is within the 10-mT isomagnetic line, computer-assisted site modeling is required.

A more difficult problem results from moving masses of iron. Vehicular traffic, elevators, and motorized dollies in hospitals are examples of such moving masses. Protecting the B_0 magnetic field from such influences is difficult, and this aspect of site selection is therefore critical. Figure 13-8 illustrates what general objects should remain outside fringe magnetic fields.

Radiofrequency Interference.   Equally critical to the operation of an MRI system is isolation of the MR signal. The signal detected in the MRI system is a radiofrequency (RF) signal of extremely low intensity, usually less than 100 mV. Broadcast radio signals are orders of mag-

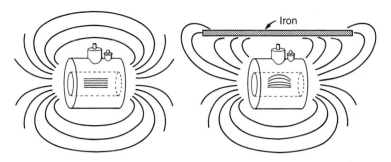

Figure 13-7 When a large, stationary ferromagnetic object is positioned near a magnetic resonance imaging system, it not only attracts the fringe magnetic field but also degrades B_0 homogeneity.

nitude higher and can substantially obscure the MR signal. These environmental RF signals represent severe noise that limits the detectability of the MR signal.

The Federal Communications Commission (FCC) identifies the RF band as frequencies ranging from 3 kHz to 300 GHz. Frequencies throughout the range are allocated by the FCC for certain purposes such as navigation, space operation, satellite communications, citizens band broadcast, cellular telephones, and commercial broadcast.

MRI operates in the RF range of approximately 1 to 200 MHz, where there is considerable RF activity (Figure 13-9). For example, television channels 2 to 6 broadcast in the 54- to 88-MHz RF band. Citizen's band broadcast is in the 30-MHz region, and much of the rest of the MRI RF band is taken by space and weather communications. Cellular phone

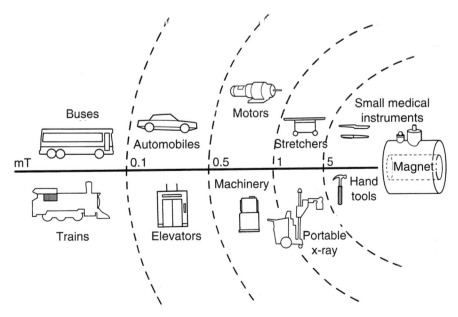

Figure 13-8 Some ferromagnetic objects should remain outside the fringe magnetic field because they may become projectiles or degrade the B_0 homogeneity in the imaging volume.

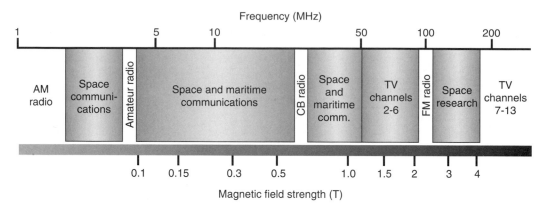

Figure 13-9 Radiofrequency allocated by the Federal Communications Commission in the magnetic resonance imaging radiofrequency band. (Courtesy Stanley Hames, Phoenix, AZ.)

communication is in the gigahertz region and therefore is not a problem for MRI.

When an x-ray examination room is designed, shielding the environment from the potentially harmful electromagnetic radiation (x-rays) produced inside the room is necessary. With MRI, the opposite is required. The MRI system must be shielded from the electromagnetic radiation (RF) that exists outside the room.

In an x-ray room, lead sheeting up to $\frac{1}{16}$ inch thick is installed to attenuate the x-radiation. In MRI, the room is lined with copper or aluminum mesh or sheets to absorb external RF.

MRI rooms are shielded completely by a continuous sheeting or wire mesh of copper or aluminum to improve the MR signal detection by reduction of environmental RF. Such a design feature is called a *Faraday cage,* for Michael Faraday, the English physicist who first described electromagnetic induction in the 1850s.

 The MRI system is housed in a Faraday cage.

The shielding must be continuous and include both the ceiling and the floor. Secure continuous electrical contact must also be provided. Any breach of electrical continuity

allows environmental RF to leak into the room and interfere with the MR signal. MRI shielding should attain at least a 90-dB reduction in signal intensity in the RF range from 1 to 200 MHz.

Figure 13-10 illustrates a Faraday cage. The entire room, including the doors and windows, is shielded from RF. The RF enclosure is often a room built within a room. All wiring and cables that enter the imaging room must be properly filtered to exclude environmental RF. View windows should be fabricated with sufficiently large mesh so that vision is not compromised and at the same time a continuous RF shield is provided.

Several manufacturers have successfully used self-shielded magnets (Figure 13-11). The telescoping cage can make RF shielding of the total room unnecessary. This approach is not acceptable at all sites, particularly at higher B_0 field strengths.

DESIGNING THE FACILITY

Once an MRI system has been selected and the site identified, the facility can be designed. Many design features are independent of the type of MRI system selected. Others must take into account certain characteristics of the type of MRI system. Because many characteristics

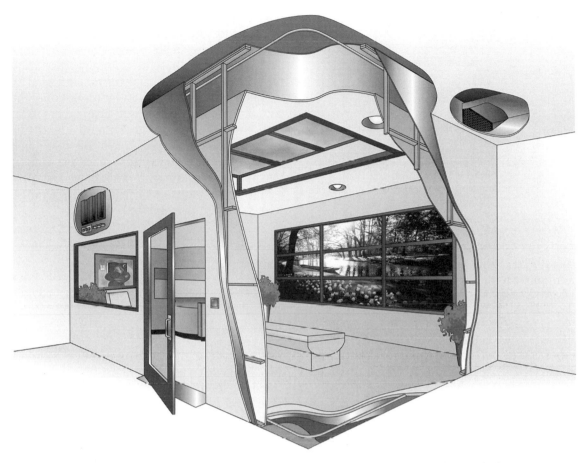

Figure 13-10 A cutaway of a magnetic resonance imaging room shielded to exclude environmental radiofrequency (RF) by a continuous enclosure of sheet or wire mesh of copper or aluminum. The windows and door are specifically designed to be part of the shield. Penetrations into the room are designed to attenuate RF. (Courtesy ETS Lindgren.)

are shared by each type of MRI system, general design criteria can be used.

General Design Criteria

Figure 13-12 is a typical plan layout of an MRI facility as part of an imaging center. A similar layout can be proposed for an existing hospital. Within the immediate imaging area, space must be allocated for the imaging room, computer room, control room, viewing room, and cryogen storage area. A minimum of approximately 150 m² is required. In addition, a reception area, an office space, and a physics/engineering space are necessary.

Reception. Most MRI facilities are not going to be an integral part of an existing radiology department. Therefore a reception and waiting area common with radiology may not be available. In such situations a separate reception area must be provided.

Many MRI examinations are conducted on an outpatient basis, so the patient is examined in street clothes, eliminating the need for change rooms. However, some sort of security

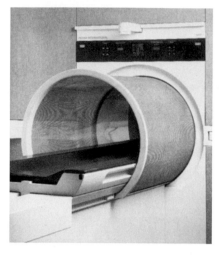

Figure 13-11 The telescoping Faraday cage has been satisfactorily used by several manufacturers. (Courtesy Philips Medical Systems.)

area is required so that the patient can remove metal objects and valuables before the examination. Often patients are asked to wear scrubs so the technologist can be confident that their clothes are not conductive or magnetic.

Metal Detection. At the threshold of the examination area, space must be reserved for metal detection. Most facilities choose to simply instruct the patient to remove all metal. However, a threshold-type metal surveillance device similar to those used for airport security or a wand-type metal detector may be used.

Metal detection is important for not only the patient before imaging but also others who may enter the facility. Physicians, attendants, and custodial personnel must be instructed about potential hazards from metal projectiles. Magnets and people can be damaged by projectiles from individuals who may not otherwise be adequately advised.

Office Support. Office space for radiologists, imaging technologists, and medical physicists is required. A darkroom may be needed for processing images. However, most facilities now use self-contained processors or dry process printers.

Patient Access. The position of the entrance door to the imaging room must be considered. The door should be positioned so that a patient in distress can be quickly and easily removed from the room without undue manipulation. Such a design feature also permits the easy

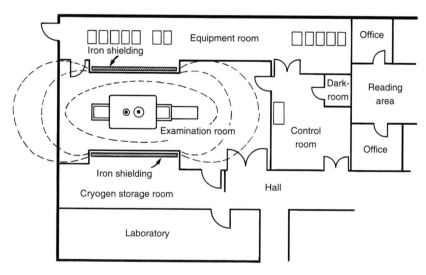

Figure 13-12 A representative plan layout for a magnetic resonance imaging facility showing the required support areas.

access of a crash cart, whose implements must be confirmed nonmagnetic. The door should also be positioned so that access cannot be gained without knowledge of the staff.

Power Requirements. Regardless of the type of MRI system selected, approximately 10 kW of power is required for computers, operating consoles, and other electronic devices. An additional 10 to 20 kW is required to power the shim coils, gradient coils, and RF network. Beyond that, a superconducting MRI system requires an additional 20 to 30 kW but only while the imaging system is being brought up to the design B_0 field strength. During operation, no power is required for the primary magnet coils.

Construction Materials and Techniques

Because the presence of external ferromagnetic material can degrade the homogeneity of the B_0 magnetic field, construction materials must be selected carefully. Large existing metal objects such as cast-iron waste water lines and electrical machinery may have to be moved. In general, the site should be metal free and vibration stable. This requires special material and construction techniques.

It is particularly important that the RF shielding of the imaging room remain at least 90-dB attenuation. This presents special problems for all penetrations through the RF shield.

All wires and cables for power or data must be fitted with appropriate RF filters. Heating, ventilation, and air conditioning (HVAC) ducts must be of nonconducting material, such as polyvinyl chloride (PVC), and maintain length-to-diameter ratio in all sections to provide an RF waveguide of infinite impedance.

Foundation. The weight of most imaging systems requires a substantial concrete pad with reinforcing. Instead of iron reinforcing rods and corrugated iron sheets, some of the available fiberglass-impregnated reinforcing rods and epoxy concrete should be used.

A sufficient structural foundation is required not only in the imaging room but also along the route for installation. Posttension or other techniques may be necessary to ensure that the foundation is vibration free. Even subtle vibration can encourage cryogen to boil off and degrade image quality.

Normal construction techniques for walls and ceilings are generally acceptable. Unreinforced concrete or wood stud construction with standard nails is acceptable.

Electrical Service. Electrical conduits in the MRI room should be made of either PVC or aluminum. Electrical receptacles and fixtures should be aluminum or ceramic. Electrical distribution transformers should not be located within the 1-mT fringe magnetic field.

Lighting in the imaging room must be incandescent; no fluorescent lamps are allowed. The supply should be direct current or properly filtered. Dimmer controls should not be mounted within the room. Fixtures should be brass or ceramic.

Plumbing. Supply lines, floor drains, and soil pipes should be nonferrous. Copper or PVC is acceptable. If building codes require a sprinkler system, only brass or copper components should be used. All sprinkler heads that penetrate the RF shielding must be completely electrically grounded.

Patient Viewing. The ability to view the patient during the examination is mandatory. Although closed-circuit television capable of operating in the magnetic field of the room has been developed, it is expensive and not totally satisfactory. Most facilities find that a direct-view window incorporating a wire mesh as an RF shield is better.

HVAC. Heating, ventilation, and air conditioning are important engineering considerations for an MRI site. The HVAC design must deal with not only the normal space-occupying activities of a conventional office or laboratory but also the special requirements of the MRI system.

Constant temperature is essential for the stability of the magnet and associated electronic components. The B_0 field of a permanent magnet increases approximately 0.1% per degree. A 10° drift could cause an electronic frequency mismatch that would destroy the tuned response at the Larmor frequency.

Any computer that accompanies MRI must be in a cool, dry environment. Temperature must be maintained between 18° C and 20° C at a relative humidity of not more than 40%.

Magnet Cooling. Permanent magnet imaging systems have no special cooling requirements beyond those normally needed for electronic and computer components. This feature contributes to the relatively low capital cost and site preparation requirements.

A superconducting magnet requires cryogens (liquid helium and sometimes liquid nitrogen). Up to 0.5 l/hr of helium and 2 l/hr of liquid nitrogen may be required to maintain the low temperature to support superconductivity. Superconducting magnets require aluminum venting, usually through the ceiling, for cryogen exhaust. It is desirable to have the liquid nitrogen piped in from a storage tank.

Additional Features. In addition to the preceding design features that are appropriate for any MRI facility, there are special considerations attendant to each type of imaging system concerning the design of the facility.

Permanent magnets are small but heavy. A 0.3-T whole-body imaging system can weigh 40,000 kg. Such a mass will probably preempt its placement anywhere but on the ground level. Smaller head and neck imaging systems weigh no more than 5000 kg and can be located on any level.

Superconducting magnet imaging systems require cryogenic support. Loading, handling, and storage space for cryogens must also be provided. The loading dock for cryogen dewars should be outside the 1.0-mT isomagnetic line and easily accessible to the magnet room.

CHALLENGE QUESTIONS

1. What is the main consideration given to the proper location of a permanent magnet MRI system?
2. What is the recommended isotesla exclusion line for cryogenic dewars?
3. What is the principal advantage to siting a permanent magnet MRI system?
4. When constructing the facility to house an MRI system, what are the principal considerations to heating, ventilation, electrical, and plumbing installations?
5. What are the principal advantages and the principal disadvantage to a superconducting MRI system?
6. Why is metal detection essential in an MRI suite?
7. What are the two principal concerns to be considered for siting an MRI system?
8. What is a Faraday cage?
9. What is the difference between a passive shield and an active shield?
10. What is the range of the RF band according to the FCC?

Part III

Image Formation

Chapter 14

Digital Imaging

OBJECTIVES

At the completion of this chapter, the student should be able to do the following:

1. Discuss the difference between binary and decimal number systems.
2. Convert binary numbers to decimal and decimal numbers to binary.
3. Distinguish between bits, bytes, and words.
4. Discuss the requirements on signal sampling to avoid the aliasing artifact.
5. Identify spatial frequency domain (k-space).
6. Describe spatial localization in a magnetic resonance (MR) image.

OUTLINE

When it is applied to medical imaging, the term **digital imaging** implies that a digital computer is used and that the image is composed of discrete **pic**ture **el**ements, that is, **pixels.**

Magnetic resonance imaging (MRI) could not be performed without the digital computer because the magnetic resonance (MR) signal does not interact directly with a viewable medium as x-rays do with a radiographic intensifying screen phosphor. The MR signal does not present information in a form that can be directly viewed electronically, as does ultrasound.

The MR signal provides information about the spatial frequency content of the image rather than directly about the spatial positioning of information in the image. Figure 14-1, *A*, is a computer-generated image of two bright balls on a dark background. Figure 14-1, *B*, is a set of projections called a *sinogram* from that image of the two balls. This type of data set is obtained from a parallel beam x-ray computed tomography (CT) image. The positions and the objects may be inferred at least to a limited extent from the projection data because the data are in the spatial domain, which means that the data are related directly to coordinates in space.

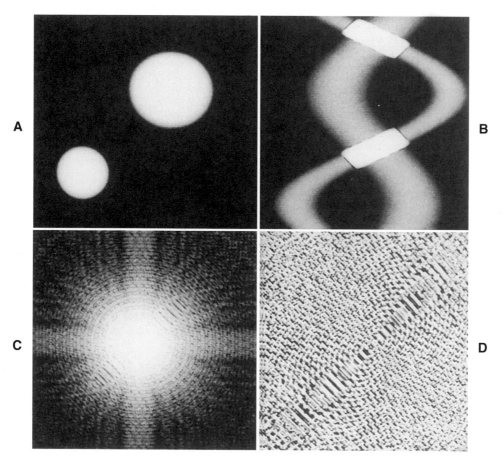

Figure 14-1   A, A plane image of two balls. **B,** The sinogram of the two balls. **C,** The magnitude of the spatial frequency representation of the image. **D,** The phase of the spatial frequency representation of the image. **C** and **D** together are the data set that is actually received in magnetic resonance imaging.

The magnitude of the spatial frequency of the image is shown in Figure 14-1, *C*. Figure 14-1, *D*, shows the phase data from the representation of the two balls. Because the MRI data are in the spatial frequency domain, making sense of the raw data from such an MR image is much more difficult than that from a projection radiograph or a CT sinogram.

 The MR image is acquired in the spatial frequency domain (k-space).

The digital computer converts this information about the spatial frequency domain into the spatial domain of the MR signal within the patient to produce the image. In this chapter some characteristics of the digital computer are reviewed and the details of the formation of MR images are examined to explain the reason why MRI is inherently digital.

THE COMPUTER'S VIEW OF THE WORLD

The digital computer works with numbers, specifically, binary numbers. The binary number set consists of 0 and 1. Perhaps, if humans had only 2 fingers instead of 10, the binary number system would seem to be more natural than the decimal number system.

A single number in the decimal system is called a **digit,** as are the fingers shown in Figure 14-2. A single number in the binary system is called a **bit,** which is short for **bi**nary digi**t.**

The digital computer uses the binary number system because it is so easy to implement with real-world components. A 1 is simply defined to be any voltage above a specified value and 0 to be any voltage below a specified value.

Binary Number System

In the binary number system, counting is done by counting 0 and 1 and then over again (Table 14-1). There are only two binary digits,

0 and 1, and the computer performs all operations by converting alphabetic characters, decimal values, and logical functions to binary values.

In the binary system, 0 is 0 and 1 is 1. The 1 is actually 2^0. Any number raised to the zero power is 1; therefore 2^0 equals 1. In binary notation, the number 2 equals 1 times 2^1 plus no 2^0. This is expressed as 10.

The decimal 3 equals 1 times 2^1 plus 1 times 2^0 or 11 in binary form. The decimal 4 is 1 times 2^2 plus no 2^1 plus no 2^0 or 100 in binary form. As shown in Table 14-1, each time 2 is raised to an additional power to express a number, the number of binary digits increases by 1.

Easily recognizing the powers of 2 is essential. Power-of-2 notation is used in radiologic imaging to describe image size, image dynamic range (shades of gray), and image storage capacity. Table 14-2 reviews these power notations. In both power notations, the number of zeros to the right of 1 equals the value of the exponent.

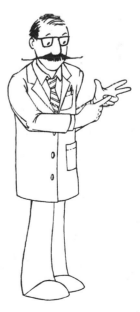

Figure 14-2 The origin of the decimal number system is obvious.

TABLE 14-1	Organization of Binary Number System	
Decimal Number	**Binary Equivalent**	**Binary Number**
0	0	0
1	2^0	1
2	$2^1 + 0$	10
3	$2^1 + 2^0$	11
4	$2^2 + 0 + 0$	100
5	$2^2 + 0 + 2^0$	101
6	$2^2 + 2^1 + 0$	110
7	$2^2 + 2^1 + 2^0$	111
8	$2^3 + 0 + 0 + 0$	1000
9	$2^3 + 0 + 0 + 2^0$	1001
10	$2^3 + 0 + 2^1 + 0$	1010
11	$2^3 + 0 + 2^1 + 2^0$	1011
12	$2^3 + 2^2 + 0 + 0$	1100
13	$2^3 + 2^2 + 0 + 2^0$	1101
14	$2^3 + 2^2 + 2^1 + 0$	1110
15	$2^3 + 2^2 + 2^1 + 2^0$	1111
16	$2^4 + 0 + 0 + 0 + 0$	10000

Question: How is the number 193 expressed in binary form?

Answer: Because 193 falls between 2^7 and 2^8, it will be expressed as 1 followed by seven binary digits. Simply add the decimal equivalents of each binary digit from left to right.

Yes 2^7 = 1 = 128
Yes 2^6 = 1 = 64
No 2^5 = 0 = No 32
No 2^4 = 0 = No 16
No 2^3 = 0 = No 8
No 2^2 = 0 = No 4
No 2^1 = 0 = No 2
Yes 2^0 = 1 = 1
11000001 = 193

Digital medical images are made of discrete numerical values arranged in a matrix. The size of the image is described in the binary system of numbers by power of 2 equivalents. The most popular MR image matrix sizes are 256 × 256 ($2^8 × 2^8$) and 512 × 512 ($2^9 × 2^9$).

Bits, Bytes, and Words

The computer will use as many bits (zeros and ones) as necessary to express a decimal number. The 26 uppercase and 26 lowercase characters of the alphabet and other special characters are usually encoded by 7 bits. The use of 8 bits by newer extended character sets doubles the possible number of characters. Depending on the computer, a string of 8, 16, 32, 64, or possibly some other number of bits is manipulated simultaneously.

 To encode is to translate from ordinary characters to computer-compatible characters (binary codes).

Bits are grouped into bunches of 8 called **bytes (B).** Computer capacity is expressed by the number of bytes that the memory of the computer can accommodate. For example, 1 kilobyte (kB) is 2^{10} or 1024 bytes; 1 megabyte (MB) is 2^{20} or 1,048,576 bytes.

Prefixes such as *kilo* and *mega* are not metric in computer use but refer to the nearest power of 2. Popular personal computers have

TABLE 14-2	Power of 10, Power of 2, and Binary Notation	
Power of 10	**Power of 2**	**Binary Notation**
$10^0 = 1$	$2^0 = 1$	1
$10^1 = 10$	$2^1 = 2$	10
$10^2 = 100$	$2^2 = 4$	100
$10^3 = 1000$	$2^3 = 8$	1000
$10^4 = 10,000$	$2^4 = 16$	10000
$10^5 = 100,000$	$2^5 = 32$	100000
$10^6 = 1,000,000$	$2^6 = 64$	1000000
	$2^7 = 128$	10000000
	$2^8 = 256$	100000000
	$2^9 = 512$	1000000000
	$2^{10} = 1024$	10000000000

16-bit or 32-bit microprocessors and contain 256 MB of main memory. The workstations and minicomputers used in radiology have main memory capacities of gigabytes, and these values are continuously increasing. Secondary memory in the form of magnetic and optical disks can have memory measured in gigabytes (GB) (1 GB $= 2^{30} = 1,073,741,824$ bytes).

Question: How many bits can be stored on a 4-MB chip whose byte size is 8 bits?
Answer: 1,048,576 bytes/MB × 8 bits/byte × 4 MB
   or
   2^{20} bytes/MB × 2^3 bits/byte × 2^2 MB
   33,554,432 bits

Depending on the computer configuration, 1, 2, or 4 bytes usually constitute a word. In the case of a 16-bit microprocessor, a word is 16 consecutive bits of information that are interpreted and shuffled about the computer as a unit. Each word of data in memory has its own address. Often each byte is addressable.

The number of bits determines the resolution or precision of the numbers that the computer manipulates. This means that the number of bits determines the total number of elements that the computer can count.

This is similar to the U.S. Postal Service zip codes. When the Postal Service wanted to add resolution to the zip codes, it added four more numbers at the end of the five-numeral zip code to define the carrier route and the postal zone to which a letter is addressed.

An 8-bit computer number can count from 0 through 255 and thus can represent 256 (2^8) different values. A 16-bit number can count from 0 through 65,535 and thus can represent 65,536 (2^{16}) different values.

Regardless of the number of bits that the computer uses, it is limited in the number of distinct values that it can represent. It cannot hold continuous data the way a tape recording, a photograph, or a radiograph can. In the digital computer, limited resolution and limited storage affect the manipulation of data. MRI is limited in the same way.

Quantization or Resolution

Precision. The limited number of elements that the computer can count restricts the precision with which the computer can store values. For proper interpretation, some quantities must be specified with great precision. However, imprecision is a fact of life, and people live comfortably with acceptable degrees of imprecision.

When someone asks, "How far is it to Dallas?" a satisfactory answer is to the nearest mile or so. An answer to the nearest foot or inch is unnecessary. When a person gets a driver's license, the person's height is required to the nearest inch, not the nearest quarter inch. Age is not given precisely to the minute but usually only to the year. Such limits of precision are totally satisfactory in everyday life. Considerably more precision is required for MRI.

In the design of a computer system, the required resolution of the data is determined first. For example, differences of 0.01 V may be distinguished in an MR signal—a free induction decay (FID), a spin echo (SE), or a gradient echo (GRE). An 8-bit computer word allows for 256 discrete steps or a voltage range from 0 to 2.55 V. A 16-bit computer word gives a voltage range from 0 to 655.35 V.

A voltage range of 24 V is typically used in MRI. Thus, 12 bits (2^{12} = 4096) is required because 12 bits allow a range from 0 to 41.96 V; 11 bits (2^{11} = 2048) provides a range of only 0 to 20.48 V, which would not be sufficient.

A total of 16 or 24 bits are commonly used to allow extra bits for computations. For example, a 22-V signal and 23-V signal are added; 12 bits would not be enough to hold the result, 45 V. An additional bit is required. Although more than ample, computers with word lengths of 32 and 64 bits are becoming more popular as the prices of the computers decrease because they typically offer other attractive features such as faster computation.

Dynamic Range.   One area in which the resolution of the data affects medical images is in the number of gray levels used to display an image. This is referred to as the **dynamic range** or **gray scale resolution** of an imaging system. An imaging system that displays only black or white has a gray scale resolution of 2^1 (1 bit) or 2. Such an image is of very high contrast but displays little information. Although the value of each pixel is unimportant, the number of values is extremely important in determining the final image.

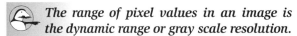 *The range of pixel values in an image is the dynamic range or gray scale resolution.*

In MR images, gray scale resolution refers to how small a difference in pixel intensity corre-

sponds to a 1-bit difference in pixel value. Visually, gray scale resolution refers to the number of different shades of gray that can be perceived.

The gray scale resolution of the human eye is somewhere between 2^4 (4 bits) and 2^5 (5 bits) or 16 to 32, shades of gray, stretching from black to white. The gray scale resolution of the MR signal from the patient exceeds 2^{10} (10 bits).

Although humans cannot perceive such a fine gray scale resolution, a computer with sufficient capacity can store that much information. The finer the steps within the span from black to white, the more gradual the gray scale representing the range from minimum to maximum intensity. Therefore the finer the gray scale resolution, the better the image.

Early image display devices were capable of only 4 bits (2^4) or 16 gray levels. Current displays provide 10 bits or 12 bits or 1024 or 4096 gray levels, respectively.

In CT the Hounsfield units have a range of 2000. In radioisotope scintigraphic imaging, thousands of counts in a pixel may occur in a first-pass study, and in MRI, T1 and T2 values may have ranges of several thousand milliseconds. Despite this, the human visual system can resolve no more than 32 different shades of gray, and so in a display system, somewhere between 32 and 256 gray levels are sufficient to ensure no loss of visual information.

However, just as CT images are displayed with bone or soft tissue windows to evade the mismatch between the resolution in Hounsfield units and the gray scale resolution of the observer, the 32 or so perceptible shades of gray in the human visual system must be used to full advantage. This is done by adjusting the brightness and contrast of the MR image so that all the gray scale information available can be perceived.

The full dynamic range of a 12-bit display is visible with **window level** and **window width** postprocessing (Figure 14-3). With variation of the window level and width, the entire 4096 gray scale can be viewed for diagnosis.

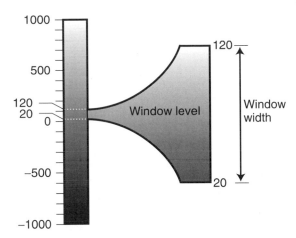

Figure 14-3 Postprocessing an image for various combinations of window level and window width allows the entire gray scale to be viewed.

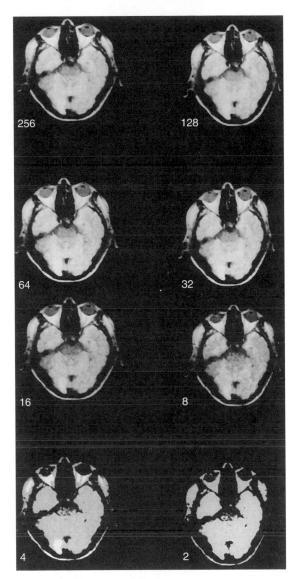

Figure 14-4 Different gray scale resolutions in an image display. For many people, the loss of gray scale resolution does not become visible until only about 16 shades of gray are present. At that point, apparent edges or contours are seen in the image where there should be none.

It is necessary to consider an MR image displayed with different numbers of gray levels to understand the significance of the concept of an acceptable degree of imprecision. In Figure 14-4, the same image is displayed with 8, 7, 6, 5, 4, 3, 2, and 1 bit of gray scale resolution. These bit values correspond to 256, 128, 64, 32, 16, 8, 4, and 2 shades of gray, respectively. With an insufficient number of gray levels available, there is a visual loss of gray scale resolution.

That loss may be perceived as **false contouring,** in which boundaries appear in the image where there should be none. However, gray scale resolution is not the only limitation implicit in working with digital computers. Limited storage capacity also leads to limitations on spatial resolution.

Question: How many bytes are required for a 256 × 256 MR image having a 12-bit dynamic range?

Answer: 12 bit ÷ 8 bit/byte = 1.5 byte/pixel
256 × 256 × 1.5 = 98,304 bytes
or 98 kB

Sampling

When the computer stores data, it must be able to address the data. In the same way that there is a limited number of postal zones in the United States that can have a unique five-digit zip code, there is a limited number of memory locations that can be used for image storage. This limitation is imposed by the limited number of bits in the memory address.

Consequently, for the image to be stored in the computer, the continuous object to be imaged must be sampled.

The process of **sampling** involves taking occasional values, or samples, of information from the MR signal. This is illustrated in Figure 14-5, in which a continuous FID is represented by a set of values taken at a regular interval. In this instance, the sampled data set is similar to a connect-the-dots picture.

> *Sampling is the rate at which a continuous signal is digitized.*

Sampling is a familiar process. The business pages of the newspapers give closing prices for stocks each day. Even though the price of a stock may change during the day, only its price at the end of the day and the range of its price during the day are given.

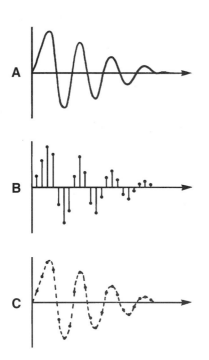

Figure 14-5   A, A continuous free induction decay (FID). **B,** A sampled version of the FID. The computer stores only the values taken at the regularly spaced indicated points along the horizontal axis. **C,** The connect-the-dots reconstruction of the original signal from the sampled values.

A television picture is not a continuously changing image, but rather, a rapid succession of still images displayed at the rate of 30 images each second. Obviously, there is no loss of important information about the action on the television screen, even though only 30 samples a second are seen, rather than continuous motion.

There is a direct relationship between the speed with which changes are occurring and the rate at which sampling is performed so that no useful information is lost. The faster the signal changes, the faster it must be sampled to describe all of the details of that change accurately with the data stored in the computer.

Signals and image patterns that change rapidly are described as containing high frequencies. Signals and image patterns that change slowly are described as containing low frequencies.

Sampling must be rapid enough so that the signal being sampled does not change direction more than once between samples. If the sampling is not quick enough, a rapidly changing process may appear to change slowly (Figure 14-6).

When a rapidly changing signal is undersampled and appears to change slowly, the process is said to be **aliased** because of the misleading nature of the sampled data. The stagecoach in a Wild West movie appears as though its wheels are moving backwards because the spokes appear to rotate backwards (Figure 14-7). The movie frame rate (sampling rate) was not fast enough to capture the true motion of the wheels. The result is an aliased image.

Aliasing results in a permanent loss of information. An example of an aliasing artifact, not uncommon in CT, appears as streaks from a very sharp interface (Figure 14-8). Aliasing artifacts in MR images appear as "wraparound" structures (Figure 14-9). MR artifacts are described more completely in Chapter 27.

Using a digital computer creates two opposing constraints. The limited amount of data storage capacity argues for taking as few samples as

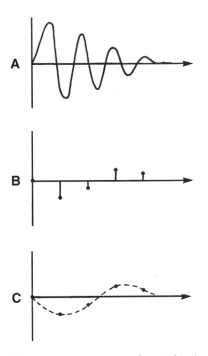

The lower limit on sampling is determined by the data because enough samples must be acquired to avoid aliasing. The upper limit is determined by the capacity of the computer.

MRI must also sample the information about the patient. The number of samples in MRI is limited by the time available to collect the data from a very short signal. The changes of the signal are changes in not only time but also space because the signal originates from various regions of the body. Thus the frequencies to be observed are those of spatial frequency.

THE SPATIAL FREQUENCY DOMAIN

Spatial resolution is measured in line pairs per centimeter (lp/cm) or line pairs per millimeter (lp/mm). Spatial frequency is measured in cycles per unit distance (e.g., cycles/cm or cycles/mm). The two are nearly identical in meaning and intuition because line pairs per unit distance applies to cycles per unit distance as well.

The ability to image high spatial frequencies is the ability to image very small objects. Five line pair patterns and five spatial frequency patterns are shown in Figure 14-10. The larger

Figure 14-6 **A,** A continuous free induction decay (FID). **B,** A sampled version of the FID in which the samples are taken too far apart in time. **C,** The connect-the-dots representation of the undersampling shows that the higher frequency has been aliased into a lower frequency.

possible. The desire for high spatial resolution argues for taking as many samples as possible.

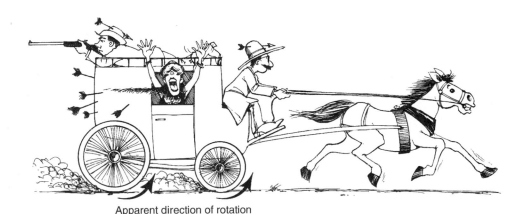

Apparent direction of rotation

Figure 14-7 The apparent backward rotation of wagon wheels in Wild West movies is due to aliasing. The frame rate is not fast enough to record the actual motion. Aliasing in magnetic resonance imaging results in a "wraparound" artifact.

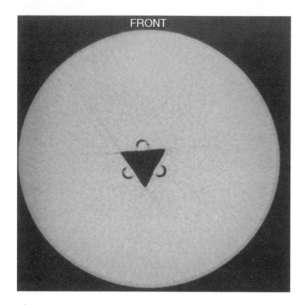

Figure 14-8 This is a computed tomography image of a plastic cylinder containing an air-filled triangular section. The dark streaks appearing off the edges of the triangles are the result of aliasing. (Courtesy Edward Nickoloff, New York, NY.)

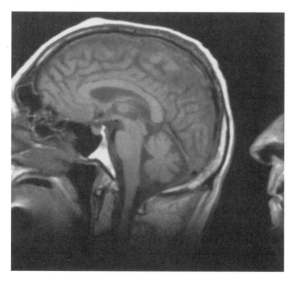

Figure 14-9 This patient was positioned too far anteriorly in the head coil; the result was wrap-around posteriorly. (Courtesy Errol Candy, Dallas, TX.)

patterns are represented by smaller numbers. As spatial frequency increases, object size decreases and becomes more difficult to image.

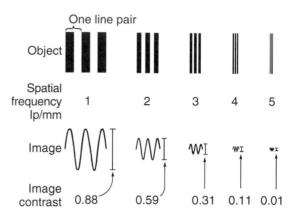

Figure 14-10 These five line pair patterns are spatial frequency patterns used to demonstrate spatial resolution.

The spatial resolution of the best clinical MRI system is approximately 10 lp/cm or 1 lp/mm. Table 14-3 shows the approximate spatial resolution for some other medical imaging modalities.

Space—Spatial Frequency
$cm = 1/2 \left[\dfrac{1}{lp/cm} \right]$
$lp/cm = 1/2 \left[\dfrac{1}{cm} \right]$

Question: An MRI system is capable of 10 lp/cm resolution. What pixel size does this represent?

Answer: 10 lp/cm = 20 objects/cm, therefore
$$1 \text{ object} = 1/20 \text{ cm}$$
$$= 0.05 \text{ cm}$$
$$= 0.5 \text{ mm}$$

Question: A 256 × 256 MR image is acquired over a 10-cm field of view (FOV). What is the limiting spatial frequency?

Answer: pixel size $= \dfrac{100 \text{ mm}}{256} = 0.4 \text{ mm}$

$$2 \text{ pixels} = 1 \text{ lp}$$
$$\text{therefore } 0.8 \text{ mm} = 1 \text{ lp}$$
$$\text{and } \dfrac{1 \text{ lp}}{0.8 \text{ mm}} = 1.25 \text{ lp/mm}$$

TABLE 14-3	Approximate Spatial Resolution Capability of Several Medical Imaging Modalities	
Imaging Modality	**Object Size (mm)**	**Spatial Frequency (lp/mm)**
Radioisotope scan	10.0	0.05
Ultrasound	2.0	0.25
Computed tomography	0.5	1.0
Magnetic resonance imaging	0.5	1.0
Intensified fluoroscopy	0.15	3.0
Screen-film	0.05	10
Human eye	0.05	10.0
Direct exposure film	0.02	25.0

A high spatial frequency reflects many changes in the intensity of the MR signal. This is a function of location within the patient. A low spatial frequency arises from few or no changes in the intensity of the MR signal across the patient.

An example of different spatial frequencies can be illustrated by the three businessmen shown in Figure 14-11: a used car salesman, an undertaker, and a banker. The used car salesman is wearing a loud plaid jacket, the undertaker is wearing a plain black suit, and the banker is wearing a pinstripe suit.

The pattern of the fabric of the used car salesman's plaid jacket has many abrupt changes in any square centimeter. Thus there are many high spatial frequencies in that jacket because there are many changes per centimeter, whether the jacket is sampled horizontally across the cloth or vertically. Whether the operator samples vertically or horizontally, there are no changes in the pattern of the fabric of the undertaker's solid black suit, and thus the jacket has very low spatial frequencies.

Between these extremes is the banker's pinstripe suit. A vertical sample on the back of the jacket reveals no change. Therefore the jacket has very low spatial frequencies vertically. On the other hand, when the jacket is sampled horizontally across the fabric, the pinstripes are crossed, and some relatively high spatial frequencies are observed. The more closely spaced the pinstripes, the higher the horizontal spatial frequency.

Image Matrix

Because the computer has a limited amount of memory in which an image can be stored, the image must be sampled in space as well as in time. For the sampling of an image in space, the values are selected at the intersections of an imaginary grid, which is superimposed on the image (Figure 14-12), and the values represent a small region of the image.

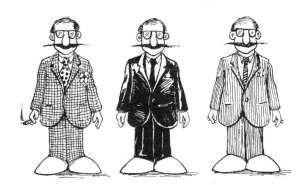

Figure 14-11   Three entrepreneurs and their working attire demonstrate the concept of spatial frequency. The used car salesman's plaid jacket contains high spatial frequencies both horizontally and vertically. The undertaker's plain black jacket has zero spatial frequency. The banker's pinstripe suit has zero vertical spatial frequency but higher horizontal spatial frequency.

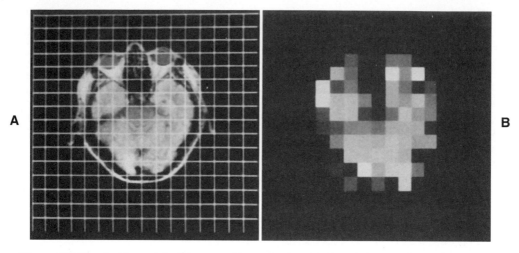

Figure 14-12 **A,** The original image with a sampling grid superimposed. **B,** The sampled values of the original image. Because of sampling in space, the resulting computer image may look blocky.

The term *image matrix* refers to a layout of rows and columns, usually containing numbers representing intensity in boxes or cells. Figure 14-13 shows a 10 × 10 matrix of cells, a 5 × 5 matrix of cells, and a 5 × 5 matrix of numbers in imaginary cells. Each MR image consists of a matrix of imaginary cells, each having various brightness levels (the gray scale). The brightness of a cell is determined by the computer-generated number in that cell.

The size of the image matrix is determined by characteristics of the imaging system and the capacity of the computer. Most MRI systems provide image matrix sizes of 256 × 256, although often other sizes such as 192 × 256 and 512 × 512 are available. Sometimes, an arbitrary acquisition matrix, such as 384 × 512, is placed in the center of the nearest larger power-of-2 matrix, 512 × 512 in this case, with the unused cells at minimum intensity.

The spatial resolution of any digital image is limited by pixel size. Therefore spatial resolution is improved with a larger image matrix,

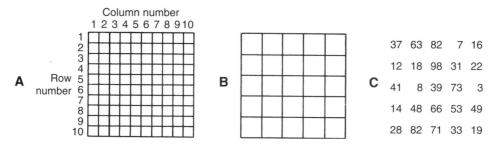

Figure 14-13 **A,** 10 × 10 matrix of cells. **B,** 5 × 5 matrix of cells. **C,** 5 × 5 matrix of numbers in imaginary cells.

assuming that the FOV of the image is held constant.

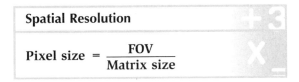

| **Spatial Resolution** |
| Pixel size $= \dfrac{\text{FOV}}{\text{Matrix size}}$ |

Figure 14-14 illustrates the influence of matrix size on image quality when the FOV remains fixed. A 64 × 64 cell matrix appears definitely "blocky," whereas a 128 × 128 matrix is a fairly good representation of the original image.

In theory, the sampled value represents the intensity of the original continuous image at an infinitesimally small point. Such a point would be invisible, so each point is represented by a pixel of the displayed image.

 Spatial resolution is limited by pixel size.

A sampled image is just like a mosaic. Each pixel is a small tile having a brightness equal to that of the sampled value at that point in the image. This accounts for the possible blocky appearance of some computer-displayed digital images.

The spacing of the samples must be sufficiently close so that there are no surprises between samples. For example, if there were a small structure in the patient and the samples were far apart, it would be difficult to say precisely where the structure should be located in the image and the precise shape of the structure. Sharp edges and small structures contain high spatial frequencies.

Frequency Domain Map

The spatial frequency content of an image is displayed in two dimensions, just the way the image itself is displayed. Low frequencies are near the center of the spatial frequency display and higher spatial frequencies are toward the edges (Figure 14-15).

Horizontal spatial frequencies appear along horizontal lines, and vertical spatial frequencies appear along vertical lines. The intensity of an arbitrary point represents the strength of a particular combination of horizontal and vertical spatial frequencies. For example, the banker's pinstripe suit was a combination of low vertical

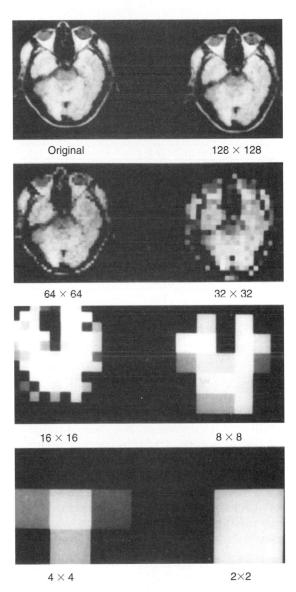

Figure 14-14   The small features and sharp edges in the image that contain much of the high spatial frequency information are progressively obscured as the sampling rate and image matrix are reduced. The fine structures become blurred as their high spatial frequencies are aliased into lower spatial frequencies.

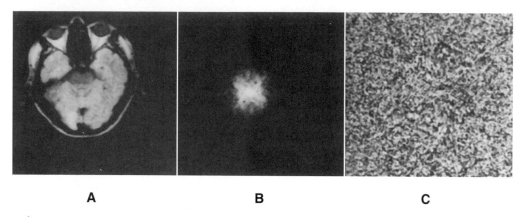

A   **B**   **C**

Figure 14-15   The spatial frequency representation of an image. **A,** The original image. **B,** The magnitude map of the spatial frequencies. **C,** The phase map of the spatial frequencies. The image is predominately positive in intensity, and the center of **B** is therefore very bright because the average value in the image is quite large.

spatial frequency and higher horizontal spatial frequency.

The information in the spatial frequency representation of the image is exactly the same as the information in the image; it is just being represented in a different way. There are examples of this concept in everyday life. Scheduled patients appear on the MRI system worksheets in chronological order. However, when they are billed for the procedure, the list is likely to be in alphabetical order or arranged by hospital number.

The same information is present; a group of patients received MRI examinations. The manner in which the data are presented is different for different purposes. Whether the information in an image is organized by horizontal and vertical position or by horizontal and vertical spatial frequency does not affect the information itself but only how it is presented.

SPATIAL LOCALIZATION AND MAGNETIC RESONANCE IMAGING

Although the topic of this book is MRI, computers, spatial frequency, and sampling are emphasized because MRI samples the strengths of the spatial frequencies of the MR signal in the patient to get the image information. The

computer then converts that information from its spatial frequency representation to a representation in the spatial domain or position. The latter is the usual definition of an image, but the former is the way in which the raw data are presented to the computer.

Several MRI techniques have been developed. However, the two-dimensional Fourier transform (2DFT) method has led people to concentrate on the spatial frequency domain, or "k-space" (see Chapter 15). What once seemed to be very different methods of imaging, projection reconstruction and 2DFT, are just different methods of measuring the spatial frequency domain. They have been joined by some other methods, all of which are easily understood in the spatial frequency domain.

 The spatial frequency information of the patient is sampled into the spatial frequency domain and ordered in the computer as k-space.

Projection reconstruction, 2DFT, and three-dimensional Fourier transform (3DFT) MRIs are digital imaging techniques. They differ in how they sample the spatial frequencies of the patient. The principles of spatial localization demonstrate why MRI is inherently digital, regardless of the particular technique used.

In a homogenous magnetic field all of the spins precess at exactly the same rate. This rate equals the Larmor frequency. The Larmor equation asserts that the frequency of precession is directly proportional to the strength of the magnetic field, B_0. Because the frequency, phase, and amplitude of the signal are all that can be measured, it becomes necessary to modify the magnetic field so that the MR signal can reflect its spatial origin.

 The difference between a nuclear magnetic resonance spectrometer and an MRI system is the presence of gradient magnetic fields in MRI.

Gradient magnetic fields are used to achieve spatial localization. When the strength of the magnetic field varies linearly across the patient, the frequency of the signal does also. Spins on one side of the patient precess faster than spins on the other side. When the MR signal is received, the range of frequencies in the patient will be detected and clearly distinguished. As shown in Figure 14-16, the MR signal from the patient's head is of lower frequency than that from the abdomen.

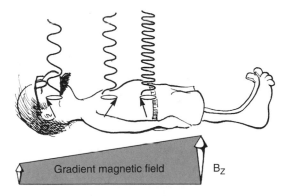

Figure 14-16 The effect of a gradient magnetic field, B_Z, on the resonant frequency of spins within the patient. Note that the spins in the head precess more slowly than those in the belly.

Gradient magnetic fields also provide the means to distinguish left from right within the slice of the image but do not yield any information about the distribution of intensity along the direction at right angles to the gradient. For information to be obtained throughout the plane of the object, two gradient magnetic fields must be used.

The two gradients are applied **simultaneously** in projection reconstruction imaging and **sequentially** in 2DFT imaging. These approaches to MRI reflect different ways of coordinating the effect of the two orthogonal gradient magnetic fields. The combination of the two gradients allows the whole slice to be sampled. Sampling the spatial frequency representation of the image slice makes MRI inherently digital imaging.

Projection Reconstruction Magnetic Resonance Imaging

The projection reconstruction MRI technique is the easiest to understand because it resembles the way in which data are collected in parallel beam, x-ray CT. As two orthogonal gradient magnetic fields are applied simultaneously, the direction of the resulting gradient is the vector sum of these two orthogonal gradients. The direction of the resultant vector sum gradient may be rotated in the imaging slice by varying the relative strengths of the two orthogonal gradient magnetic fields, B_X and B_Y (Figure 14-17).

A separate MR signal is acquired for each orientation of the resultant vector sum gradient. This MR signal is a sample of the two-dimensional spatial frequency representation of the image. As the resultant vector sum gradient is rotated from acquisition to acquisition, the orientation of the samples in the spatial frequency domain rotates. Thus the spatial frequencies in the image are sampled on a polar grid (Figure 14-18).

Back projection is a time-consuming computational chore that tends to emphasize the noise in the projections. For these reasons, the

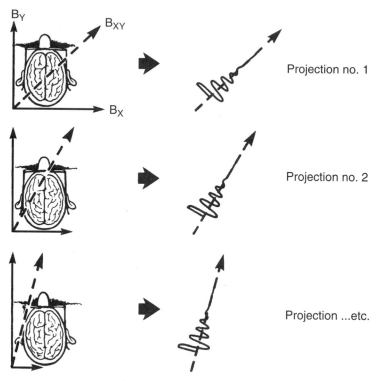

Figure 14-17 The vector sum of two simultaneously applied gradient magnetic fields can be rotated by varying the strength of each gradient. Note that the strengths of the X and Y gradients are chosen so that their strength always remains the same, even though the angle of the resultant B_{XY} changes.

2DFT and 3DFT techniques have become the methods of choice for MRI.

Two-Dimensional Fourier Transform Magnetic Resonance Imaging

The 2DFT approach also samples the spatial frequency domain of the image but does so on a rectangular grid instead of a polar grid (Figure 14-19). The 2DFT technique consists of a basic cycle that is repeated many times, typically 256. This cycle consists of radiofrequency (RF) excitation pulse (RF_t), followed by a magnetic field pulse from the phase-encoding gradient (B_Φ) and then by a steady application of an orthogonal gradient called the *read* or *frequency-encoding gradient magnetic field* (B_R), during which time the MR signal is detected.

 From one signal acquisition to the next, only the strength of the phase-encoding gradient magnetic field is changed.

After a suitable delay, the cycle is repeated. The phase-encoding gradient magnetic field selects a single line in the k-space representation of the image. Then the frequency-encoding gradient magnetic field forms the MR signal along this line. Instead of rotating the sampling line around the center of k-space, the phase-encoding gradient magnetic field shifts the MR signal so that it samples a different line of spatial frequencies parallel to the others. When the strength of the phase-encoding gradient magnetic field is changed in following cycles, other lines in k-space are measured.

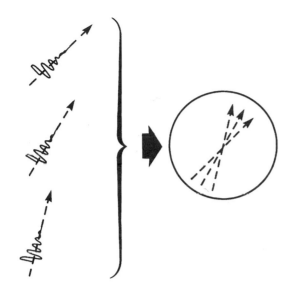

Figure 14-18 Polar sampling of the spatial frequency domain of the image. Note that the angle of the resultant B_{XY} gradient determines the angle of the sample line in the spatial frequency domain.

A family of lines in k-space has been selected, and the frequency information along those lines has been measured. This rectangular sampling is Fourier transformed to yield the image. Because the k-space data are already sampled on a rectangular grid, 2DFT replaces the filtering and back projection steps of projection reconstruction with a second Fourier transform.

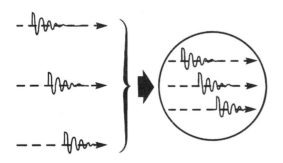

Figure 14-19 Rectangular sampling of the spatial frequency domain. The phase-encoding gradient is changed during each signal acquisition, which determines the horizontal line of the spatial frequency domain.

 The two most common artifacts peculiar to 2DFT images are the consequences of undersampling and motion.

Undersampling means that not enough points are used in the data collection. This results in the samples not being sufficiently close in the frequency representation of the data. When this happens, the image is aliased, and the bottom of the image appears to wraparound the top (Figure 14-20).

The cure for aliasing is to increase the number of samples in the data collection stage or reduce the FOV. Both of these solutions increase the sampling frequency.

The effects of the subject's motion on the 2DFT image are complicated. Most of the visible effects are in the phase-encoded direction of the image. This is because the frequency-encoding gradient magnetic field remains the same for every cycle, whereas the phase-encoding gradient magnetic field is different for each cycle.

The motion effect is related to the strength of the gradient magnetic fields, and only the phase-encoding gradient changes in strength; therefore the motion effects are only visible in the phase-encoded direction. The line between the successive application of the phase-encoding gradient is hundreds to thousands of milliseconds, repetition time (TR), whereas the time between sampling data points along the frequency-encoding gradient, B_R, is microseconds.

The motion effect is sometimes useful in identifying the phase-encoding direction. This is important to know because motion can still produce artifacts even when the image is cardiac gated and respiratory gated (Figure 14-21). Through correct selection of the phase-encoding direction, the overlap of the artifacts and organs of interest can be minimized.

Three-Dimensional Fourier Transform Magnetic Resonance Imaging

Bigger and faster computers have made it possible to store contiguous 2DFT slices and display them as an apparent three-dimensional

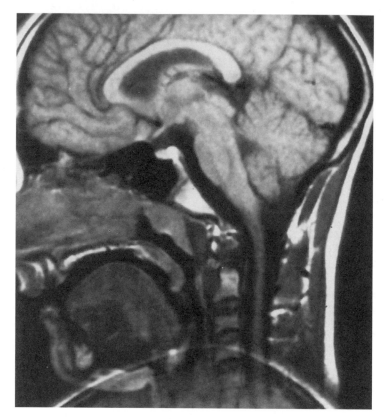

Figure 14-20   Aliasing in two-dimensional Fourier transform images can result in "wrap-around" of tissues in the patient. (Courtesy R. Mark Henkelman, Toronto, Canada.)

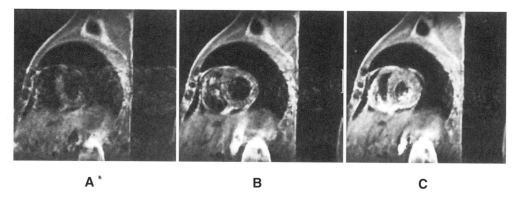

A   **B**   **C**

Figure 14-21   The effects of motion on two-dimensional Fourier transform (2DFT) images. **A,** An ungated cardiac image. **B,** End diastolic image of a heart. **C,** End systolic image of a heart (**B** and **C** are of the same heart). The ungated image has extremely poor definition of the myocardium and prominent streaking artifacts in the phase-encoded direction. The gated images show improvement in the motion artifacts, but these artifacts are not eliminated because the motion, even when gated, causes phase errors that mislead the 2DFT reconstruction algorithm.

image. A faster way of acquiring data for three-dimensional display is to follow the second Fourier transform, which produces a slice image, with yet another Fourier transform. With this method, a three-dimensional image is obtained more quickly and with improved spatial resolution.

CHALLENGE QUESTIONS

1. What is the best spatial resolution possible with any digital image?
2. What is the difference between a digit and a bit?
3. When acquiring data for an MR image, what must change from one signal acquisition to the next?
4. What would one have to do to turn a nuclear magnetic resonance (NMR) spectrometer into an MRI system?
5. An MRI system is set to have a 12-bit dynamic range. How many gray levels can that imaging system display?
6. The best resolution MRI systems can obtain is approximately 2 lp/cm. What is the equivalent spatial resolution expressed in size?
7. The patient aperture for most MRI gantries is approximately 60 cm. Express this in binary form.
8. An MRI examination results in 32 images of 256 matrix size and 12-bit gray scale. How much disk space will be required to store these images, uncompressed?
9. Explain why a 12-bit dynamic range is useful for MRI when the dynamic range of the human eye does not exceed 5 bits.
10. As spatial frequency increases, what happens to object size, spatial resolution, and the contrast resolution?

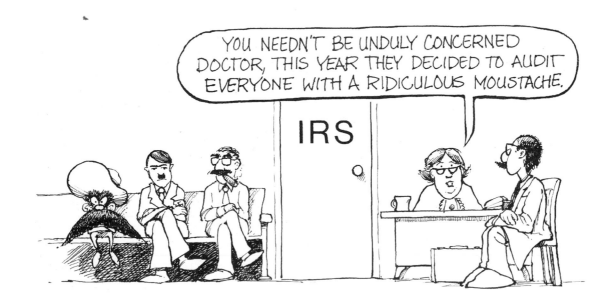

Chapter 15

A Walk Through the Spatial Frequency Domain

OBJECTIVES

At the completion of this chapter, the student should be able to do the following:

1. Define spatial frequency, spatial frequency domain, and k-space.
2. Relate the forward and inverse Fourier transforms to their place in two-dimensional Fourier transform (2DFT) magnetic resonance imaging (MRI).
3. Draw several graphic representations of a Fourier transform.
4. Identify a sinc pulse and its appearance graphically.
5. Describe the relationships among receiver bandwidth, signal-to-noise ratio, and field of view.

OUTLINE

The spatial frequency domain is crucial to magnetic resonance imaging (MRI) because all but the very earliest methods of MRI (such as the sensitive point method) scan the spatial frequency information about the image, not the image plane itself.

A useful analogy is the human auditory system. When a microphone is attached to a strip chart recorder and is used to listen to a musical ensemble, the result is a tracing of sound intensity as a function of time; the microphone simply responds to changes in air pressure at its sensor.

When a member of the audience hears the same performance, the individual instruments of the ensemble are perceived as they play in concert (Figure 15-1). This is because the human auditory system converts the variations of loudness observed by the microphone into a temporal frequency representation from which the brain extracts higher level information about the instrumentation.

In MRI, the imaging system measures the information about the image slice differently than the human visual system would if the slice were directly visible. A method of analyzing the spatial frequency components and converting them into spatial location information is needed to reconstruct the image. The usual method is the Fourier transform (FT).

The purpose of this chapter is to extend the introduction to spatial frequency in the preceding chapter and to discuss the FT. Chapter 16 demonstrates how the MRI system actually measures spatial frequencies.

SPATIAL FREQUENCY

The term *spatial frequency domain* comes from the field of electrical engineering. The term *k-space* comes from physics. They refer to the same thing. Either is correct and both are in common use. The former is far more descriptive; however, k-space is firmly entrenched in MRI and therefore used here to emphasize the subject under discussion.

 Spatial frequency has units of line pair/cm or line pair/mm—10 lp/mm = 1 lp/cm.

Consider a series of high contrast bar patterns to be imaged (Figure 15-2). One bar and its equal width interspace are called a **line pair**.

The number of line pairs per unit length is the spatial frequency, and for MRI systems it is expressed in line pair per centimeter (lp/cm). A low spatial frequency represents large objects, and a high spatial frequency represents small objects.

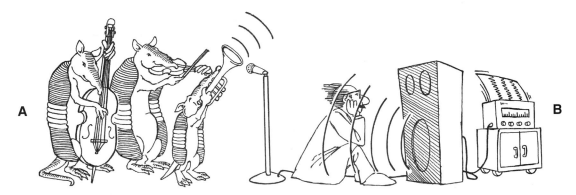

Figure 15-1   **A,** The tracing of the output of a microphone picking up the performance of ensemble. The instruments in the ensemble produce a combined sound that is recorded as a single signal. **B,** A listener enjoys the performance of the ensemble and hears each instrument individually. This is because of the human auditory system's ability to perform a real-time frequency analysis.

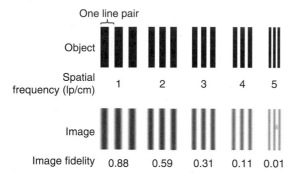

Figure 15-2 The fidelity of the image of a bar pattern decreases with increasing spatial frequency. This loss of fidelity of a high contrast object results in a low contrast image.

The image obtained from the low-frequency bar pattern more faithfully reproduces the object than that of the high spatial frequency bar pattern. The less faithful reproduction with increasing spatial frequency describes the limitation of spatial resolution of an imaging system and is indicated graphically as a modulation transfer function (MTF).

A graph of the ratio of image-to-object at the spatial frequencies in Figure 15-2 results in the MTF curve of Figure 15-3. For MRI, the MTF is obtained from the FT of an edge or impulse. The 10% MTF value is usually stated as the

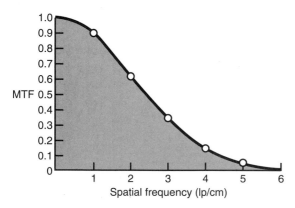

Figure 15-3 Modulation transfer function *(MTF)* is a plot of the image fidelity versus spatial frequency. The five data points plotted here are from the analysis of Figure 15-2.

limiting spatial resolution of an MRI system, and that value depends on matrix size and field of view (FOV). Limiting spatial resolution is approximately 10 lp/cm for head/body images and 20 lp/cm for surface coil imaging.

A *spatial frequency* is a number of cycles in space or per unit distance. Cycles of what? The answer is a bit tricky. In the previous chapter, the complex nature of the magnetic resonance (MR) image was not emphasized, but now it is very important.

A complex number is one that has two dimensions, such as north-south and east-west or azimuth and range. The two dimensions are called the *real part* and the *imaginary part*. These names are unfortunate; there is nothing more or less tangible about one part than the other, at least in the MRI context. This is simply a mathematical convenience.

Complex numbers are important in MRI. For example, as the net magnetization vector precesses in the XY plane, it takes two numbers to specify where it points at any given time. One number gives the X coordinate and the other number gives the Y coordinate. Thus if the X-axis value is assigned to the real part of a complex number and the Y-axis value to the imaginary part of a complex number, the position of the net magnetization vector can be represented by a single complex number.

Two coordinate systems are commonly taught in geometry. One is the Cartesian coordinate system, in which a point in a plane is represented by its X and Y coordinates. The other system is polar coordinates, in which a point is represented by its distance from the origin and the angle that the line connecting it to the origin makes with the X-axis (Figure 15-4). Polar coordinates fit MRI naturally.

When the net magnetization vector precesses in the XY plane, its length is essentially constant when compared with its rotation (change in angular orientation) in the XY plane. If polar coordinates are used to describe the position of the net magnetization vector in the XY plane, the length of the vector is constant but the angle changes as the vector pre-

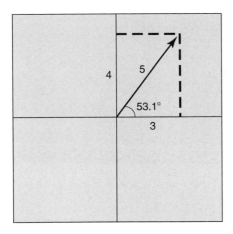

Figure 15-4   A net magnetization vector in the XY plane, as represented in polar coordinates.

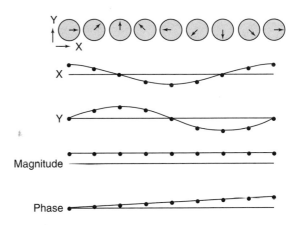

Figure 15-5   The XY plane component of the net magnetization vector of each voxel is plotted. The orientation of the net magnetization vector describes a spiral in space. The pitch of the spiral is proportional to the spatial frequency.

cesses. Temporal frequency is measured in cycles per second (hertz [Hz]). One cycle equals 360°.

It is relatively easy to imagine the net magnetization vector rotating as a function of time as it precesses. If the net magnetization vectors positioned along the patient have different angles, that represents a spatial frequency (Figure 15-5).

Any object can be viewed as a weighted sum of spatial frequencies. There are mathematical conditions under which this statement is not true, but any patient who met those conditions would have an acute need for treatment far in excess of an MRI.

A few examples of real and imaginary FT pairs are shown in Figure 15-6. The important thing to notice about these examples is that if the spatial frequencies in an object can be measured, the object can be described. In a formal sense, that is usually done by the FT.

During imaging, each MR signal is Fourier transformed to fill a single line of k-space (Figure 15-7). High amplitude phase-encoding gradients fill the periphery of k-space and contribute to spatial resolution. Low amplitude phase-encoding gradients fill the center of k-space and contribute to contrast resolution.

The low amplitude phase-encoding gradients result in high intensity MR signals. The zero phase-encoding gradient that fills the central line of k-space produces the highest intensity signal line of k-space.

When k-space is filled, there exists a matrix array of cells, each containing a real and an imaginary number. These two number arrays result in the magnitude and phase maps present before the second FT.

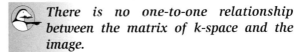

There is no one-to-one relationship between the matrix of k-space and the image.

Each matrix cell in k-space contains information about image pixels. Also, each image pixel contains information obtained from each matrix cell.

THE FOURIER TRANSFORM

The FT is a mathematical method for analyzing the frequency content of something. In the current discussion, it applies to the spatial frequency content of a patient.

The inverse FT analyzes the set of spatial frequency values given to it and indicates the

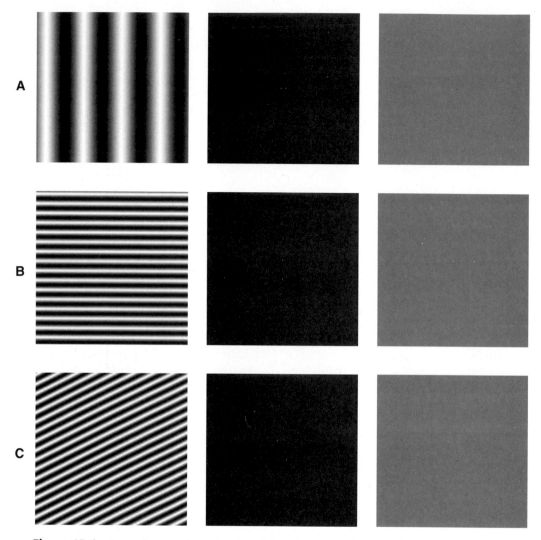

Figure 15-6 Several examples of real and imaginary Fourier transform pairs. **A,** 8 horizontal cycles. **B,** 16 vertical cycles. **C,** 16 cycles + 18° phase shift. (Courtesy Bud Wendt, Houston, TX.)

object corresponding to those frequencies. Technically, the inverse FT is used to reconstruct an MR image; that is, to convert the spatial frequency information measured by the imaging system into an image.

The FT converts a time-varying signal into its frequency components. Figure 15-8 shows this relationship for several functions important to MRI. Note the two lower functions. The FT of a rectangular function is an oscillating

frequency spectrum called a *sinc function.* The FT of a sinc function is a band of frequencies of equal intensity.

This sinc function is of particular importance to MRI because its FT is rectangular, as in a rectangular slice. Most MRI radiofrequency (RF) pulses are sinc functions for this reason. That is why the RF_t shape in Figure 15-9 is used throughout this text.

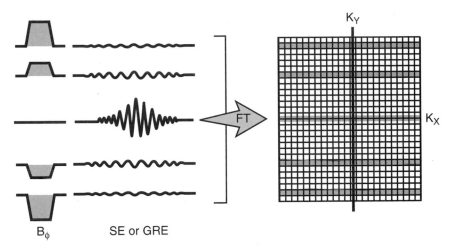

Figure 15-7   During spin echo *(SE)* magnetic resonance imaging, each SE is sampled and Fourier transformed to fill one line in k-space. *FT,* Fourier transform; *GRE,* gradient echo.

The FT (sometimes called the *forward transform* to distinguish it from the inverse transform) is involved mathematically but is simple conceptually. The FT compares the object with a set of test functions and reports how similar the object is to each test function. When combined, the test functions are defined by the FT and have the property that they can completely describe all possible objects.

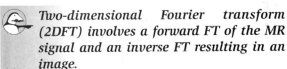

Figure 15-8   When the signal or mathematical function on the left is Fourier transformed, the result is to the right. The Fourier transform *(FT)* of the right is the inverse Fourier transform (FT^{-1}) and results in the function to the left.

The purpose of the comparison is to determine the exact details of the combination. Each of the test functions represents a different spatial frequency. The two parameters determined by the comparison are the magnitude, that is, how much of that spatial frequency is contained in the object and the phase or what is the starting angle for that spatial frequency.

Two-dimensional Fourier transform (2DFT) involves a forward FT of the MR signal and an inverse FT resulting in an image.

The inverse transform takes the magnitude and phase information for each spatial frequency

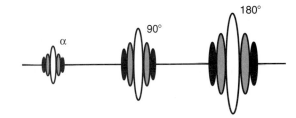

Figure 15-9   The magnetic resonance imaging broadband sinc pulse is symbolized as shown for the three types of RF_t.

and by knowing what the appearance of the test function associated with those data looks like, reconstructs the object. Because the MRI raw data are the magnitudes and phases of the spatial frequencies, the inverse FT is used to reconstruct the image.

IMPACT OF SPATIAL FREQUENCIES

Spatial Resolution

The basic rule of thumb is that higher spatial frequencies result in better spatial resolution. Thus if a sharp, crisp image is desired, it is necessary to measure not only the low spatial frequencies but high spatial frequencies as well. For example, if two objects separated by 1 mm need to be resolved, a resolution of 1 line pair per millimeter (lp/mm) is necessary. This implies that the spatial frequencies must be measured to at least 1 cycle/mm.

Figure 15-10 illustrates the same image measured with different numbers of spatial frequencies. The importance of the higher spatial frequencies to spatial resolution is obvious. The way to improve the spatial resolution is not to increase the density of the measure-

ments of spatial frequency, but rather, to measure higher spatial frequencies.

Field of View

Generally, FOV is an operator-defined parameter that controls the apparent size of the patient in the image. The matrix size is the operator-defined parameter that, with the FOV, controls the pixel size in the image.

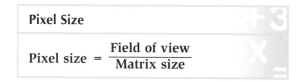

Pixel Size
$$\text{Pixel size} = \frac{\text{Field of view}}{\text{Matrix size}}$$

The pixel size is the dimension of the FOV divided by the number of points in the acquisition matrix in that direction. It takes two pixels to define a line pair, so the resolution is one line pair per the width of two pixels, and the highest spatial frequency is one cycle per width of two pixels.

Question: A 256 (wide) × 128 (high) acquisition matrix has a 25.6-cm FOV. What is the spatial resolution and maximum spatial frequency in each direction?

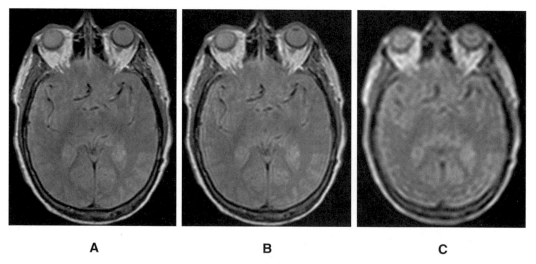

A   **B**   **C**

Figure 15-10   256, 128, and 64 phase-encoding step acquisitions of a transverse image of the head.

Answer: Horizontally, each pixel is 256 mm/256 pixels = 1 mm wide. Thus there is 1 line pair per 2 mm or 0.5 lp/mm horizontal resolution, and the maximum unaliased spatial frequency is 0.5 cycle/mm. Vertically, each pixel is 256 mm/128 pixels = 2 mm high. Thus there is 1 line pair per 4 mm or 0.25 lp/mm vertical resolution, and the maximum unaliased spatial frequency is 0.25 cycle/mm.

The image in the this example may be interpolated to a 256 × 256 matrix for viewing, but that does not alter the actual resolution, which is determined by the data acquisition.

Signal-to-Noise Ratio

The signal-to-noise ratio (SNR) is a comparison of the intensity of the information (signal) in the image to the intensity of the noise in the image. Most images have more signal strength at low spatial frequencies and less signal strength at high spatial frequencies. Most noise is uniformly distributed in spatial frequency. Thus, if SNR is considered as a function of spatial frequency, it is much better at low spatial frequencies than at high spatial frequencies (Figure 15-11).

 High SNR improves image contrast and contrast resolution.

This is not to say that high spatial frequencies are unimportant visually. Sometimes small structures and fine detail are the reasons to acquire the image. Often mathematical importance and clinical importance are two separate issues. It should be kept in mind, however, that the higher spatial frequencies are typically more noisy, and thus improving the spatial

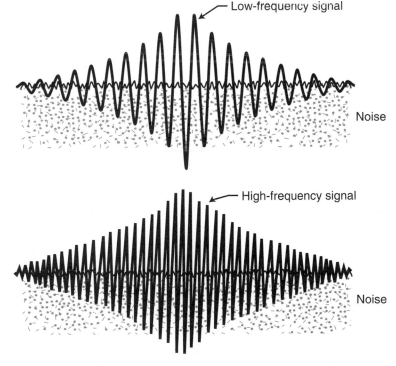

Figure 15-11 Signal-to-noise ratio is usually higher with low-frequency signals.

resolution of the image results in a noisier looking image.

Usually the radiologist makes the determination of the relative importance of resolution and SNR for each protocol. Some types of images have more inherent SNR than others, therefore allowing more flexibility in trading off spatial resolution and noise.

 Narrow receiver bandwidth results in better SNR.

The term *bandwidth* refers to the range of frequencies contained in an RF pulse. There are two RF bandwidths of importance to MRI: transmitted (RF_t) and received (RF_s). The RF_t is involved in slice thickness and image weighting and does refer to a range of frequencies.

Receiver bandwidth is principally involved with SNR and FOV. The receiver bandwidth refers to the sampling rate of the MR signal (RF_s).

The SNR is higher with narrow bandwidth than wide bandwidth. This is because noise is nearly uniform regardless of frequency and is therefore called *white noise* (Figure 15-12). A signal with narrow bandwidth contains relatively less noise than a signal with wide bandwidth.

At a fixed gradient magnetic field, receiver bandwidth determines FOV. If the read gradient magnetic field (B_R) is constant, a narrow bandwidth will result in a proportionally reduced FOV and a proportionally reduced pixel size. For a fixed FOV the read gradient magnetic field is lower, the receiver bandwidth is lower, and the resulting SNR is higher (Figure 15-13).

Contrast

Contrast is a property of the spatial domain. For example, two pixels, one of which has twice the brightness of the other, have contrast ratio of 2:1. If the pixels are far apart, they represent a low spatial frequency. If they are adjacent, they represent a high spatial frequency.

Thus the relationship between contrast and spatial frequency depends on the particular image. However, most of the amplitude in k-space is concentrated in the low spatial frequencies for most typical clinical imaging situations (with MR angiography being one notable exception), and thus the contrast in an image lies in the low spatial frequencies.

Artifacts

MRI artifacts result from a variety of characteristics of the imaging system and the imaging process (see Chapter 27). However, there is one example, sometimes called a *spark arti-*

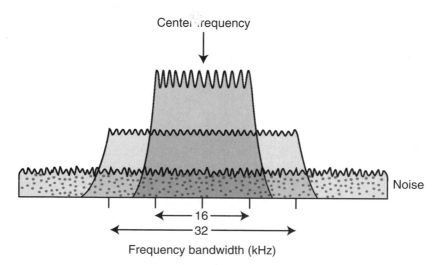

Figure 15-12 Narrow receiver bandwidth results in higher signal-to-noise ratio.

fact, that actually helps to illustrate the points of this chapter. The spark artifact is a spike of noise, perhaps from the discharge of a static buildup in the imaging system, which appears as an isolated bright spot in k-space because it was a momentary occurrence during the sampling of the spatial frequency domain. This bright spot will be treated as normal data by the reconstruction algorithm, resulting in a striped pattern (Figure 15-14).

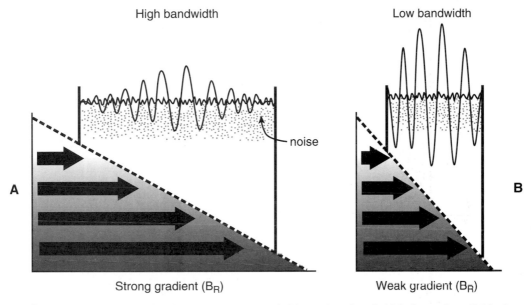

Figure 15-13   **A,** At a fixed gradient magnetic field, receiver bandwidth determines field of view (FOV). **B,** At a fixed FOV, signal-to-noise ratio improves with lower receiver bandwidth.

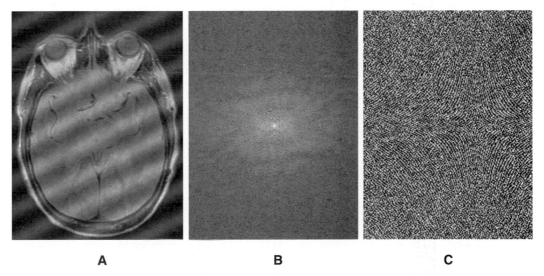

Figure 15-14   Inverse transform of a normal image contaminated with a hot spot. **A,** Image. **B,** Magnitude of Fourier transform (FT). **C,** Phase of FT.

Question: The FOV of the image in Figure 15-14 is 20 cm. What are the horizontal and vertical spatial frequencies of the spark artifact?

Answer: Count the number of cycles of the artifact horizontally and vertically and divide by the FOV to get the spatial frequencies of K_X and K_Y. This is a magnitude image, and therefore there is not enough information to know whether the spatial frequencies are positive or negative.

SPATIAL FREQUENCY PATTERNS AND ORDER

The spatial frequency domain representation of any given object exists. A variety of strategies have been developed for measuring it. The sampling concepts mentioned in Chapter 14 apply here. It is necessary to make measurements of the spatial frequency information sufficiently close together so that there are no surprises.

The easiest way to do this is with the rectangular raster image (Figure 15-15). This method is used for standard (2DFT) imaging (see Chapter 16).

The measurement points are uniformly distributed in k-space. The trajectory in k-space is sometimes used to describe the locations of the measurements in the spatial frequency domain because each sample point is measured at a slightly different time. The location of each measurement is controlled by the gradient magnetic fields.

A slightly different path through k-space is used by the blipped echo planar imaging technique. Instead of scanning every line from left to right as in 2DFT, blipped echo planar alternates the direction of the line scanning so that the pattern is a squared-off zigzag.

Projection reconstruction imaging was the first method of MRI and is still used in a few special applications, typically those requiring extremely short echo times. The sampling scheme for projection reconstruction is shown in Figure 15-16.

The density of measurements in projection reconstruction is greater in the center of the spatial frequency domain, that is, at the lowest spatial frequencies. This is the reason filtering is used in the back projection method of reconstructing these data. It compensates for the higher density of samples at low spatial fre-

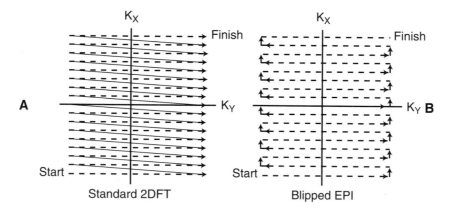

Figure 15-15   A, Diagram of the path through k-space taken by two-dimensional Fourier transform *(2DFT)* imaging. The bottom row of the spatial frequencies is sampled left-to-right, the next row is sampled left-to-right, and so on until all of the rows of k-space have been filled. **B,** A similar diagram for the blipped echo planar imaging *(EPI)* method. Note the direction of sampling alternates left-to-right then right-to-left, thereby eliminating the need to jump back to the left edge for sampling of each row.

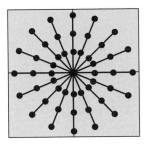

Figure 15-16 The projection reconstruction measurements of spatial frequencies. The measurements are along diameters of a circle. The scan lines pass through the origin and are equally spaced in angle.

quencies by attenuating the low spatial frequencies so that the effective density is uniform.

Another method of reconstructing projection data is to resample the spatial frequency measurements onto a rectangular grid. They look like 2DFT data and can be reconstructed by an inverse FT.

There are a number of relatively exotic methods of sampling k-space. These include spiral scanning, square spiral scanning, and interleaved spiral scanning (Figure 15-17). In general, these data are resampled onto a rectangular grid and then reconstructed with the inverse FT. The actual reconstruction algorithms are complicated because of a variety of technical factors including correcting for residual inhomogeneities of the magnetic field.

The order in which the spatial frequencies are sampled is a parameter over which the operator has some control in many MRI system software releases. Ordinarily, k-space is sampled from bottom to top (see Figure 15-15). There is a class of MR data acquisition protocols, however, in which the relative contrast among organs changes during the data acquisition. In these images, it is usual to sample from the middle of k-space outward. This is based on the premise that the low spatial frequencies contain most of the contrast information and should be measured early while the contrast among organs is greatest.

Another type of protocol is referred to as *segmented k-space*. Only a portion of k-space is sampled in each of several acquisitions that are then combined into a complete measurement of k-space. The idea of this approach is to sample as many rows of k-space as time permits, for example, the end-systolic period of the cardiac cycle, and then to measure some more rows of spatial frequency the next time conditions are appropriate.

This chapter has covered only the basics of sampling the k-space. Researchers are discovering more imaginative and productive ways of sampling k-space information in the imaging slice or volume. Chapter 16 discusses the way MRI actually measures spatial frequency.

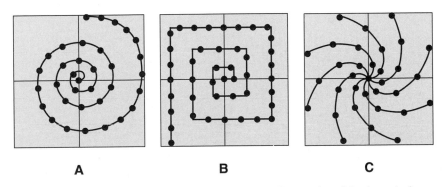

A   **B**   **C**

Figure 15-17 Diagrams of the spatial frequency sampling paths of **A,** the spiral sampling method; **B,** the square spiral sampling method; and **C,** the interleaved spiral sampling method.

CHALLENGE QUESTIONS

1. What is the measure of spatial frequency in MRI?
2. MR image data are stored mathematically in something called *k-space*. Explain another term in which it is described.
3. What is the approximate limiting spatial resolution expressed in spatial frequency for an MRI system?
4. What is meant by trajectory through k-space?
5. A picture of k-space shows 256 lines. What does that tell you about the image and the imaging process?
6. As a general rule, when comparing a 256 matrix image with a 512 matrix image, what can be said regarding spatial resolution and contrast resolution?
7. Which region of k-space, if any, is most important to the final image?
8. Because k-space is filled digitally, what is the relationship between one pixel of k-space and one pixel of the image?
9. Describe the relationship of signal and of noise across a range of spatial frequencies in MRI.
10. How does a receiver bandwidth affect SNR and therefore contrast resolution?

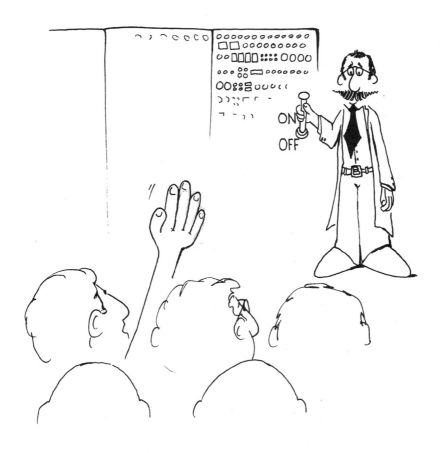

Chapter 16

The Musical Score

OBJECTIVES

At the completion of this chapter, the student should be able to do the following:

1. Identify the five lines of a magnetic resonance imaging (MRI) pulse sequence.
2. Recognize the various symbols used to diagram an MRI pulse sequence.
3. Describe how a slice is selected for imaging.
4. Describe how a pixel is located within a slice
5. Relate two ways that slice thickness can be changed.
6. Draw the MRI pulse sequence diagrams for partial saturation, inversion recovery, and spin echo.

OUTLINE

THE PURPOSE OF THE PULSE SEQUENCES
GRADIENT COIL FUNCTION
SLICE SELECTION
PIXEL LOCATION WITHIN A SLICE
THE EFFECT OF A GRADIENT ON PRECESSION
    Phase-Encoding
    Frequency-Encoding

PULSE SEQUENCE DIAGRAMS
    Partial Saturation
    Inversion Recovery
    Spin Echo

The magnetic resonance imaging (MRI) system operates like a player piano. The control program for the MRI system is a **pulse sequence.** The pulse sequence diagram is a complicated schematic containing graphs that show what each major component of the MRI system should be doing at each moment.

The pulse sequence diagram is analogous to the musical score used by a conductor to lead an orchestra. Just as each instrument follows its own line of music in the conductor's score, each component of the MRI system (i.e., the transmitted radiofrequency [RF_t], the received MRI signal [RF_s], and the three gradient magnetic fields coils, B_{SS}, B_Φ, B_R) has its own row of timing information in the pulse sequence diagram.

Fortunately, routine imaging uses preprogrammed pulse sequences, so the MRI technologist needs only to select a programmed technique.

THE PURPOSE OF THE PULSE SEQUENCES

After the preceding discussions of the physics of MRI and the necessary equipment for MRI, discussion can turn to how magnetic resonance (MR) signals (RF_s) make an image and what characterizes the image.

In MRI, a pulse sequence is a set of instructions given to the imaging system to tell it how to make an image. In radiography, instructions are given to the x-ray imaging system by setting the kilovolt peak (kVp) and the milliampere-second (mAs). The manner in which these controls, especially the kilovolt peak control, are positioned influences the contrast of the resulting image.

In x-ray imaging, the relative order of the gray scale remains unchanged. Regardless of the kVp, bone always appears brighter than soft tissue. However, with MRI, the relative brightness of different tissues and the contrast rendition can be reversed by changing the timing and magnitude of the radiofrequency (RF) pulses (Figure 16-1).

 The MRI pulse sequence diagram details the timing pattern for the RF pulses and gradient magnetic fields.

In computed tomography (CT), the image time, slice thickness, kVp, field of view, matrix size, and the reconstruction algorithm are selected by the technologist. These choices influence the contrast and spatial resolution of the image.

MRI pulse sequences are analogous to the radiographic and CT selections made by the technologist. The pulse sequences specify the timing and magnitude of the RF pulses and the gradient magnetic fields. The amplitude and timing of the RF pulses affect the image contrast. The pulsed gradient magnetic fields provide spatial localization and influence the spatial resolution of the image.

As in CT, the MR image is formed digitally. In conventional radiography, the image is analog. The MR image is a mosaic of pixels. Each pixel has two properties: character and position. *Character* refers to the intensity of the pixel.

In a CT image, shades of gray are assigned on the basis of Hounsfield units (HU), which relate to x-ray attenuation values (Figure 16-2). White is assigned to pixels with high attenuation values (e.g., bone); black is assigned to pixels with low attenuation values (e.g., air).

In MRI, the gray scale is assigned on the basis of the intensity of the MR signal emitted from a given voxel (Figure 16-2). That intensity, in turn, is dependent on the T1, T2, and proton density (PD) of tissue. White is assigned to pixels with high signal intensity; black is assigned to those with low signal intensity. Subsequent chapters fully discuss pixel character and therefore image contrast. This chapter focuses on spatial localization.

 Gradient magnetic fields provide spatial localization of the MR signal (RF_s).

The intensity of the received MR signal (RF_s) as it is apportioned among the pixels of the image determines its spatial location. A single

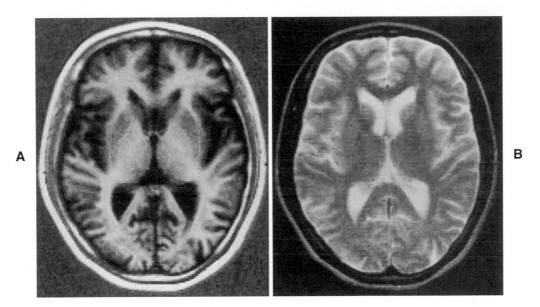

Figure 16-1 These images of the same slice in the same patient illustrate that the timing of radiofrequency pulses not only controls contrast but also can reverse contrast. **A,** A T1 weighted inversion recovery image. **B,** A T2 weighted spin echo image.

signal is emitted from the entire slice after excitation by a slice-selective pulse, (RF_t, B_{SS}).

Even though each voxel has its own net magnetization that produces an MR signal, the signal received by the imaging system (RF_s) combines the signals from each voxel (Figure 16-3). This differs from radiography, which is basically a projection shadowgram.

In most MRI systems, the main magnetic field (B_0) is horizontal and aligned with the bore of the magnet and the longitudinal axis of the patient. This is true for most superconducting and resistive magnets but not for most permanent magnets. In keeping with earlier discussions, a horizontal orientation is assumed for the following discussion.

The Z-axis, which is parallel to B_0, runs through the center of the magnet in the direction of the long axis of the patient. The X- and Y-axes are perpendicular to Z. X is horizontal and Y is vertical (Figure 16-4).

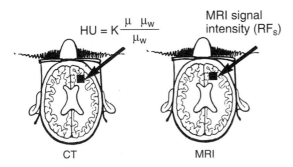

Figure 16-2 Pixel brightness in CT is determined by the x-ray attenuation coefficient, and in MRI, it is determined by T1, T2, and proton density.

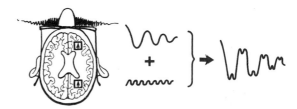

Figure 16-3 During proton relaxation, a complicated magnetic resonance signal is received and computer processed to form an image.

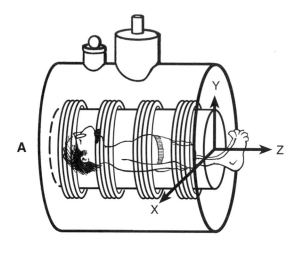

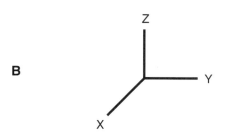

Figure 16-4 **A,** Axis orientation in the gantry. **B,** Axis orientation for vector diagrams.

B_0 is intense and is energized throughout the MRI examination. Vendors go to great lengths to ensure that this B_0 field is not only intense, but also uniform throughout the imaging volume. Purposefully, the vendors also provide a means of disturbing the field homogeneity systematically and orderly.

This disturbance of field homogeneity is achieved through the use of paired gradient coils. These paired gradient coils are the key features distinguishing an MRI system from a nuclear magnetic resonance (NMR) spectrometer (see Chapter 12).

The gradient coils produce weak magnetic fields superimposed on the B_0 field. These gradient coils are intermittently pulsed for milliseconds each time. Each pair of coils produces a small gradient magnetic field along one of the axes.

These small gradient magnetic fields are either parallel or perpendicular to B_0. Because the gradient magnetic field varies in intensity along the direction of the axis of the gradient coils, the combined magnetic field is stronger at one end of an axis than at the other.

GRADIENT COIL FUNCTION

The purpose of the gradient magnetic field is twofold: slice selection and pixel localization within the slice. The gradient coils identify which part of the signal belongs in each pixel.

The Larmor equation ($f = \gamma B$) states that hydrogen nuclei in a magnetic field precess at a frequency (f) that depends on the strength of the magnetic field (B). The constant γ is characteristic of a given nuclear species. For hydrogen, the constant equals 42 MHz/T. If the magnetic field is not homogeneous, protons in a slightly stronger field precess faster than those in a weaker magnetic field (Figure 16-5).

For protons to be excited in an area with a stronger magnetic field, a higher frequency, RF_t, is required to match the resonance frequency of those protons. The combination of the magnetic field inhomogeneity produced by the gradient coils and the excitation by a specific RF frequency permits slice selection.

During relaxation, the frequencies of the signals from the protons also depend on the magnetic field strength at the location of each excited proton. When the RF_t is turned off and the excited protons relax back to equilibrium, the free induction decay (FID) at the strong end of a gradient magnetic field has higher frequencies than the FID at the weak end of the field. Consequently, the presence of a gradient magnetic field during signal reception helps localize the protons within the slice that was selected during excitation.

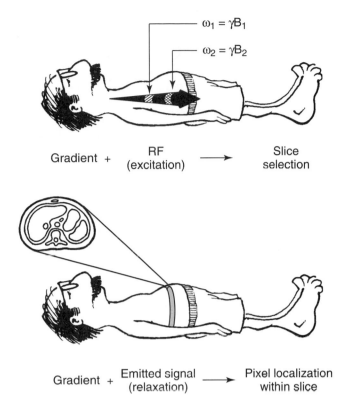

Figure 16-5 Gradient magnetic fields cause slight differences in proton resonant frequencies, which can be used for selective excitation of a slice and for localization of protons in that slice.

SLICE SELECTION

If the Z gradient coils are on, the magnetic field intensity varies linearly from one end of the patient to the other (Figure 16-6). At one end of the magnet, the magnetic field is stronger than at the other end. The proton precessional frequency for a 1-T magnet is 42 MHz. A proton at the strong end may precess at 43 MHz, whereas one at the weak end may precess at 41 MHz.

An RF pulse of exactly 42.7 MHz excites all of the protons in the plane perpendicular to the Z-axis at the 42-MHz position along the gradient magnetic field. At all other points along the gradient magnetic field, the protons remain unaffected by the 42-MHz RF pulse because they do not resonate at that frequency. They

are insensitive to it. In this way, the Z gradient performs slice selection (G_{SS}), and a single transverse slice is selectively excited.

If a gradient along the X-axis were used instead of the Z gradient, the slice selected would be in a sagittal plane. Similarly, a Y gradient would select a coronal plane. In fact, with the X, Y, and Z gradients turned on together, any plane in the body may be chosen (Figure 16-6). All subsequent discussions assume transverse slice selection; however, the principles apply to slices in any orientation.

The steepness, or slope, of the gradient magnetic field and the range of frequencies, or bandwidth, of the RF pulse determine the thickness of the selected slice. The steeper the gradient magnetic field, the thinner the slice.

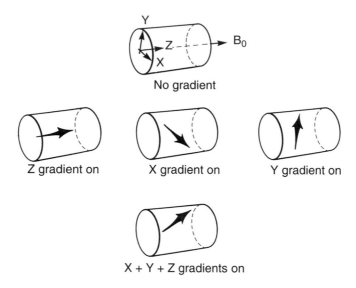

Figure 16-6 Selective excitation along the Z-axis results in a transverse plane. Excitation along the X and Y axes results in parasagittal and paracoronal planes, respectively. When the three gradients are energized at the same time, any oblique plane can be selected.

The narrower the bandwidth of the RF pulse, the thinner the slice.

The purity of an RF pulse is identified by its quality value (Q). The Q of a pulse is the center frequency divided by the bandwidth. As bandwidth becomes more narrow, the Q of an RF pulse becomes higher.

Quality Value
$Q = \dfrac{f}{\Delta f}$

Bandwidth is the range of frequencies contained within the RF pulse (RF_t). This is different from the receiver bandwidth, which was discussed in Chapter 15. If a pure 42-MHz pulse could be produced, it would have a Q of infinity. However, this would result in an infinitely thin slice, so the MR signal would be weak and noisy.

Question: Suppose a 42-MHz RF pulse contained frequencies ranging from 41.4 to 42.6 MHz. What is the Q of that RF pulse?

Answer: The frequency bandwidth is 42.6 − 41.4 = 1.2 MHz.

The Q Value $= \dfrac{42}{1.2} = 35$

In the presence of a fixed Z gradient magnetic field, slice thickness can be selected by changing the bandwidth of the excitation RF pulse (Figure 16-7). Alternately, slice thickness can be selected by changing the intensity of the gradient magnetic field in the presence of a constant Q RF excitation pulse (Figure 16-8).

Gradient magnetic field intensity ranges from approximately 10 mT/m to 40 mT/m. The difference is due to the power supply that drives the direct current through the gradient coils. The steeper the applied gradient magnetic field, the thinner the imaged slice.

Usually the frequency width of the RF excitation pulse is fixed for a range of slice thicknesses (e.g., 1 to 10 mm), and the strength of the slice selection gradient magnetic field, B_{SS},

42 ± 0.5 MHz

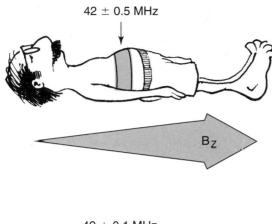

42 ± 0.1 MHz

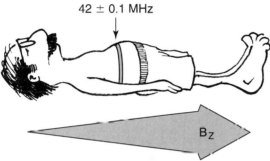

Figure 16-7 In the presence of a fixed Z gradient magnetic field, reducing the radiofrequency (RF) bandwidth increases the RF Q value, which results in thinner image slices.

is adjusted to fine-tune the slice thickness within the range allowed by the particular RF excitation pulse.

PIXEL LOCATION WITHIN A SLICE

Perhaps the most difficult concept to grasp in MRI is how to determine the location of each pixel within a slice. This is because the MR data are acquired in the spatial frequency domain, k-space, whereas radiologists visualize the patient in the spatial domain or pixel position (see Chapter 15).

MRI does not measure spatial location directly like most medical imaging modalities. Instead, it measures spatial frequency content directly. Spatial location must be determined

by analyzing the spatial frequencies during the image reconstruction process.

 Pixel location is determined by the inverse Fourier transform of k-space.

The spatial frequencies of the FIDs from the two highlighted voxels shown in Figure 16-9 have the same frequency but different amplitudes. The frequencies are the same because the voxels are in a uniform magnetic field. A gradient magnetic field is not present. The higher amplitude signal occurs because of either a higher PD or a different relaxation time (T1 or T2).

When a gradient magnetic field is energized during relaxation, pixels can be localized by their characteristic frequency along the X-axis (Figure 16-10). In the same way, columns are localized within a slice by energizing a frequency-encoding gradient (Figure 16-11).

The frequency-encoding gradient magnetic field or read gradient (B_R) is energized during signal reception.

This discussion concentrates on the two-dimensional Fourier transform (2DFT) imaging technique, which is the predominantly used method in clinical MRI. In 2DFT imaging, k-space is sampled more quickly, much as a television picture is displayed line by line on the television tube.

Similarly, the phase-encoding gradient magnetic field (B_Φ) localizes pixels into rows (Figure 16-12). The phase-encoding gradient controls which horizontal line of k-space is to be sampled; the frequency-encoding gradient accomplishes the actual sampling across the line of data.

THE EFFECT OF A GRADIENT ON PRECESSION

In the discussion regarding how protons precess in the presence of a magnetic field, the effect of the static magnetic field (B_0) is ignored. This viewpoint is called the *rotating frame of reference* (see Chapter 3).

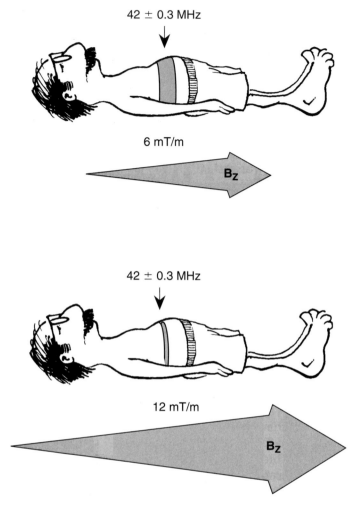

Figure 16-8 For a given radiofrequency pulse, slice thickness is thinner with stronger gradient magnetic fields.

In the rotating frame of reference, all protons are stationary unless in a magnetic field that is stronger or weaker than B_0, such as a gradient magnetic field. If protons are in a field stronger than B_0, they precess at a higher frequency. If the protons are in a field weaker than B_0, they precess with lower frequency (Figure 16-13).

Consider the evolution of the net magnetization vectors of the voxels along the direction of the gradient magnetic field. The voxels on

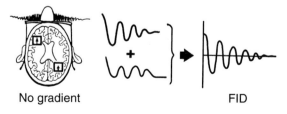

Figure 16-9 Without a gradient magnetic field present, signal frequency from all voxels is the same and spatial localization of the signal is impossible.

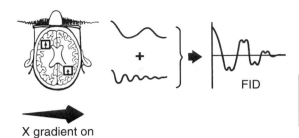

X gradient on

Figure 16-10 With the X gradient magnetic field energized during relaxation while receiving a free induction decay *(FID)*, frequency differences make pixel location by column possible.

the positive end of the gradient precess counterclockwise; voxels on the negative end of the gradient precess clockwise. Voxels further from the center of the gradient precess faster. Each point along the gradient has a unique precessional frequency.

Phase-Encoding

What happens to the net magnetization vectors of each voxel if a gradient magnetic field is applied for only a short time—a pulse? Before the application of the gradient, all magnetization vectors precess in phase at the same frequency (Figure 16-14).

During the application of the pulsed gradient magnetic field, the net magnetization vector of each voxel precesses with a frequency determined by its position along the gradient. When the pulsed gradient is turned off, all magnetization vectors return to pre-

cessing at the same frequency. The effect of the pulsed gradient is still present in the form of a difference in phase for each net magnetization vector.

 The phase-encoding gradient magnetic field, B_Φ, is energized as a pulse before signal reception.

The phase shift in the voxels changes as a result of their position. This is a spatial frequency. The originators of the 2DFT method, William Edelstein and James Hutchinson, called it the **spin warp** method because the phases of the net magnetization vectors twist along the direction of the gradient, just as a warped piece of lumber twists along its length.

An object can be viewed as a sum of objects, each of which has a single spatial frequency (Chapters 14 and 15). When one of these frequencies is phase-encoded, the twist or warp, from the phase-encoding is added to the twist inherent in that spatial frequency.

If the original twist equals and opposes the phase-encoding twist, then the resulting object is straight as if the warped board was ironed flat. If the original twist and the twist from phase-encoding are not equal and opposite, the resulting object is twisted even more.

Remember that the MR signal is a bulk signal from the excited spins in the sensitive volume of the receiver coil (Chapter 5). The signal from each voxel adds vectorially to produce a single signal for the entire excited slice.

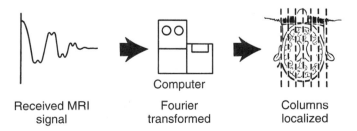

Received MRI signal

Computer Fourier transformed

Columns localized

Figure 16-11 The free induction decay received while the X gradient magnetic field is energized is Fourier transformed to provide information about the column of origin of the signal contribution.

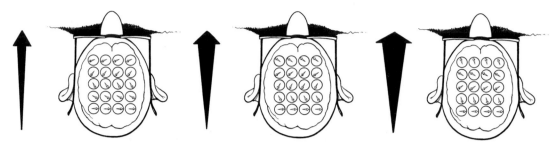

Figure 16-12 As the Y gradient magnetic field increases in intensity, the phase shift between adjacent rows also increases.

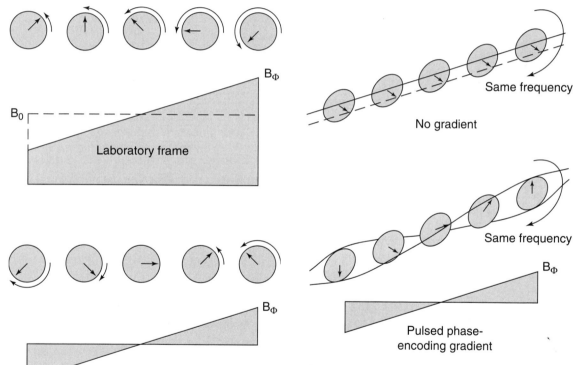

Figure 16-13 Proton spins precess with increasing frequency in the presence of a gradient magnetic field in the laboratory frame representation. Such spins precess with either positive or negative frequency from the average in the rotating frame representation.

Figure 16-14 Each spin system precesses at the same frequency but with different phase after a pulsed phase-encoding gradient.

This signal has profound implications for imaging. If an object has a phase twist in it, the phase shifts of the voxels are different. When the phase shifts are added vectorially, the result is essentially nil. However, if a twist is not present, then the vector sum of the signals from each voxel reinforce each other, resulting in a signal of significant amplitude.

Ordinarily, the only spatial frequency observed is the zero-frequency component because it does not have an inherent phase twist. When phase-encoding is applied, the spatial frequency with no net twist and therefore no signal cancellation is controlled by the phase-encoding gradient pulse.

 The duration of the phase-encoding gradient pulse is fixed, and the amplitude is varied.

A stronger gradient magnetic field pulse makes all of the spins precess proportionately faster. In a fixed amount of time, more twist per unit distance along the direction of the gradient is produced.

For a particular spatial frequency with the phase-encoding gradient pulse to be measured, its amplitude is chosen so that the desired spatial frequency is exactly untwisted. In actual imaging pulse sequences, the phase-encoding gradient pulse is stepped through the spatial frequencies so that they are measured individually. As a result, the resolution in the phase-encoded direction of the image directly relates to the number of measurements made with different phase-encoding values resulting from different intensities of the phase-encoding gradient magnetic field.

Frequency-Encoding

Phase-encoding takes care of one direction within the slice but the slice is two-dimensional. As a result, it is necessary to measure the spatial frequencies in the direction perpendicular to the phase-encoded direction. This is done by applying a gradient magnetic field in the direction within the slice that is perpendicular to the direction of the phase-encoding gradient.

This second gradient is left on while acquiring the MR signal (RF_s) and is called the *read gradient* (B_R). For the following discussion, ignore any previous phase-encoding and consider only the effect of frequency-encoding.

When a gradient magnetic field is first applied, the voxels have net magnetization vectors that are all aligned and also have spatial frequencies with the normal inherent twist per unit distance. As the frequency-encoding gradient is applied, the net magnetization vectors begin to precess faster or slower proportional to their locations along that axis. In other words, the phases of the voxels begin to twist.

Throughout the duration of the frequency-encoding gradient pulse, the amount of twist increases linearly with time. Recall from phase-encoding that applying a phase twist causes a different spatial frequency to be untwisted and measurable.

In the case of the frequency-encoding gradient, the twist is applied continuously, thereby changing the measurable spatial frequency constantly. This means that if the signal throughout the duration of the frequency-encoding gradient pulse is measured, a sampling of all spatial frequencies along the frequency-encoded direction results.

Note that only half of the spatial frequencies are observed because the sweep starts at zero spatial frequency. For the measurement to be started at the edge of the spatial frequency plane rather than in the middle, a pretwist is applied to the object before the actual frequency-encoded measurement is made.

If a gradient pulse of half the duration and opposite amplitude is applied, the phase shifts of the object in the frequency-encoded direction are initialized to the maximum negative spatial frequency, so that the sweep covers both halves of the spatial frequency information.

Phase-encoding selects a particular spatial frequency in one direction within the selected slice—the vertical direction. Frequency-encoding then scans all of the spatial frequencies perpendicular to the phase-encoded direction, horizontally. As a result, all of the horizontal spatial frequencies at a particular vertical spatial frequency have been sampled.

For the entire k-space to be measured, this process is repeated with different amplitudes of the phase-encoding gradient each time. The sweep of horizontal spatial frequencies associated with each row is measured with different vertical spatial frequencies.

 The application of the three gradient magnetic fields—B_{SS} for slice selection, B_{Φ} for phase-encoding, and B_R for frequency-encoding (the read gradient)—provides the spatial localization necessary to identify each voxel.

This process is similar to that used to prepare a potato (Figure 16-15). First the Z gradient is used to select a slice, like slicing a potato to make potato chips (B_{SS}). Next, the phase-encoding gradient is energized momentarily, allowing the columns to be identified within the slice (B_{Φ}). If the potato slice is thick enough, these columns would become french fries. Finally, the frequency-encoding gradient is energized during signal acquisition, which identifies the rows in each column (B_R). For the potato analogy, the result is diced potatoes.

PULSE SEQUENCE DIAGRAMS

This chapter started by suggesting the analogy between the musical score used to conduct an orchestra and the pulse sequence diagrams of the MRI system. Then, for a continuation of the analogy, the piece of music itself was explained. The last section of this chapter discusses some of the different types of pulse sequences (i.e., different musical forms).

Partial Saturation

The simplest pulse sequence is called **partial saturation**. In a diagram of this pulse sequence, the top line indicates when to turn on the RF transmitter, specifying a 90° RF exciting pulse (RF_t). The symbol for this RF pulse, called a *sinc pulse*, is shown in Figure 15-9. The numerical notation above the sinc symbol indicates the magnetization flip angle.

For a single transverse slice excitation the Z gradient magnetic field, B_{SS}, must occur at the same time as the RF_t, and the frequency of the RF_t must be specified. This is indicated by the trapezoid shape in Figure 16-16.

Although the gradient magnetic fields are thought to be turned on and off instantaneously, they are not. Some finite time is required to rise to maximum intensity (i.e., slew rate) and then return to zero again. These rise and fall times result in the trapezoid symbol, rather than, a rectangular shape.

The FID is immediately observed after turning off the RF_T. This is the third line of the musical score, and it is labeled RF_S for the MR signal. The phase-encoding gradient is briefly pulsed at the beginning of the FID. This is shown on the fourth line of the musical score as B_{Φ}.

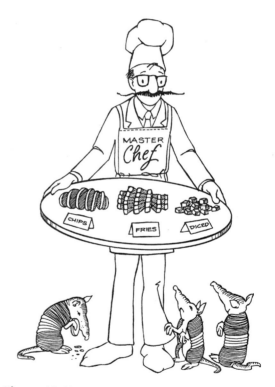

Figure 16-15 Preparing a potato for potato chips, french fries, and diced potatoes is similar to the application of the three gradient magnetic fields.

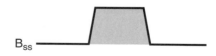

Figure 16-16 A shaded trapezoid is used to symbolize the gradient magnetic fields.

During the signal acquisition, the phase-encoding gradient magnetic field (B_Φ) is turned off, and the frequency-encoding read gradient, (B_R), is turned on. The result is the five-line pulse sequence diagram shown in Figure 16-17.

One signal acquisition samples only one row of k-space. Typically, 256 such acquisitions are needed to make an image. Each time a new signal is acquired, the strength of the phase-encoding gradient changes (Figure 16-18).

Because the only change from one signal acquisition to the next is the intensity of the phase-encoding gradient magnetic field, the phase-encoding gradient is represented as a stepped-pulse envelope (Figure 16-19). This implies a repetitive application of this basic pulse sequence with variation only in the amplitude of the phase-encoding gradient pulse.

 The RF_t pulse sequence for partial saturation imaging is $90°\ldots//\ldots 90°\ldots//\ldots 90°\ldots//\ldots \rightarrow$.

Finally, the time interval between each $90°$ pulse, called the *repetition time* (TR), must be specified. The TR can last for any length of time, and its value typically ranges up 10,000 ms; this time interval substantially influences the character of the pixels and the image contrast. It also has the dominant influence on the overall time required to acquire the image.

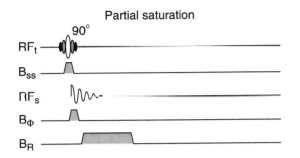

Figure 16-17 The first signal acquisition of a partial saturation pulse sequence.

Imaging Time		
Time = TR × # B_Φ × ACQ where TR = repetition time, # B_Φ = number of phase-encoding steps, and ACQ = number of signals acquired per phase-encoding step		

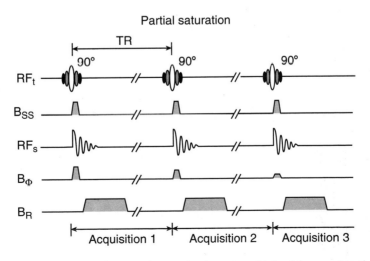

Figure 16-18 Multiple partial saturation projections are obtained by varying the strength of the phase-encoding gradient magnetic field.

Question: How long does it take to make an image, assuming a TR of 2500 ms, 1 signal acquisition per phase-encoded step, and a 256 × 256 matrix?

Answer: Image time per slice = (TR) × (number of signals acquired each phase-encoding step) × (number of phase-encoding steps) = (2500 ms) × 1 × 256 = 640 s or almost 11 minutes

If the resulting image appears too noisy, the whole sequence can be repeated, and both sets of data can be combined to make one image. This procedure is called **signal averaging.**

Image quality can be improved if several acquisitions are combined at the expense of increasing the overall imaging time. The number of signals averaged is symbolized by **ACQ,** for the number of signals acquired, or **NEX,** for the number of excitations, or **NSA,** for the number of signals acquired. If the number of signals acquired in the example above were doubled, the signal-to-noise ratio (SNR) would improve by 41% ($\frac{1}{\sqrt{2}}$ = 1.41), but the examination time would double to nearly 22 minutes.

Signal-to-Noise Ratio

$S = 1, N = 1$ $\therefore$ SNR $= \frac{1}{1} = 1$

$S = 2, N = \sqrt{2}$ $\therefore$ SNR $= \frac{2}{\sqrt{2}} = 1.41$

$S = 4, N = \sqrt{4}$ $\therefore$ SNR $= \frac{4}{\sqrt{4}} = 2$

Question: A given pulse sequence is repeated four times to improve contrast resolution by increasing SNR. How much is SNR improved?

Answer: At the expense of quadrupling examination time, signal(s) is also quadrupled to 4 s. Noise (N) is only doubled $\sqrt{4N} = 2N$.

Therefore SNR $= \frac{4S}{2N} = 2$

For a 10-slice head image, 11 minutes per slice would require nearly 2 hours of imaging time.

Although TR might be shortened to reduce the imaging time, that would alter the contrast in the image. The number of phase-encoding steps could be reduced, but that would reduce the spatial resolution.

It is possible to interleave the acquisition of data from many different slices so that the overall acquisition time equals that of a single slice, a technique called **multislice imaging.** Note that Figure 16-20 shows a significant time between signal acquisitions during which nothing happens.

That dead time during TR can be used to acquire data from other slices. This is similar to a musical round, that is, a song sung by several people who each start and end the same song at different times.

If the TR is 1000 ms and the FID for the first projection is gone after a few milliseconds, there is a long waiting period while the excited protons relax to equilibrium. Interleaved multislice acquisition takes advantage of that time by energizing the RF transmitter with a different frequency to excite a different tissue slice.

This RF pulse does not disturb the first slice because the frequency is inappropriate for the first slice. Because each slice excitation and data measurement only require a few milliseconds, the procedure can be repeated many times before the TR of the first slice is finished

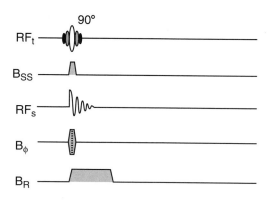

Figure 16-19 The change in intensity of the phase-encoding gradient magnetic field is represented symbolically in a single pulse sequence.

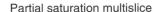

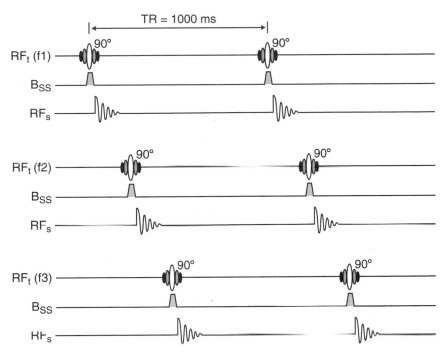

Figure 16-20 Multislice techniques used to reduce total imaging time.

and must be restimulated to acquire the next signal.

Unfortunately, it is impossible to confine the RF excitation to a defined slice. The edges of the slice usually receive less RF energy than the middle of the slice. As a result, protons outside of the effective slice thickness receive a slight exposure to RF excitation.

The significance of this broadened excitation is that when the time comes to excite the adjacent slice, some of the protons have already been excited and are undergoing relaxation. This leads to a degradation of the image contrast.

This problem of slice overlap can be avoided with a nonimaged gap specified between slices. If contiguous slices are needed, the multislice acquisition is specifically designed for maximum time between excita-

tion of adjacent slices, given the constraints of the prescribed TR.

Inversion Recovery

The inversion recovery pulse sequence has inherently long imaging time because TR is long (Figure 16-21). This pulse sequence helps to better understand MRI contrast mechanisms. Inversion recovery is also used in combination with fast imaging techniques, such as STIR and FLAIR (Chapters 21 and 22).

This pulse sequence, as its name implies, inverts the net magnetization vector by applying a 180° RF pulse. This inverting pulse takes the net magnetization vector, which lies parallel to the Z-axis at equilibrium, and rotates the vector so that it points in the opposite direction along the Z-axis. The spin-lattice relaxation

Inversion recovery

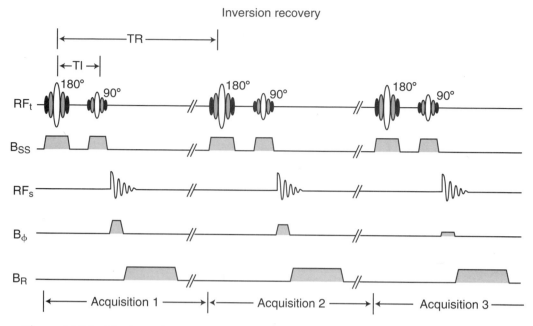

Figure 16-21 The inversion recovery pulse sequence requires a 180°RF pulse followed by a 90° RF pulse.

time (T1) can be determined by timing how long it takes the inverted net magnetization vector to relax to equilibrium (Chapter 7).

To determine T1 after the 180° inverting pulse, apply a 90° pulse after waiting a time interval equal to the inversion time (TI). Because the magnetization parallel to the Z-axis cannot be measured directly, the 90° RF pulse must be used to rotate the Z-axis magnetization (M_Z) to XY magnetization (M_{XY}) so that it can be observed as it creates an FID.

The time interval between the 180° RF pulse and the 90° RF pulse is the TI. As with other time intervals, the duration of the TI interval influences image contrast considerably.

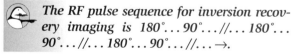

The RF pulse sequence for inversion recovery imaging is 180°...90°...//...180°... 90°...//...180°...90°...//...→.

As with the partial saturation pulse sequence, the Z gradient magnetic field (B_{SS}) must be on during the 180° and 90° RF pulses for proper slice selection. The B_ϕ is pulsed and the B_R is

on while receiving the FID to provide spatial localization within the slice. Although any time interval shorter than TR can be used for TI, typical durations range from 100 to 2000 ms.

Multislice techniques can also be used with the inversion recovery pulse sequence (Figure 16-22). However, the long TI interval severely restricts the number of slices that can be obtained during a TR interval. For example, if the TR is 2500 ms and the TI is 400 ms, only five slices can be interleaved.

For instructional simplification, the pulse sequences were introduced with the assumption that FIDs are collected to make MR images. However, the switching on and off of the gradient magnetic fields and other practical timing considerations make it difficult to acquire a true FID, so an MR signal called a **spin echo** is used instead.

The spin echo is the most common signal echo. In fact, a partial saturation pulse sequence is actually a partial saturation spin echo sequence and differs from the true spin echo sequence only in that the echo time (TE) lasts as

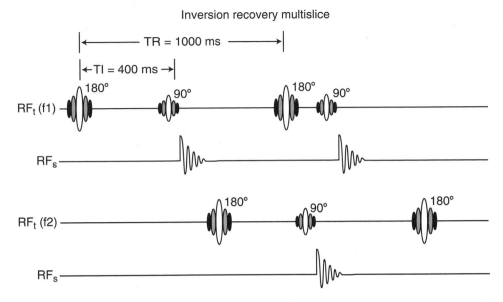

Figure 16-22 Multislice techniques can be used with the inversion recovery pulse sequence; however, the number of slices is limited.

short as possible. Similarly, inversion recovery pulse sequences are actually inversion recovery spin echo sequences with short TE.

The use of the FID as the MR signal in gradient echo (GRE) imaging will be revisited in Chapter 20.

Spin Echo

The spin echo pulse sequence is the most commonly used MRI pulse sequence (Figure 16-23). In spin echo imaging, the proton spins are pretwisted as the first step of frequency-encoding in the 2DFT method. For a spin echo to be obtained, first, a 90° excitation RF pulse is used to flip the magnetization into the XY plane. This is followed by a 180° refocusing RF pulse that flips the vectors about an axis in the XY plane. After time, an echo forms.

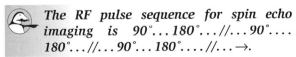 *The RF pulse sequence for spin echo imaging is $90°\dots180°\dots//\dots90°\dots.$ $180°\dots//\dots90°\dots180°\dots.//\dots\rightarrow.$*

For the spin echo pulse sequence and most other pulse sequences, spin echoes are the MR

signals used to make an image. As before, the slice selection gradient magnetic field (B_{SS}) remains on during the 90° excitation RF pulse for slice selection. When the 90° pulse is turned off, an FID is formed but ignored.

After $\frac{1}{2}$TE, a 180° refocusing RF pulse is applied. The slice selection gradient is turned on again during the 180° pulse so that only those protons in the slice of interest are affected. At TE the spin echo forms.

The spin echo forms at TE after the 90° RF pulse. Because the spin echoes are the MR signals acquired to make the image, the read gradient (B_R) must be on during the spin echo to encode spatial localization information.

 The time interval between the 90° RF pulse and the spin echo is the TE.

Once again, the interval from one 90° RF pulse to the next, the TR, must be specified and is important for pixel character. The TE must also be specified because it too is an important determinant of image contrast. TEs range from approximately 2 to 120 ms.

Spin echo

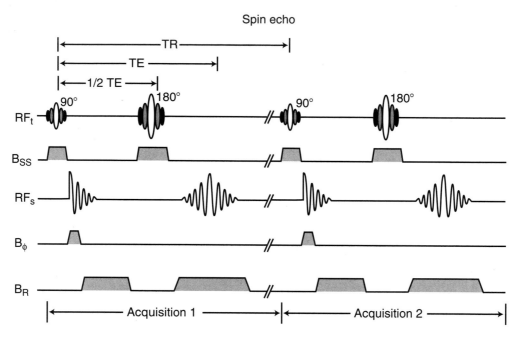

Figure 16-23 The spin echo pulse sequence requires a 90° RF excitation pulse followed by a 180° refocusing RF pulse.

Question: What is the imaging time for a spin echo pulse sequence with TR = 2500 ms, TE = 60 ms, ACQ = 4, and a 256 × 256 image?

Answer: Image time = (TR) × (number of signal acquisitions) × (number of phase-encoding steps)

= 2500 ms × 4 × 256

= 2560 s

= 42 min 40 s

For multislice imaging, the spin echo must be obtained before exciting the next slice (Figure 16-24). If TR equals 1000 ms and TE equals 30 ms, excitation of the next slice can be implemented after about 50 ms; for this situation, a maximum of 20 slices can be excited before returning to the first slice for the second phase-encoding step.

It is often clinically useful to make images with different spin echo times, a technique called **multiecho imaging.** A pulse sequence with TR equal to 2500 ms, TE equal to 30 ms, 256 projections, and 1 signal average takes 10 min, 40 s. It may be useful to have another image made with the same parameters except for making TE equal to 60 ms, which would take an additional 10 min, 40 s.

However, both images can be obtained in one pulse sequence by taking advantage of the echo formed by a second 180° RF refocusing pulse (Figure 16-25). At 15 ms after the 90° RF excitation pulse, a 180° RF refocusing pulse is applied to produce a spin echo with a TE of 30 ms; after an additional 15 ms, another 180° RF refocusing pulse produces a second spin echo with a TE of 60 ms.

The 256 × 30 ms spin echoes are collected to make one image; the 256 × 60 ms spin echoes are collected separately to make another image. This results in two separate images with different image contrast because of the different TEs.

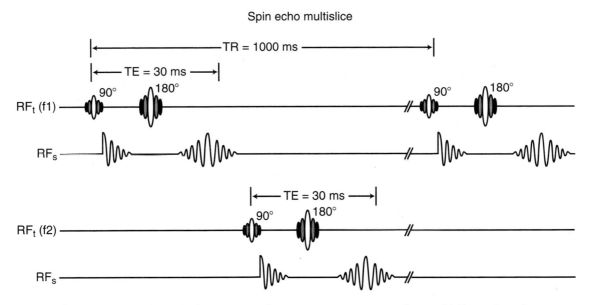

Figure 16-24 The radiofrequency pulse sequences necessary for multislice spin echo imaging.

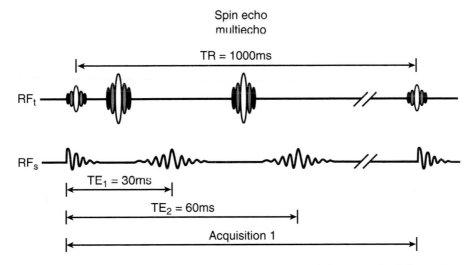

Figure 16-25 Multiecho imaging allows the acquisition of distinctively different images formed at different echo times.

Because both echoes are collected within 60 ms, excitation of another slice can begin at approximately 100 ms; therefore 25 slices can be excited within the 2500-ms TR interval. In this way, it is possible to generate 50 images in the time previously required to make one.

This common imaging technique is called **multislice, multiecho spin echo imaging.** The musical score* is complete (Figure 16-26).

---

*Susan Weathers, MD, is the author of this felicitous metaphor.

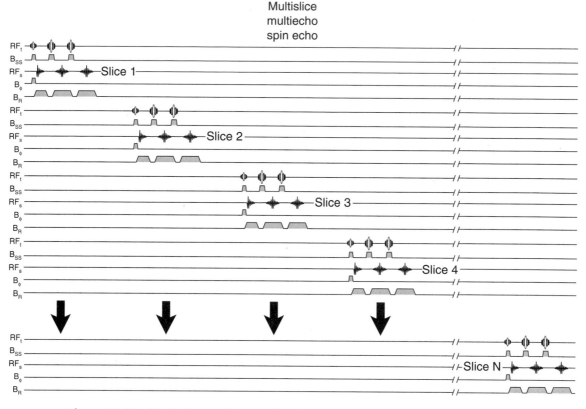

Figure 16-26 Multislice, multiecho spin echo imaging involves an amazing arrangement of radiofrequency and gradient magnetic field pulses.

CHALLENGE QUESTIONS

1. How many lines of information are there in an MRI pulse sequence diagram and what are they?

2. How long does it take to acquire a gradient echo (GRE) image having the following characteristics: TR = 20 ms, TE = 6 ms, number of acquisitions = 2, and the matrix size is 512 × 512?

3. In radiography, kVp controls image contrast. What principally controls contrast in MRI?

4. Diagram the RF pulse sequence for an inversion recovery image and indicate the timing for the appearance of the MR signal.

5. For 2DFT MRI, why are contiguous slices not obtained as in CT?

6. Three signals are acquired and summed to improve SNR. How much improvement will be realized?

7. When is the slice selection gradient coil (G_{SS}) energized?

8. How does the vector diagram appear when an ensemble of spins are partially saturated?

9. For most superconducting MRI systems, the B_0 field is horizontal. For most permanent magnet MRI systems, the B_0 field is vertical. For all MRI vector diagrams, the Z-axis is vertical. What is the relationship between B_0 and the Z-axis?

10. What is the difference between a gradient coil (G_{XYZ}) and a gradient magnetic field (B_{SS}, B_Φ, B_R)?

Chapter 17

Magnetic Resonance Images

OBJECTIVES

At the completion of this chapter, the student should be able to do the following:

1. Describe the features of a visual image.
2. Define representational image and cite three examples.
3. Discuss the pixel character of a magnetic resonance (MR) image.
4. Identify the three principal magnetic resonance imaging (MRI) parameters.
5. Name the primary and secondary MR signals.
6. Relate the approximate spin echo pulse sequences necessary to obtain proton density weighted (PDW), T1 weighted (T1W), and T2 weighted (T2W) images.

OUTLINE

WHAT IS AN IMAGE?

In the most general sense an image is a mental picture. It may be a visual image based on direct observation, such as, the viewing of the Grand Canyon, or an imaginary image, such as the duck elicited by the sound of the oboe in Prokofiev's *Peter and the Wolf*. An image can also be abstract, such as the famous painting by Tanner (Figure 17-1).

Medical images generally fall into the category of visual images; they attempt to represent real objects accurately. A brief discussion of some basic concepts of visual images is helpful in explaining magnetic resonance (MR) images.

Visual Images

All visual images are initially detected by the eye and are the result of stimulation of receptor cells in the retina by electromagnetic radiation in the visible region of the spectrum. The two types of receptor cells are rods and cones. These receptor cells can be considered digital detectors that are stimulated by the input of light photons. They respond to such stimulation with an output of discrete electrical impulses called **action potentials.**

Each retinal receptor is arranged by the optical structure of the eye to be sensitive to light coming from a specific region of the visual field and to characterize the nature of that light as to intensity and color. This initial information about the source and character of light is then relayed through complex visual pathways to the occipital lobe, where the most complex processing and analysis of these data are performed (Figure 17-2).

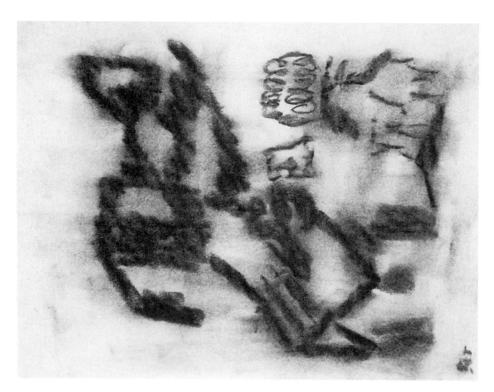

Figure 17-1   This famous painting by Tanner, entitled *Stampede across the Pecos,* is an example of an abstract image. (Courtesy Raymond Tanner, Memphis, TN.)

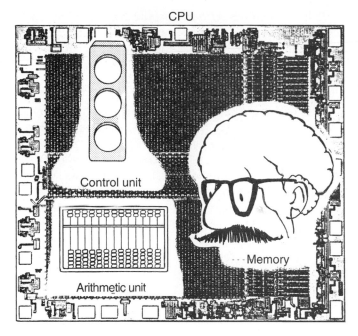

Figure 17-2 Processing and analysis of signals from the visual receptors occur in the occipital lobe. This occurs much like a computer.

In the occipital lobe, the myriad of discrete data concerning light impinging on the retina is reconstructed into the perceived image. Although the final image is often considered to be a continuum of information about light, it is initially detected, processed, and conceived as a high-resolution digital image.

Optical Receptors

When light arrives at the retina, it is detected by the rods and the cones. Rods and cones are small structures; there are more than 100,000 of them per square millimeter of the retina.

The cones are concentrated on the center of the retina in an area called the *fovea centralis.* On the other hand, rods are most numerous on the periphery of the retina. There are no rods at the fovea centralis.

The rods are very sensitive to light and are used in dim-lighting situations. The threshold for rod vision is approximately 10^{-6} ml. However, cones are less sensitive to light; their threshold is only 5×10^{-3} ml, but they can respond to intense light levels, whereas rods cannot. Consequently, cones are used primarily for daylight vision, called *photopic vision,* and rods are used for night vision, called *scotopic vision.*

This aspect of visual physiology explains the reason dim objects are more readily viewed if they are not looked at directly. Astronomers and radiologists are familiar with the fact that a dim object can be seen better if viewed peripherally, in which case rod vision dominates.

The ability of the rods to visualize small objects is much worse than that of the cones. This ability to perceive fine detail is called **visual acuity.** Cones are also much more able than rods to detect differences in brightness levels. This property of vision is termed **contrast perception.** Furthermore, cones are sensitive to a wide range of wavelengths of light.

Cones perceive color; rods are essentially color-blind.

The cones of the eye are color receptors of three types, each stimulated by relatively narrow bandwidths of light generally referred to as *red, blue* and *green.* They are sensitive to brightness (number of light photons), hue (wavelength), and saturation (ratio of monochromatic to white light). The human eye can detect approximately 2000 different color combinations or hues compared with perhaps only 20 shades of gray.

Therefore color images contain significantly more information than black and white images. Imaging techniques, such as magnetic resonance imaging (MRI), intrinsically contain more information and are more naturally adaptable to color imaging.

In a standard clinical setting, when someone views a 14 × 17 inch chest radiograph at 50 cm, the eye can spatially resolve 0.5 to 1 mm, 20 shades of gray, and 1000 different colors. Optimal medical imaging should take maximum advantage of this basic physiological capability. Functional MRI (fMRI) is the first step in this direction.

Pattern Recognition

The spatial map of light that is a visual image does not have any intrinsic intellectual significance. The intellectual value of such an image primarily depends on the mental comparison of an image with the large library of images stored within the brain and the subsequent evaluation of the meaning of the image.

Most medical imaging is a process of pattern recognition, which basically involves comparing one image pattern with another. Evaluation for similarities and differences with known patterns results in a "best fit" conclusion or "most likely" diagnosis (Figure 17-3).

This leads to the inescapable fact that a major factor in diagnostic efficiency is the observer's development of a large image memory bank, which at least partially comes from viewing many images. Such a memory bank is currently implemented and supplemented in CAD (computer-assisted detection).

Regardless of the significance of an image, visual images can be evaluated on the basis of **spatial resolution** and **contrast resolution.** That is, the perception and interpretation of an image depend on the location of light photons and the differences in character of those photons.

LOCATION AND CHARACTER

Therefore an image consists of discrete spatial points, each having different light characteristics. This concept was appreciated and emphasized by a group of Postimpressionist painters called **pointillists,** who painted pictures made up of dots of different colors. When they are viewed at close range, the dots are obvious, but at a distance, they appear to merge into a continuum of space and color.

The painting shown in Figure 17-4 is patterned after the work of a famous pointillist, Georges Seurat, and illustrates this concept. When it is viewed at a distance, the painting is of a picnic in the Texas hill country and elicits the psychological impression of such a real scene. When it is viewed at close range, the painting loses its totality and becomes simply a matrix of dots.

Such artists called these dots **points,** but these dots are perfectly analogous to what we call pixels. Each pixel has a unique location and character. The location is the position of each pixel in relationship to others. The character is represented by brightness, color, or both.

Most medical images differ from paintings in what the character of the pixel means. When an object is directly viewed, the pixel character is the actual brightness and wavelength of light reflected to the eye. When a representational image is viewed, the pixel character still primarily reflects the light incident onto the eye, but this initial character of light represents or stands for something else. In a realistic painting, the pixel character represents the visual light characteristics of actual objects.

 Medical images are representational.

Medical images represent something else and are not realistic. They do not attempt to copy a

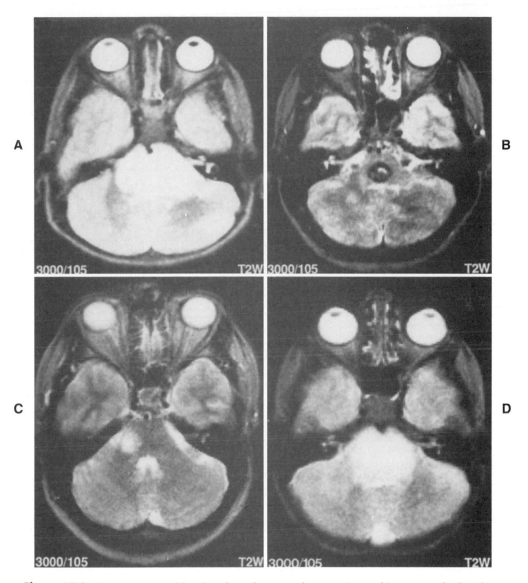

Figure 17-3   Pattern recognition involves the mental comparison of images to fit the "best fit" pattern for diagnosis. **A,** A clinically unknown case with high signal mass in the brain stem. **B,** Comparison pattern 1—low signal brain stem lesion without mass, indicating a hematoma. **C,** Comparison pattern 2—excentric, high signal brain stem lesion without mass, indicating multiple sclerosis. **D,** Comparison pattern 3—high signal brain stem mass, indicating a brain stem glioma.

real, directly visualized object. For example, in the infrared images shown in Figure 17-5, the pixel character represents the radiant heat of an object, a feature that cannot be seen directly.

Equally representational is the temperature map shown in Figure 17-6 in which the various pixels stand for the temperature of a region rather than any geographic feature; such a

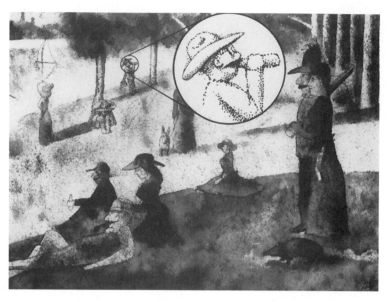

Figure 17-4   This scene of a picnic in the Texas hill country is patterned after the pointillist Seurat's *Sunday Afternoon on the Island of La Grande Jatte.* Essentially, it is a digital image. (Courtesy Frank Scalfano, Decatur, AL.)

representational image can be made whenever any parameter can be measured as a function of location.

Representational Images

Medical images are representational because the character of the pixel does not attempt to reflect the actual visual light feature of the tissue, but rather, some other physical parameter that has been measured and transformed into the image. The character of a pixel can be made to stand for essentially any measurable quantity that can be spatially defined. Examples include electron density maps (radiographs), radioactive decay maps (radionuclide images), and hydrogen concentration maps (MR images).

Another obvious difference between most directly observed images and medical images is that medical images are of the interior of a body rather than the surface. The primary clinician does the medical imaging of the surface of the body by direct observation,

whereas the radiologist images the inside of the body.

Radiographic Images

Imaging the inside of the body was a major problem in early medicine. Before Roentgen's discovery of x-rays in 1895, the only way medical images of the interior of the body were made was by direct visualization. This obviously required cutting into the subject and viewing the organ or tissue of interest in the form of traditional medical illustration (Figure 17-7).

With the discovery of x-rays, it became possible to make images of the interior of the body in a relatively noninvasive fashion. Radiographic images have features comparable to the representational images discussed. A radiographic image has pixels (groups of silver grains) with unique location and concentration differences that account for pixel character or brightness.

The basic difference between the radiographic image and a direct visual image of

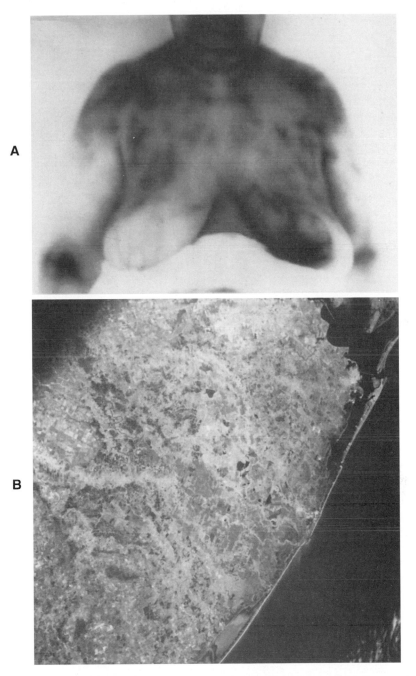

Figure 17-5 These infrared images represent emitted radiant heat, which is something the optical receptors cannot detect. **A,** A thermogram of a patient. **B,** An infrared photograph of the Texas gulf coast shows Houston at the top of the photo and Galveston Bay at the upper right. (**A,** Courtesy Alphonso Zermeno, Austin, TX; **B,** Courtesy NASA.)

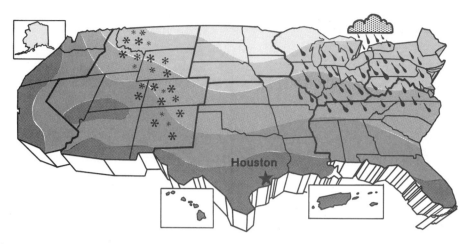

Figure 17-6 This weather map is normally published in multicolor and shows regional temperatures.

the body is in the devices that measure pixel character or the detectors. In the case of direct visualization, the detectors are the rods and cones of the retina. In the case of a radiograph, the detectors are the silver halide grains of the film emulsion that are sensitive to short-wavelength electromagnetic radiation.

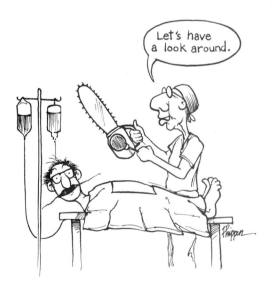

Figure 17-7 Before radiography, the interior of the body could only be viewed directly during surgery.

The number of x-rays detected determines pixel character. The amount of x-rays absorbed by the body is physically determined by the x-ray attenuation coefficient, which is principally related to the density of electrons in different tissues.

 A radiograph is essentially an electron density map of the body.

However, a radiograph does not relay any numerical information about the electron density (Figure 17-8). The informed observer knows only that the blackness or whiteness on the image is related to electron density. The whiter the image, the higher the electron density.

This gray scale information is very useful, even if the physics of x-ray interaction and electron density are not considered. This concept is used empirically to evaluate the internal structure of the anatomy.

Radiographic contrast resolution among tissues is determined principally by differences in electron density. For example, bone has a much higher electron density than soft tissue and is therefore highly contrasted to soft tissues on a radiograph. The evaluation of bone remains one of the main uses of radiography.

Radiographs differentiate among tissues and therefore report gross anatomy. However, radio-

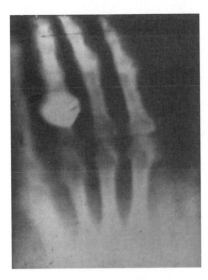

Figure 17-8 Radiographs are electron density maps of tissue, but they do not provide numerical data. This famous radiograph was taken by Roentgen and shows his wife's hand. (Courtesy Deutsches Roentgen-Museum.)

graphs can also relate pathological anatomy by showing abnormal gross anatomy, as reflected by deformities, distortions, absence, enlargement, and reduction of organs and tissues.

In addition to providing information about normal and abnormal gross anatomy, radiographs can provide some information about physiology, such as the healing of fractures reflected by calcium deposition in callus formation or the abnormal deposition of calcium in the basal ganglia in patients with hypercalcemia.

Magnetic Resonance Images

Unfortunately, most anatomical or physiological implications of radiographic images are indirect because there is no intrinsic biological significance to electron density. The clinical significance of an x-ray image is based on the recognition of patterns from accumulated experience of empirically evaluated radiographs.

Essentially, all forms of medical imaging use the substitution of some primary physical detector system other than the human visual system. The visual system becomes a second-

ary receptor that interprets the representational images created by the primary receptor system.

All medical image detector systems create a spatially defined map of the human body as a function of some particular physical parameter. Such medical images, then, are really three-dimensional images. Two dimensions define pixel location, and the third dimension, represented by brightness or color, contains information about the physical character of the tissue.

 An MR image is essentially a map of the nuclear characteristics of atoms in the body.

The physical character of the pixels in an MR image is multidimensional. The numerical value of an MRI pixel is principally determined by the MRI parameters: proton density (PD), spin-lattice relaxation time (T1), and spin-spin relaxation time (T2).

Secondary determinants of MRI pixel values are chemical shift, magnetic susceptibility, and motion. The weighting given to each of these parameters can vary greatly depending on the timing of the radiofrequency (RF) pulses and the gradient magnetic fields.

IMAGE EVALUATION CRITERIA

Spatial Criteria

The primary value of pixel location is to display geometry or gross anatomy. The display of gross anatomy requires not only appropriate pixel positioning but also adequate differences in pixel character to produce sufficient contrast between tissues to allow their separation and recognition.

However, most evaluation of gross anatomy is geographical and therefore relatively independent of the imaging technique. For instance, once the lateral ventricles have been displayed on an image (Figure 17-9), the character of the pixels becomes largely irrelevant.

 The three principal spatial criteria are size, shape, and position.

The relevant factors for the evaluation of the gross anatomy of the lateral ventricles or any other structure are basically the geometrical factors: size, shape, and position. In the viewing of the image, the size, shape, and position of the lateral ventricles are referenced to normal, which is based on experience.

Evaluation of the spatial aspects of an image is relatively straightforward. The specific possibilities in terms of size are normal, large, and small (Figure 17-10).

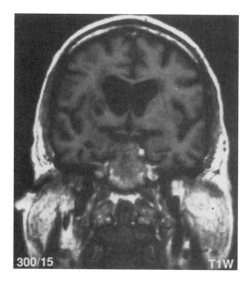

Figure 17-9 The lateral ventricles in this magnetic resonance image show such high contrast from surrounding brain tissue that further pixel characterization is largely irrelevant. (Courtesy Pedro Diaz-Marchan, Houston, TX.)

The main classifications regarding the shape of a tissue are normal (Figure 17-11, *A*), intrinsically deformed, and extrinsically compressed. For example, Figure 17-11, *B*, shows the beak deformity of the quadrigeminal plate in a patient with the Arnold-Chiari malformation. This is an intrinsic deformity, whereas the flattening of the quadrigeminal plate from a pineal tumor seen in Figure 17-11, *C*, is an extrinsic compression.

In terms of position, the main categories are normal, intrinsically malpositioned, and extrinsically displaced. For example, the low position of the cerebellar tonsils in the Arnold-Chiari malformation is an intrinsic malposition, usually indicating a congenital anomaly. On the other hand, the caudal herniation of the tonsils from a posterior fossa mass is an extrinsic displacement, indicating the presence of a distant mass in addition to the malpositioned tonsil.

Pixel Character

Unexpected pixel brightness indicates abnormal tissue character. The significance of this is entirely dependent on the imaging technique. Pixels that are abnormally bright in the brain on a computed tomography (CT) image suggest either blood or calcium, whereas abnormally bright pixels on T2 weighted MR images suggest multiple sclerosis or tumor but not blood or calcium.

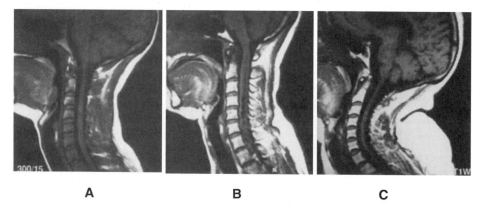

A	B	C

Figure 17-10 These three spinal cord images demonstrate image evaluation according to object size. **A,** Normal. **B,** Large. **C,** Small. (Courtesy Pedro Diaz-Marchan, Houston, TX.)

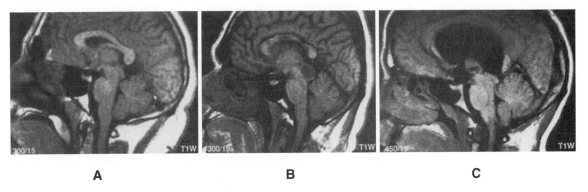

A   **B**   **C**

Figure 17-11 **A,** Normal quadrigeminal plate. **B,** An intrinsic deformity (glioma). **C,** An extrinsic deformity (hydrocephalus). (Courtesy R. Nick Bryan, Philadelphia, PA.)

As with spatial criteria of an image, evaluation of pixel character requires knowledge of what is normal. There are basically two ways to determine such normalcy. The first and most commonly used is the subjective, empirical visual interpretation of the image. In this case, the interpreter looks to see whether the pixels simply appear to be brighter than expected (Figure 17-12).

 The three principal character properties are normal, bright, and dark.

This technique works relatively well for experienced individuals looking at focal abnormalities. Here, the abnormal pixel brightness of the focal lesion is referenced to the presumed normal pixel brightness of the adjacent normal tissue. If the organ is symmetrical, such as the brain, the normal reference tissue does not have to be adjacent but can be in an equivalent position on the opposite side of the body.

This subjective approach depends on appropriate selection of pixel display values, windowing, and the presence of appropriate normal reference tissue somewhere on the image. If inappropriate pixel values are chosen for display, the lesion may be excluded or windowed out of the image (Figure 17-13). If an organ is diffusely involved by disease, the abnormality may not be obvious even if appropriately windowed because there is no normal reference density (Figure 17-14).

In general, observers have more difficulty detecting a minor overall change in pixel brightness than detecting focal lesions. Despite the lack of objectivity in the empirical evaluation of images, it is still the primary interpretative skill used.

The visual system is extremely well designed for such empirical analysis. It is quick, and its use in training is relatively inexpensive. Little or

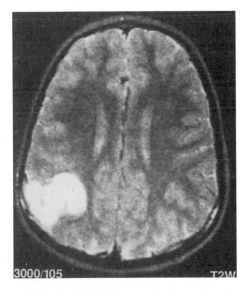

Figure 17-12 Subjective evaluation of an image recognizes brighter regions more easily than expected, as in the case of cerebral glioma. (Courtesy R. Nick Bryan, Philadelphia, PA)

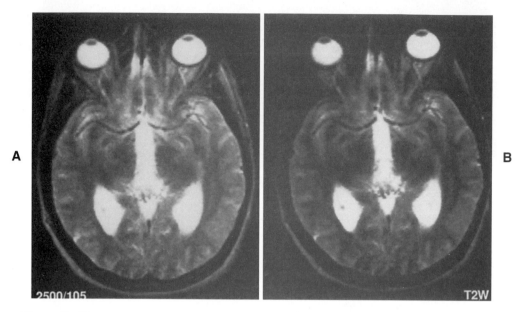

Figure 17-13 Improper windowing (**A,** width 849, center 469) may obscure an otherwise obvious lesion such as this pinealoma (**B,** width 849, center 757). (Courtesy Michael Mawad, Houston, TX.)

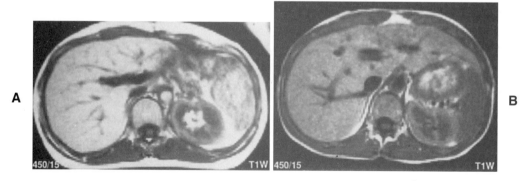

Figure 17-14 Even with proper windowing, diffuse disease may be missed because of a lack of adjacent normal tissue. **A,** Fatty liver. **B,** Normal liver. (Courtesy Tom Hedrick, Houston, TX.)

no direct interaction is required between the observer and the instrument. More detailed, objective, and computer-assisted evaluation of images (CAD) is now affecting and improving clinical diagnosis.

Quantitative interpretation of medical images requires knowledge of pixel values. This is an additional analytical step that can slow the interpretive process and increase the complexity of instrumentation. Interpretation of the quantitative data also requires knowledge of the actual normal range of numbers for the particular examining technique. This is not necessarily required in the more subjective approach.

Obtaining quantitative data in a small portion of an image by defining a region of interest (ROI) is relatively easy and requires little interaction and instrument complexity. It is the most common type of objective evaluation of an image.

Magnetic Resonance Images

The significance of abnormal pixel brightness in terms of tissue characteristics is directly a function of the imaging technique, which for MR images is the choice of RF pulses and gradient magnetic fields. Therefore, for each imaging technique, the interpreter must know which pathophysiological processes increase pixel brightness versus those lesions that diminish pixel brightness.

At the subjective, empirical level, it often comes down to those lesions that appear very bright versus slightly bright versus slightly dark or very dark. With a quantitative approach, the observer has to know the disease processes that produce pixel values within specific ranges. In general, lesions that increase pixel values are distinctly different from those that decrease pixel values.

A number of practical things must be understood in the daily practice of MRI. Perhaps most important are characteristics of an image and the way they are influenced by MRI technique. The location of a pixel is usually well defined. The gradient magnetic fields are responsible for pixel location. Without the gradients, there is no spatial localization in MRI.

The MRI technologist has little or no control over pixel location. However, the MRI technologist is directly responsible for determining the character or brightness of pixels.

 The RF pulse sequence determines pixel character and therefore contrast rendition and contrast resolution.

Pixel character can be appreciated in two fashions: black-and-white or color. In most medical imaging, black and white is used, but a color image can provide a great deal more information, as in fMRI.

In x-ray, gamma ray, and ultrasound images, the physical information that determines pixel character can be adequately conveyed by a black-and-white format because only one parameter, electron density, radioisotope construction, or reflectivity, respectively, is involved.

An MR image can be displayed in black and white, but a color rendition may potentially convey more information because three parameters (PD, T1, and T2) are involved. Nevertheless, at the present time, color MR images are rarely produced except for fMRI.

MAGNETIC RESONANCE IMAGE CHARACTER

A radiograph is a flat, gray image with low contrast resolution and therefore has relatively little detail. The tissue parameter that determines brightness in this image is electron density, which varies by no more than 1% for most soft tissues. Therefore the inherent subject contrast is very low. Radiographic contrast is improved with grids, with the use of tomographic techniques, and with the injection of radiographic contrast material.

The CT image shown in Figure 17-15, *A*, gives even better contrast resolution than a radiograph because the x-ray beam is highly collimated. This collimation rejects scatter radiation, preventing it from reaching the detectors. In the CT image of the brain, the 0.5% difference between the electron density of gray matter (GM) and white matter (WM) can just be detected.

The principal advantage of the MR image shown in Figure 17-15, *B*, over a CT image is contrast resolution. The anatomic location of the pixels is the same, but the character of the pixels is different. The improved contrast resolution is due to the intrinsic differences in the tissue values of the MRI parameters. These parameters differ by as much as 40%.

Magnetic Resonance Imaging Parameters

The three principal MRI parameters are PD, T1, and T2. Secondary parameters such as

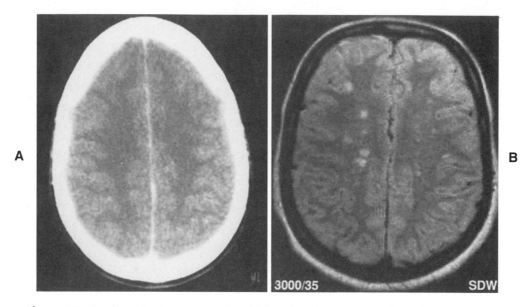

Figure 17-15   These brain images of multiple sclerosis show that the **(A)** magnetic resonance image is superior to the **(B)** computed tomography image because of better low contrast resolution.

chemical shift, paramagnetic materials, magnetic susceptibility, and motion also influence pixel character. The MR imaging system detects these parameters and converts them into pixel character.

A complete MRI examination should include images of each of these parameters. However, such a complete MRI examination is never done. With most MRI systems, chemical shift imaging cannot be done, paramagnetic materials are unnecessary, and motion imaging is a special case. This leaves three tissue characteristics, PD, T1, and T2 that MRI routinely detects to make an image.

These MRI parameters can be discussed in terms of an image without understanding PD, T1, or T2 at all. They are simply MRI characteristics of tissues. With proper technique, the MRI technologist can measure each of them as a function of location and create an anatomical map or representational image.

Figure 17-16 is a histogram of x-ray linear attenuation coefficients and the MRI parame-

ters PD, T1, and T2 for various tissues. The linear attenuation coefficient of most soft tissues is approximately the same.

However, the MRI parameters of the same tissues show a much greater variation. This variation of MRI parameters among soft tissues results in superior contrast resolution.

Pure Magnetic Resonance Images

With color as an analogy, the MRI parameters can be considered as being comparable to the three primary colors (blue, yellow, and red). All color images viewed consist of a mixture of these primary colors. Depending on the intensity of each primary color in the mix, all colors of the spectrum can be obtained.

A look at the screen of a color television confirms this. However, a magnifying glass may be necessary. The screen actually consists of only three types of dots—blue, yellow, and red. Combinations of these dots produce the full-color image seen from a distance. Regions that appear white have all dots glowing intensely.

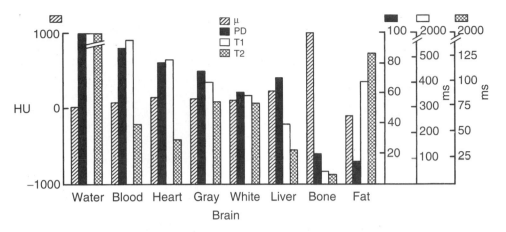

Figure 17-16 This histogram shows that the relative differences in magnetic resonance imaging parameters for various tissues are greater than the range of the x-ray linear attenuation coefficients of x-ray imaging as measured by Hounsfield units *(HU)*.

 MR images representing solely PD, T1, or T2 cannot be obtained.

MR images consist of the influences of PD, T1, and T2. Pure MR images are analogous to the primary colors because they represent only a single MRI parameter. Unfortunately, in normal practice, pure images of MRI parameters cannot be obtained. Weighted images are routinely produced, and these are analogous to color images obtained by adding the primary colors in various proportions.

PD Images. A pure PD image is shown in Figure 17-17. In this image, pixel brightness is a function only of PD. The higher the PD is, the brighter the pixel. The GM has a higher PD than WM, and therefore it is brighter.

This image shows that a high contrast MR image can be made of the brain on the basis of PD alone. There is about a 20% difference between the PD of GM and that of WM. That is a bigger difference than the 0.5% difference in the x-ray linear attenuation coefficients of the same tissues as seen on CT images.

T1 Images. Figure 17-18 shows a pure T1 image. The character of the pixels is influenced only by the T1 of the tissue. The big difference between the T1 of GM and that of WM is obvious; this is a high-contrast image.

The T1 of GM is approximately 700 to 800 ms; on the other hand, the T1 of WM varies from 500 to 600 ms, resulting in approximately a 30% difference in the T1 of these two tissues. This difference produces a high-contrast image of the brain.

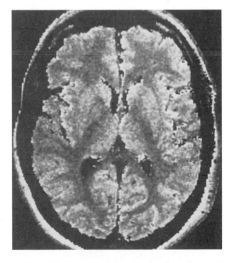

Figure 17-17 A calculated pure proton density image. (Courtesy Richard Wendt III, Houston, TX.)

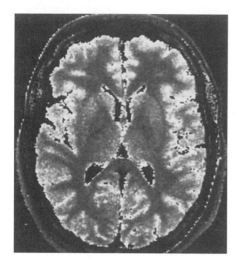

Figure 17-18 A calculated pure T1 image. (Courtesy Richard Wendt III, Houston, TX.)

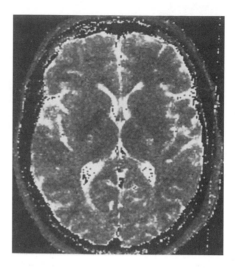

Figure 17-19 A calculated pure T2 image. (Courtesy Richard Wendt III, Houston, TX.)

T2 Images. Figure 17-19 shows a pure image of the third primary MRI parameter, T2. This looks significantly different from the other pure images even though they are of the same slice from the same patient. There is little difference between T2 of GM and T2 of WM, and the result is very little contrast. The T2 of both GM and WM is approximately 100 ms.

Routinely, these are the three primary MR images that should be obtained. Each of these three images is uniquely different from the others; they may only occasionally look similar and happen to have similar contrast.

WEIGHTED IMAGES

Clinically, RF pulse sequences are used to produce images that are a blend of the intrinsic PD, T1, and T2 characteristics of tissue. When the three primary colors are blended, hues that may obscure original information are obtained.

Similarly, such an MR image may be practical and aesthetically pleasing but may also obscure inherent tissue contrast. Such weighted-images have pixel intensity determined more strongly by one of the three MRI parameters.

 MR images are weighted by PD, T1, and T2.

The RF pulse sequences routinely used are like color filters over a color photograph; they can hide information. Sometimes that information is not needed for diagnosis, but without it, the diagnosis may not be certain. Partial saturation, inversion recovery, spin echo, and gradient echo RF pulse sequences result in weighted images.

The following discussion deals only with the RF pulse sequences because they determine image contrast. It is assumed throughout that the gradient magnetic fields have been pulsed properly to provide spatial localization and spatial resolution.

Partial Saturation

Proton spins exist in four states, as shown in Figure 17-20. The patient is at equilibrium with the B_0 field before the pulse sequence begins. After a 90° RF pulse, the spin system is saturated.

If repetition time (TR) is sufficiently long, all spins will relax to equilibrium. Such a pulse sequence is called **saturation recovery,** but it is rarely used because it takes too long to make an image. With short TR, the pulse sequence is **partial saturation.**

The partial saturation pulse sequence is the simplest way to obtain weighted images. It consists of a chain of 90° RF pulses (Figure 17-21). Before the first pulse, net magnetization (M_Z) is at maximum value (M_0), in equilibrium with the external magnetic field (B_0).

The 90° RF pulse rotates the M_Z onto the XY plane so that M_Z is now zero and M_{XY} is at a maximum value determined by M_0. Because M_Z equals zero, the proton spins are said to be **saturated.** They recover longitudinal magnetization according to the T1 relaxation time. Because M_0 is directly proportional to the PD, the initial amplitude of the free induction decay (FID) depends on PD.

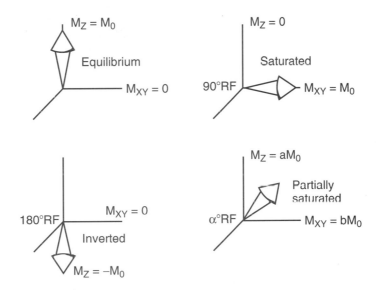

Figure 17-20 These vector diagrams represent the four spin states: equilibrium, saturation, inversion, and partial saturation.

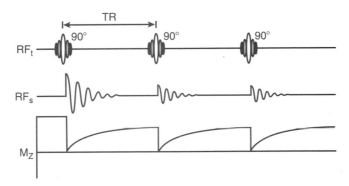

Figure 17-21 A partial saturation radiofrequency *(RF)* pulse sequence is the simplest imaging sequence. Free induction decays after the first repetition time *(TR)* have lower intensity because the proton spins remain partially saturated; that is, all of them have not relaxed to equilibrium.

For the proton spins to recover fully from saturation, a TR equal to at least 5 times the longest T1 is required. Clinically, this would require a TR equal to many seconds, which would result in unacceptably long imaging times. However, with a very long TR, the saturated spins would fully recover, resulting in FIDs of equal amplitude each time. Such a pulse sequence is called a **saturation recovery,** and the resulting image is a PD weighted (PDW) image.

When shorter TRs are used, the amplitude of the second and subsequent FIDs is less than that of the first because enough time has not been allowed for full longitudinal relaxation. The second and subsequent 90° RF pulses excite already partially saturated proton spins, spins that have not relaxed to equilibrium, such that the FID will be of equal amplitude but less than that of the first FID. In such a partial saturation pulse sequence, the earliest FIDs are ignored.

A partial saturation pulse sequence is therefore weighted by PD but also has a contribution from T1, depending on the value of TR. Figure 17-22 shows the relaxation of M_Z to equilibrium after a 90° RF pulse. Here, three tissues are considered: cerebrospinal fluid (CSF), GM, and WM. CSF has the highest PD of the three; therefore its relative value of M_0 is the highest. It should produce the brightest pixels.

CSF also has the longest T1 relaxation time, approximately 1200 ms; it can be seen from the graph that CSF has the longest T1 because it rises from M_Z equal zero with the lowest slope. Therefore CSF proton spins relax to equilibrium more slowly than GM or WM proton spins. When equilibrium for all tissues is reached, however, M_0 will be higher for CSF, resulting in brighter pixels for CSF.

GM has a lower M_0 than CSF and a much shorter T1, approximately 700 ms. Therefore pixels representative of GM relax to equilibrium more rapidly than CSF, but the equilibrium value is lower.

WM has the shortest T1 relaxation time of the three, approximately 500 ms and the lowest PD. Therefore WM relaxes to equilibrium most quickly, but the equilibrium value is least of the three.

Figure 17-23 illustrates the necessity for selecting the proper RF pulse sequence. If a long TR is selected, the image is PDW, and CSF is bright, GM is gray, and WM is dark.

At a TR of approximately 3000 ms, CSF and GM will appear equally bright, both brighter

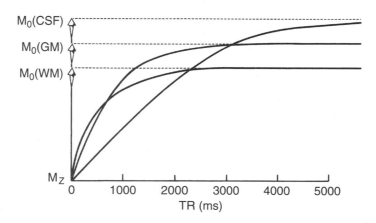

Figure 17-22   This shows relaxation of longitudinal magnetization (M_Z) during a partial saturation pulse sequence. A more rapid relaxation to equilibrium (M_0) occurs in tissues with short T1, such as white matter *(WM)* The amplitude of M_0 is a function of proton density, the gyromagnetic ratio, and B_0.

than WM. If 90° RF pulses are applied at 3000 ms intervals, the M_Z of both CSF and GM will have recovered to the same value so that the representative FIDs have the same amplitude, and there is no difference in pixel intensity. Such a TR results in a crossover on the time scale of the T1 curves and an absence of contrast on the image.

Another crossover appears at approximately 2400 ms between CSF and WM and yet a third crossover at approximately 600 ms between GM and WM. The crossover at 600 ms is clinically significant because it is within the clinically acceptable TR of approximately 1000 ms, ensuring reasonable imaging time.

At this 600 ms crossover, contrast reversal occurs. Below 600 ms, WM appears brighter than GM; above 600 ms, GM appears brighter than WM. Tissue contrast is lost completely at the crossover. Furthermore, at a TR of less than approximately 2000 ms, CSF appears darker than either GM or WM. This represents another contrast reversal.

Table 17-1 summarizes pixel appearance for various ranges of TR. A partial saturation image made with a long TR is PDW; with a short TR, less than 500 ms, it is T1 weighted (T1W).

Figure 17-23 shows a series of partial saturation images in which pixel character is a function of both PD and T1. There is little contrast between the GM and WM in these images.

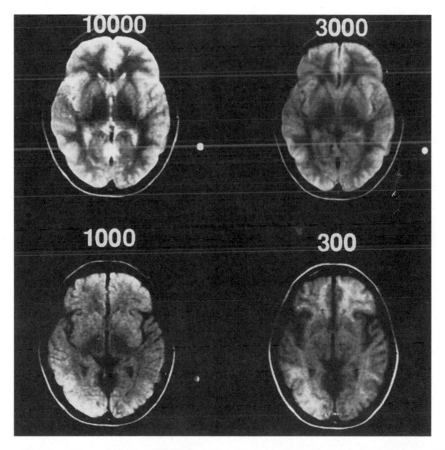

Figure 17-23 This series of partial saturation images obtained at the indicated repetition times demonstrates contrast reversal as a result of changes in proton density and T1 influence.

| TABLE 17-1 | Pixel Appearance for Cerebrospinal Fluid, Gray Matter, and White Matter as a Function of Repetition Time in a Partial Saturation or Inversion Recovery Image |

Tissue	Repetition Time		
	Very Long	**Long**	**Short**
CSF	Bright	Dark	Dark
GM	Gray	Bright	Gray
WM	Dark	Gray	Bright

These are not bad images in terms of signal-to-noise ratio (SNR) and spatial resolution, but they are poor images in terms of contrast resolution and visualization of brain anatomy. This lack of contrast may seem peculiar because the pixel brightness is a function of PD and T1, both of which differ significantly between GM and WM.

This is the problem with MRI pulse sequences; contrast information can be lost. Brain contrast due to PD can be viewed as making GM bright and WM dark and the tissue contrast due to T1 as making GM dark and WM bright. The contrast rendition is reversed between these two tissues.

Therefore when an image is made that puts the two together, it is like doing a subtraction film in angiography. Positive and negative images of the brain together result in a flat image; contrast is lost. That is the case with the partial saturation image obtained with an intermediate TR.

The risk involved in doing routine MRI is that important underlying information may be lost. The MRI technologist must make sure that the information lost is not important. This phenomenon is not a function of imaging system design but a function of the MRI pulse sequence, which is under the control of the MRI technologist.

Inversion Recovery

A 180° RF pulse, rather than a 90° RF pulse, is used to expand the range of longitudinal mag-netization, M_Z. The 180° RF pulse inverts the M_Z, which immediately begins to relax to equilibrium according to the T1 relaxation time (Figure 17-24).

This relaxation of M_Z is not detectable in the presence of the B_0 field because it is too small. Therefore an additional 90° RF pulse is needed to rotate the M_Z onto the XY plane, where it will be detectable.

This two-pulse sequence, a 180° RF pulse followed by a 90° RF pulse, is called an **inversion recovery** pulse sequence, and it is used to produce predominantly T1 weighted (T1W) images. The time between the initial 180° RF pulse and the following 90° RF pulse is the inversion time (TI).

If TI is very long, M_Z will have relaxed to equilibrium, and FID amplitude will be principally determined by PD. Such imaging times would be even more objectionable than for the partial saturation sequence.

After shorter TIs, the FID amplitude is determined by the PD and T1 relaxation time because, as in the partial saturation pulse sequence, the spins have not relaxed to equilibrium but, rather, have remained partially saturated. Therefore pixel brightness will be a function of PD and T1.

There is a value of TI where M_Z equals zero. Application of a 90° RF pulse at this time results in no signal because there is no Z magnetization to rotate onto the XY plane. This value of TI is called a **null point**.

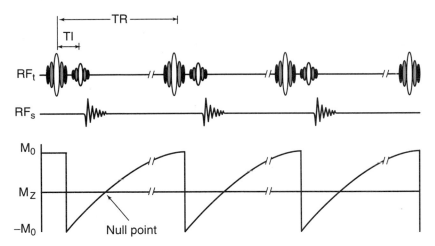

Figure 17-24 An inversion recovery radiofrequency *(RF)* pulse sequence consists of a 180° RF pulse followed by a 90° RF pulse. The inversion time *(TI)* can be programmed for any time. Here it is shown occurring before the null point.

> *At the null point, there is no transverse magnetization, hence no signal.*

The return to equilibrium magnetization after an inversion recovery pulse sequence follows a similar behavior as that from a partial saturation pulse sequence (Figure 17-25). The principal difference is that the dynamic range is twice that for a partial saturation pulse sequence, resulting in greater image contrast if the TI is properly chosen. At a TI of approximately 500 ms, the M_Z of the three tissues is more widely separated than in a partial saturation pulse sequence.

There are some problems with the inversion recovery pulse sequence. If the TI is chosen at a tissue null point, no signal is generated, and the overall SNR is poor. The negative value of M_Z after the 180° RF pulse is a problem for some MRI systems.

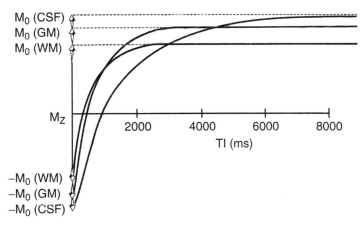

Figure 17-25 Relaxation of M_Z during an inversion recovery pulse sequence covers twice the range of the partial saturation pulse sequence. The result can be even greater image contrast.

Rather than displaying the full dynamic range of MR signals, some imaging systems display the negative magnetization as positive magnetization (Figure 17-26). This results in more crossovers for tissues and can confuse image interpretation. To prevent this confusion, the imaging system must be capable of detecting the phase of the MR signal and the amplitude so that contrast resolution following the scheme of Figure 17-26 is displayed.

Inversion recovery images are usually high-contrast images that are T1 weighted. Repetition times in excess of approximately 3000 ms are unacceptable because of low patient throughput. Inversion times of 300 to 600 ms are most often used. Such long TIs make multislice techniques limited.

Several inversion recovery images are shown in Figure 17-27. These images show good contrast between GM and WM. However, a closer look at the relative intensities of CSF, GM, and WM as a function of TR and TI demonstrates contrast reversals and null regions. Careful prescription of the RF pulse sequence is required for inversion recovery images.

Spin Echo

The pulse sequences just described for partial saturation and inversion recovery imaging sampled the primary MR signal, the FID. The MR signal detected for imaging is usually a spin echo, not an FID (see Chapter 16). Therefore a 180° RF pulse follows the 90° RF pulses in both sequences so that a spin echo is formed. This does not significantly change the analysis of an image if the time between the 90° RF pulse and the spin echo is short.

The most widely used pulse sequence, the spin echo pulse sequence, generates spin echoes at various times after the 90° RF pulse (Figure 17-28). The 90° RF pulse rotates the M_Z onto the XY plane just as in a partial saturation pulse sequence. The FID that is formed is ignored, and sometime later, at one half the echo time (TE), a 180° RF pulse is applied.

This 180° RF pulse is called a **refocusing pulse** because it causes the proton spins to rephase (Chapter 5). The rephased spins produce a spin echo with amplitude less than that of the FID because of spin-spin interactions and the resulting loss of transverse magnetization due to the T2 relaxation in the tissue.

Multiple spin echoes can be formed by multiple 180° RF pulses. Each spin echo is reduced in amplitude by T2 relaxation; therefore the overall SNR is reduced with later echoes. The relaxation curves at the bottom of Figure 17-29

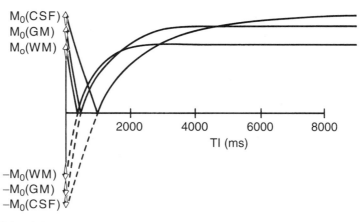

Figure 17-26 If the magnetic resonance imaging system is incapable of displaying the negative range of M_Z in the inversion recovery, image information may be obscured by reduced dynamic range and confusing crossovers.

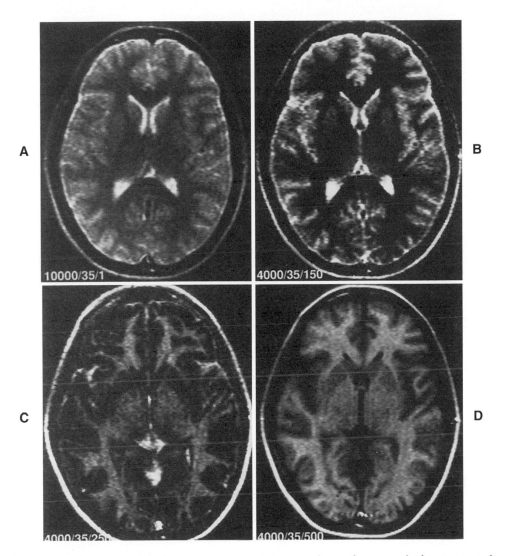

Figure 17-27   This series of inversion recovery images shows the reversal of contrast and null regions as a function of repetition time and inversion time.

plot the loss of M_{XY}, the transverse magnetization, and therefore, T2 relaxation.

Partial saturation and inversion recovery images are principally PDW and T1W. Spin echo images can be PDW, T1W, or T2W, depending on the values of TR and TE. All images have a contribution from PD.

Figure 17-29 illustrates the T2 relaxation for the three tissues CSF, GM, and WM. As with the other pulse sequences, the initial signal intensity from CSF, GM, and WM is determined by the equilibrium magnetization, M_0, for each. Loss of magnetization in the XY plane, M_{XY}, and therefore, MR signal intensity is determined by the T2 relaxation time of each tissue.

Cerebrospinal fluid has a relatively long T2, approximately 1500 ms. Gray matter and WM have shorter T2 relaxation times, both

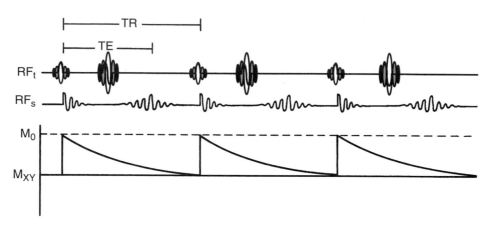

Figure 17-28 A spin echo radiofrequency *(RF)* pulse sequence showing the received magnetic resonance signals (RFs) and the loss of transverse magnetization (M_{XY}). The actual decrease in M_{XY} is much faster than shown here because it follows the T2* relaxation time (see Chapter 7).

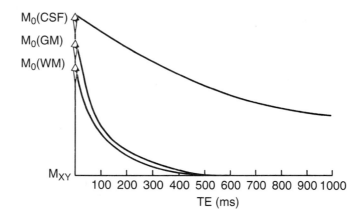

Figure 17-29 T2 relaxation curves for cerebrospinal fluid *(CSF)*, gray matter *(GM)*, and white matter *(WM)* are determined by the amplitude of M_{XY} as a function of echo time *(TE)*.

approximately 100 ms; therefore the CSF signal remains intense, resulting in a bright pixel for all TEs.

If TRs for a spin echo pulse sequence were very long, the relationship between spin echoes for the three tissues would be like that shown in Figure 17-30. CSF would always be brightest, and WM would always be darkest because with TR at least 5 times the longest Tl, all the proton spins have relaxed to equilibrium before each new pulse sequence.

Figure 17-30 shows the relaxation of M_Z back to equilibrium and the relaxation of M_{XY} to zero after a 90° RF pulse, both plotted on the same scale. It is clear that the relaxation of M_{XY} is far more rapid than the relaxation of M_Z.

At a very long TR, for example, 5000 ms, M_Z has relaxed to equilibrium for nearly all tissues. Subsequent 90° RF pulses followed by 180° RF refocusing pulses result in images that are PDW and T2W. At long TR, as the TE is reduced, the image becomes more PDW.

If the TR is shortened, more Tl relaxation influence is brought into the image because all tissues will not have recovered to M_0. A review of Figure 17-30 shows how magnetization among these tissues changes with reduced TR.

 The initial signal amplitude is reduced for subsequent 180° refocusing pulses, and the relative amplitudes among the tissues also change.

If the TR is reduced to 1000 ms, GM exhibits a higher initial MR signal than CSF or WM

(Figure 17-31). Therefore GM appears brightest on an early echo, and CSF appears brightest on a late echo. This is a contrast reversal resulting from a crossover.

If the TR is made very short, for example, 300 ms, there is little relaxation of M_Z because of the T1 relaxation times being too long (Figure 17-32). WM now appears brightest on an early echo. CSF is still brightest on a late echo. These reversals of contrast result from crossovers of the T2 relaxation curves.

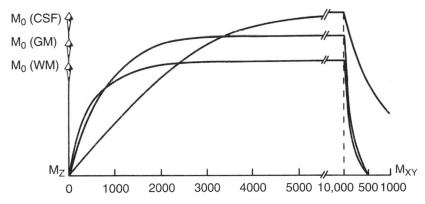

Figure 17-30 Relaxation of M_Z to equilibrium and relaxation of M_{XY} for an extremely long repetition time. If the image is formed after a short echo time (TE), it will be weighted by proton density. Use of long TE results in T2 weighted images.

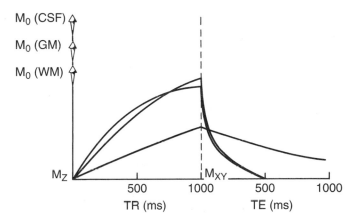

Figure 17-31 Use of an intermediate repetition time *(TR)* does not allow full regrowth of M_Z. Images formed with short echo time *(TE)* are proton density (PD) weighted and T1 weighted; images formed with long TE are PD weighted, T1 weighted, and T2 weighted.

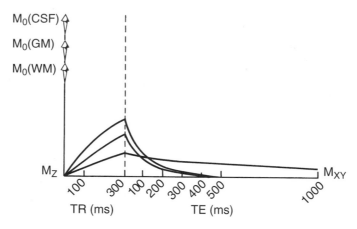

Figure 17-32 With extremely short repetition time *(TR)*, little M_Z is reformed, resulting in more T1 weighted images at all clinically used echo times *(TEs)*.

With a long TR and a long TE, the result is a T2W image. A long TR and a short TE result in a PDW image. Short TR and short TE result in T1W images (Table 17-2). Short TE produces early echoes, and long TE produces late echoes.

All spin echo images have a PD contribution. Depending on the T1 and T2 relaxation times of adjacent tissues, there will be many opportunities for obscuring contrast at crossovers.

A little thought shows that the amplitude of the spin echo from any tissue increases as the TR is lengthened, as TE is shortened, as T1 decreases, and as T2 increases. Stated differently, in general, a long T1 means less signal at a given TR, and a long T2 means more signal at a given TE.

The signal intensity of successive spin echoes decreases regardless of TR; therefore, the SNR also decreases. Long TE results in a dim, noisy image. As a general rule, short TE (early echoes) results in a T1W image, and long TE (late echoes) results in a T2W image. Both images also have some contribution from PD.

The spin echo images shown in Figure 17-33 represent variations of this most common imaging sequence. When considering spin echo imaging, the radiologist must recognize whether the image is from an "early" echo or a "late" echo. These images were made with four different TR times, ranging from 2000 ms to 4000 ms, at a TE of 130 ms; they are all late spin echo images. Late spin echoes are viewed primarily as providing a T2W image because

TABLE 17-2	**Weighting of Spin Echo Images as a Function of Repetition Times and Echo Times**		
	TR		
	Short (<300 ms)	**Intermediate (300-1000 ms)**	**Long (>2000 ms)**
Short TE (<40 ms)	T1 weighted	PD and T1 weighted	PD weighted
Long TE (>80 ms)	T1 and T2 weighted	PD, T1, and T2 weighted	T2 weighted

the character of a pixel is primarily related to the T2 relaxation of the tissue.

However, these images are considerably different from the pure T2 image discussed earlier. The pure T2 image is dull and has little contrast. On these late spin echo images, there is at least some differentiation between GM and WM. Consequently, some other parameter must contribute to contrast. The additional parameter is PD, which always influences pixel intensity. Longer TR images are brighter

because of the relaxation of all tissues to their equilibrium magnetization.

These images are examples that can be used to begin planning clinically useful spin echo pulse sequences. To view detail on normal or abnormal anatomy, the MRI technologist would not want to do heavily T2W images. Rather, a PDW or T1W image would be produced.

Figure 17-34 shows spin echo images produced at various TRs varying from 350 ms to

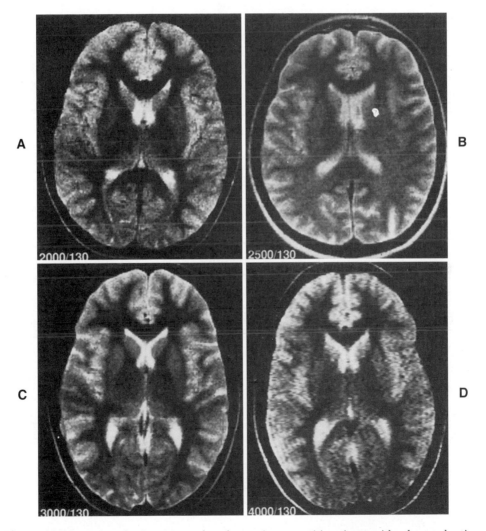

Figure 17-33 Spin echo images produced at various repetition times with a long echo time result in T2 weighted images. (Courtesy Orlando Diaz-Daza, Houston, TX.)

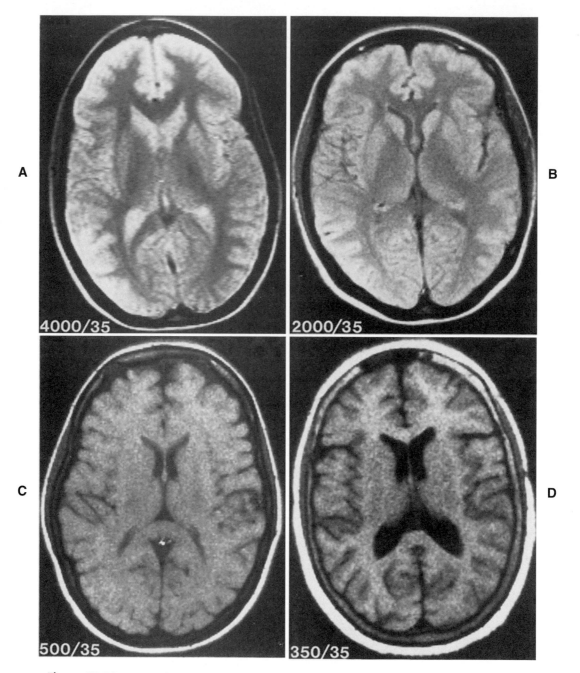

Figure 17-34 Spin echo images produced at various repetition times with short echo time result in varying proton density weighted and T1 weighted images. (Courtesy Orlando Diaz-Daza, Houston, TX.)

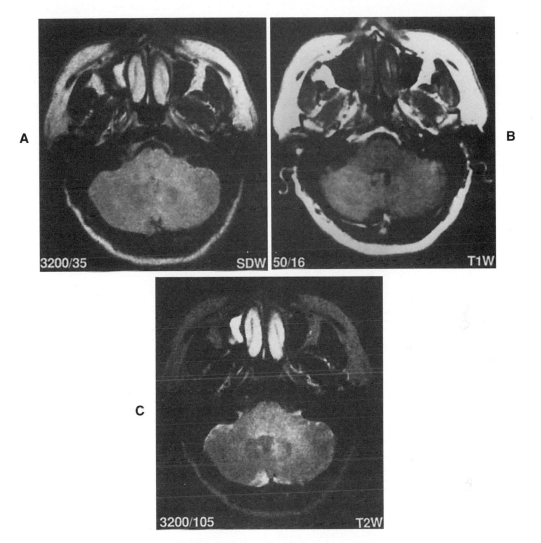

Figure 17-35 The late spin echo image seen in **C** is most useful for identifying pathologic conditions, such as this brain stem glioma. (Courtesy Orlando Diaz-Daza, Houston, TX.)

4000 ms with a short TE of 35 ms. At long TR, in excess of 1000 ms, the image is PDW. At short TR, approximately 300 ms, the image is principally T1W. If the TE is made very short (zero time), a partial saturation pulse sequence with a 270° RF pulse results.

A pathologic condition usually differs significantly with T2. Figure 17-35, *C,* shows a late spin echo image that does not have much normal brain contrast, but the lesion is very dis-

tinct. The contrast between normal tissues and pathologic tissues of the brain is usually due to differences in T2 relaxation. A heavily PDW or T1W image is nearly always needed to show correct anatomy, and a heavily T2W image is used to show disease.

CHALLENGE QUESTIONS

1. Define the term *visual acuity.* What is its relationship to viewing an MR image?

2. When a spin echo image is made with a short echo time and a long repetition time, what weighting will the image exhibit?

3. MR images are said to be representational. What does this mean?

4. When you perform a double echo, spin echo pulse sequence to produce two images, how is each weighted?

5. Which tissues have longest relaxation times?

6. Medical images can be produced with transmitted, reflected, absorbed, or emitted electromagnetic radiation. Which of these terms refers to MR images?

7. What is the principal advantage and disadvantage to inversion recovery imaging?

8. The spatial resolution of an MR image is determined by field of view and matrix size. What determines spatial localization?

9. When the image of adjacent tissue losses contrast, how can the contrast resolution be improved?

10. What are the relative values for the relaxation times of soft tissues?

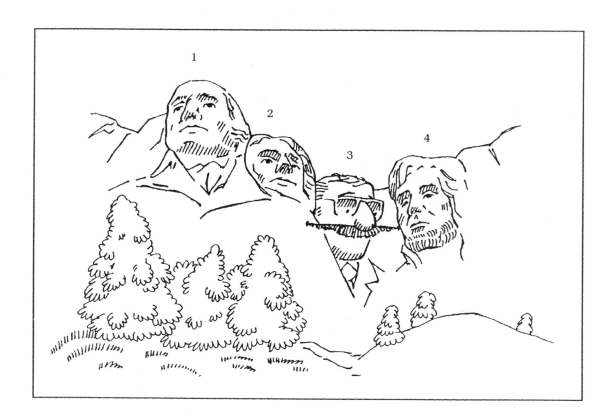

Match the face to the appropriate description.

a. Led us out of the Civil War   ____
b. Our first president   ____
c. Author of the Declaration of Independence   ____
d. Golf handicap = 23   ____

Part IV

Pulse Sequences

Chapter 18

Spin Echo Imaging

OBJECTIVES

At the completion of this chapter, the student will be able to do the following:

1. Diagram a complete spin echo pulse sequence.
2. Diagram an inversion recovery pulse sequence.
3. Define Hermitian symmetry.
4. Identify the region of k-space most responsible for contrast resolution and spatial resolution.
5. Diagram a fast spin echo pulse sequence.
6. Discuss the importance of echo train length.

OUTLINE

Since the introduction in 1980 of clinically practical two-dimensional magnetic resonance imaging (MRI) followed shortly by multiecho, multislice imaging, magnetic resonance (MR) image quality has continued to improve. In addition to better images, developments in MRI have been driven by the goal of reduced image acquisition time.

For instance, such reduced imaging time is required to image in the presence of normal tissue motion, including flowing blood (magnetic resonance angiography [MRA]). Figure 18-1 is a timeline representing the increase in temporal resolution of MRI since clinical introduction. Various tissue motion and MRI techniques are included on this timeline, along with the approximate dates of application of these techniques.

MRI development was predicted to follow a course similar to that of computed tomography (CT). An exponential introduction of new imaging techniques and clinical capabilities were expected up to a saturation point where the process would routinely remain clinical. Many predicted the death of CT because of the promise of MRI; however, MRI and CT are complementary in many respects. Advances in CT such as multislice spiral CT and computed tomography angiography (CTA) have extended the capabilities of CT.

MRI appears to be developing exponentially, not toward saturation but rather ever increasing. This chapter and the following four chapters describe the enormous advances in MRI **temporal resolution.** The term *temporal resolution* refers to resolution in time in the same way that spatial resolution refers to resolution in space and contrast resolution refers to resolution of one soft tissue from another.

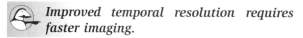

Improved temporal resolution requires faster imaging.

Although many of these MRI advances have resulted in faster imaging and increased patient throughput, they have also added new diagnostic capabilities. In addition to the imaging of cyclic motion such as respiration and heartbeat, noncyclic physiological processes, such as peristalsis, saccadic eye motion, and joint movement, are being imaged with MRI. Furthermore, MR fluoroscopy (MRF) is now possible.

Even the first paper on nuclear magnetic resonance (NMR) by Felix Bloch in 1946 considered basic concepts leading to fast imaging techniques. The current development of fast and ultrafast imaging has been accompanied by an abundance of acronyms by vendors (Table 18-1). Each technique is a development of spin echo (SE) or gradient echo (GRE) imaging.

A rare, two-stalk century plant found in the Big Bend region of west Texas is shown in Figure 18-2. The root spines represent MR image reconstruction methods and the flowering pods, imaging techniques.

SPIN ECHO PULSE SEQUENCE

The most commonly used MRI technique is based on the SE pulse sequence that was introduced in 1950 by Hahn. This was first applied to imaging in 1980 and was quickly followed by additional modifications in the pulse sequence to allow multislice imaging. The Carr-Purcell-Meiboom-Gill (CPMG) pulse sequence is an improved SE pulse sequence for producing images from multiple echoes.

The terms *radiofrequency* (RF) *pulse sequence* and *pulse sequence* are often used interchangeably. However, RF pulse sequence correctly applies only to the first line of the musical score. Therefore the term *pulse sequence* is used here to represent not only the RF pulses but also the pulsed gradient magnetic fields and the received MR signals. The basic SE pulse sequence is shown in Figure 18-3.

Often the lines of the musical score are identified as RF_t, G_z, RF_s G_Y $(_\phi)$, and G_X (ω) (Figure 18-4, *A*). These symbols identify images that are acquired in the transverse plane. Other orthogonal and oblique planes are now frequently obtained, so the symbols G_Z, G_Y, and G_X are less meaningful.

In this and successive chapters, the following symbols are used: RF_t, B_{SS}, RF_s, B_ϕ, and B_R

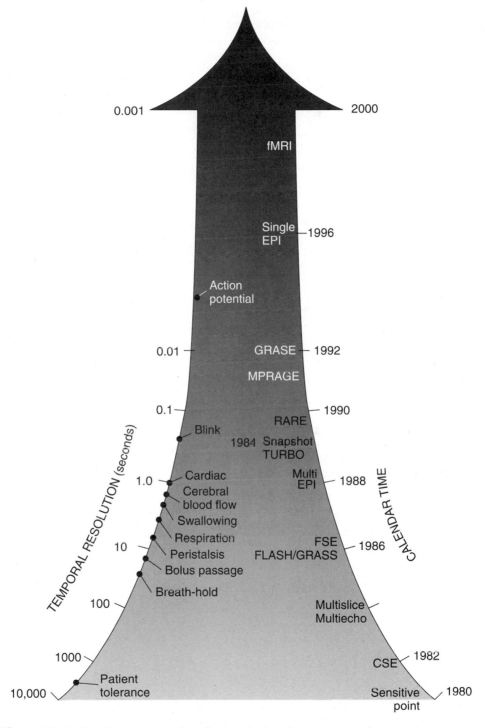

Figure 18-1 Timeline representing the continuing development of magnetic resonance imaging techniques and required temporal resolution for imaging various physiological motions.

TABLE 18-1	Acronyms Used in Spin Echo and Gradient Echo Imaging
Acronym	**Explanation**
ABSIR	Absolute inversion recovery
CE-FAST	Contrast-enhanced FAST
DEFAISED	Duel echo fast acquired interleaved spin echo
FAST	Fourier acquired steady state
FE	Field echo
FEER	Field even echo by reversal
FFE	Fast field echo
FGR	Fast GRASS
FISP	Fast imaging with steady state precision
FLAIR	Fluid attenuated inversion recovery
FLASH	Fast low angle shot
FS	Fast scan
FSE	Fast spin echo
GFE	Gradient field echo
GFEC	Gradient field echo compensation
GRASS	Gradient recalled acquisition in the steady state
HASTE	Half Fourier acquired single shot turbo spin echo
HASTIRM	HASTE inversion recovery magnitude
HFI	Half Fourier imaging
IR	Inversion recovery
IRM	Inversion recovery magnitude
MPGR	Multiplanar GRASS
MPRAGE	Magnetization prepared rapid gradient echo
PFI	Partial flip angle
PSIF	Reversed FISP
RAMFAST	Rapidly acquired magnetization prepared FAST
RARE	Rapid acquisition by repeated echo
RASE	Rapid acquired spin echo
RF-FAST	RF-spoiled FAST
RS	Rapid scan
SPGR	Spoiled GRASS
SSFP	Steady state free precession
STIR	Short time inversion recovery
TFE	Turbo field echo
TSE	Turbo spin echo
TurboFLASH	Turbo version of FLASH

(Figure 18-4, *B*). The symbol B is more appropriate for indicating a gradient magnetic field.

The slice selection gradient is represented by B_{SS}, which can define any of the three orthogonal planes. Oblique images are obtained when B_{SS} represents any combination of the three gradients energized simultaneously. The phase-encoding gradient magnetic field is B_{Φ}. The gradient magnetic field that is energized while a signal is acquired is B_R, the read gradient. Sometimes B_R is identified as the frequency-encoding gradient magnetic field.

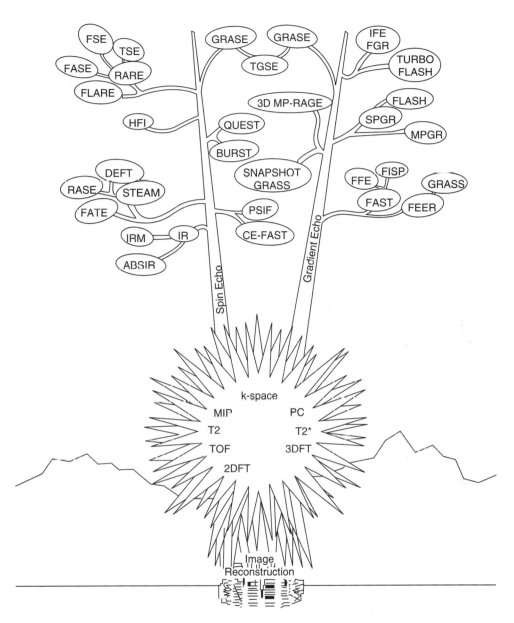

Figure 18-2 Magnetic resonance imaging techniques grouped according to the two principal schemes of image acquisition.

The B_{SS} is energized to establish a difference in resonance frequency along one axis. Usually, it is the long axis of the patient lying supine if transverse images are required. An RF pulse covering a specified frequency range excites proton spins in a slice of the patient.

The transverse magnetization of the patient (M_{XY}) is then phase-encoded, B_Φ, in a direction perpendicular to the long axis of the

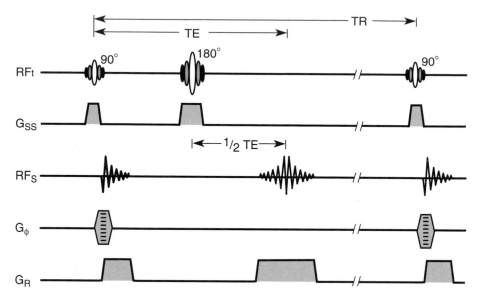

Figure 18-3   The basic spin echo pulse sequence showing the relative timing of each radiofrequency *(RF)* and gradient pulse.

patient, along either the anterior-posterior axis (Y) or the lateral axis (X). This phase-encoding is accomplished by briefly energizing either the X or Y gradient coils. When the phase-encoding gradient magnetic field is off, all spins precess with the same frequency but now have different phase shifts that depend on position along the phase-encoding gradient.

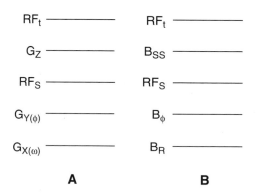

Figure 18-4   Musical score symbol **(A)** used in Chapters 1 through 17 to describe transverse plane images and **(B)** generic form used in the rest of the text.

> *Frequency-encoding of the MRI signal helps locate that signal in the patient.*

Next, the remaining gradient magnetic field, B_R, is switched on for a well-defined interval, during which time the MR signal is received. During this time interval, a difference in resonance frequencies along the direction of frequency-encoding occurs, causing the transverse magnetization to rotate with different frequency depending on location along that axis (Figure 18-5). This is often termed **frequency-encoding.**

The commonly used reconstruction algorithms can distinguish between phase positions of opposite sign. The phase-encoding gradient has to be of a defined amplitude and time duration to distinguish between adjacent voxels (Figure 18-6).

Unfortunately, with just one phase gradient amplitude, an ambiguous signal is received. The solution, as discussed in Chapters 14 through 16, requires that this pulse sequence be repeated with a number of different phase-

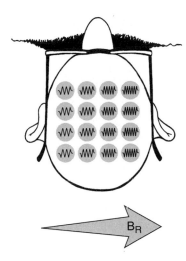

Figure 18-5 Frequency encoding with the B_R gradient magnetic field.

encoding amplitudes equal to the required matrix size.

During the time between the 90° and 180° RF pulses, the spin-spin or transverse relaxation causes a dephasing of the transverse magnetization. Other mechanisms, such as magnetic field inhomogeneities, varying magnetic susceptibility of different tissues, and chemical shift, also contribute to the dephasing of M_{XY} during this time.

The 180° RF refocusing pulse inverts the phase of the spins by putting the faster component of the transverse magnetization behind the slower. This effect should persist over time, except the dephasing caused by nonrandom processes, such as static magnetic field, B_0 inhomogeneity. Inhomogeneity is refocused after the 180° RF pulse to form the SE.

 *When refocusing is provided by a 180° RF pulse, the pulse sequence is called a **spin echo pulse sequence.***

In SE imaging, the spatial frequency domain (k-space) is filled line by line in sequential order from bottom to top (Figure 18-7). This process normally starts with large, negative phase-encoding gradient amplitudes going through zero phase-encoding gradient amplitude and then to a large, positive phase-encoding gradient amplitude.

Weak phase-encoding gradients provide information about the coarse structure of the object in the direction of phase-encoding, contrast resolution. Strong phase-encoding gradients provide information about smaller structures, spatial resolution.

The data are sorted into a raw data matrix. Each measured line of k-space consists of the analog SE sampled and converted to digital form during the read period.

This read period is the time when the frequency-encoding gradient is turned on and data are acquired. The received signal contains the phase information encoded before the read period. Therefore the central zone of the k-space contains the coarse structure of the object (Figure 18-8).

The measured lines of k-space associated with strong phase-encoding gradient pulses contain the information about the smaller details (Figure 18-9). When the entire k-space is filled (Figure 18-10), a complete MR image can be reconstructed with an inverse Fourier transform (FT^{-1}).

A significant source of artifacts in MR images is variation in the subject from one phase-encoded measurement to the next. The FT assumes that each line of k-space came

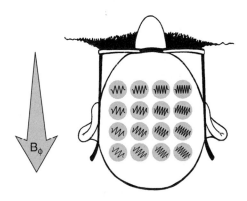

Figure 18-6 Phase-encoding with the B_ϕ gradient magnetic field.

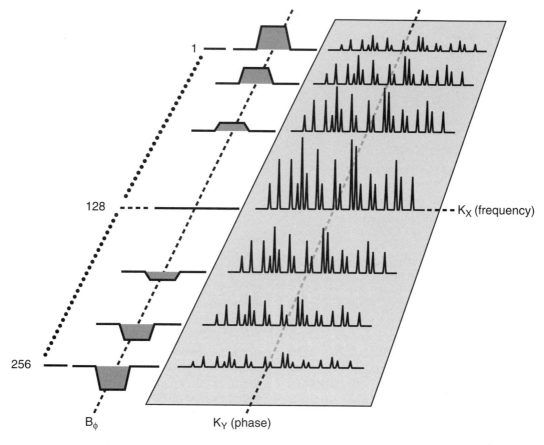

Figure 18-7 The ordering of k-space is sequential in spin echo.

from the same subject. If the subject changes from one repetition time (TR) to the next, this assumption is violated; therefore image artifacts result.

If any object moves from one TR to the next (blood flow, respiration, peristalsis, cardiac), an artifact may result. Phase alterations resulting from motion while gradients are on produce streaking artifacts.

INVERSION RECOVERY IMAGING

Inversion recovery (IR) imaging was introduced as an approach to enhance the T1 weighted (T1W) contrast in SE imaging. For the conventional IR technique, the longitudinal magnetization, M_Z, is inverted before sampling a line in k-space. The pulse sequence is shown in Figure 18-11.

After relaxation with the characteristic T1 relaxation time for each tissue, the SE pulse sequence starts following a given inversion time (TI). The differences among the longitudinal magnetization of various tissues can be larger in IR imaging than in SE imaging (Figure 18-12). The increased difference in longitudinal magnetization in the IR pulse sequence can therefore be used to increase T1W and improve the contrast between tissues with slightly different T1 values.

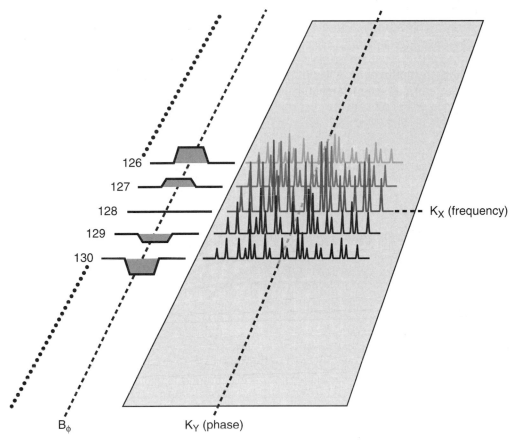

Figure 18-8 Low spatial frequencies acquired from the phase-encoding steps of weaker gradient pulses produce a higher signal-to-noise ratio and higher contrast.

 TI is the time between the 180° RF inversion pulse and the subsequent 90° RF pulse.

A valuable application of IR for some clinical situations is the nulling of signal from tissues having a specific T1 relaxation time. If the SE part of the IR pulse sequence is started so that the longitudinal magnetization of a relaxing tissue is crossing the zero line ($M_Z = 0$) at the time when the 90° RF pulse is applied, there is no net magnetization to be flipped onto the XY plane. Therefore no signal can be produced for that tissue.

For tissue with a short T1 relaxation time, such as fat, a short TI allows elimination of the high signal from fat, thereby improving the image of true abnormalities surrounded by fat. Such pulse sequences are called *short time inversion recovery* (STIR) *sequences.* Figure 18-13 is a coronal T1W, fat-suppressed image that shows right-sided optic neuritis.

Fluid has a relatively long T1, and TIs of about 2 seconds are necessary to minimize the signal from fluid structures. Such a pulse sequence is called *fluid attenuated inversion recovery* (FLAIR). This allows a better diagnosis

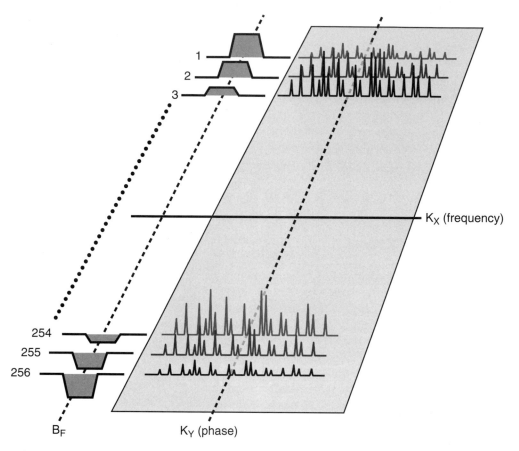

Figure 18-9 High spatial frequencies acquired with strong gradient pulses produce noisier images with better spatial resolution.

of periventricular lesions in which the bright pathological areas are close to the equally bright, fluid-filled spaces.

 STIR and FLAIR are pulse sequences designed to null the signal from fat and water, respectively.

IR techniques can distinguish between a negative net magnetization ($-M_Z$) and a positive net magnetization (M_Z) (Figure 18-14). Zero signal is usually represented as an intermediate gray in the image, whereas negative magnetization is dark and positive values are bright.

A more common technique is one that considers only the absolute value of the net magnetization. Such imaging techniques are called *inversion recovery magnitude* (IRM) or *absolute inversion recovery* (ABSIR). As with SE imaging, techniques used to produce IRM or ABSIR images represent tissue that emits no signal as dark and all other tissue with increasing brightness according to the magnitude of the received signal.

FAST SPIN ECHO IMAGING

The time-consuming part of SE imaging is the necessary repetition of B_{SS} excitation and frequency-encoding B_R with different B_Φ to collect the spatial information of the slice. The

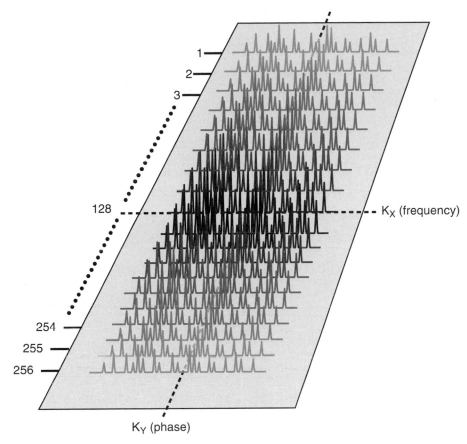

K_X (frequency)

K_Y (phase)

Figure 18-10 When k-space is filled, a magnetic resonance image with good contrast resolution and spatial resolution can be reconstructed.

need to measure k-space line by line in SE imaging is why so many repetitions are required, up to 256.

Partial Fourier Imaging

Two important statements about k-space and the principle of phase-encoding follow. First, when switched on, the phase-encoding gradient magnetic field has to be sufficiently intense and long to establish a sufficient phase shift to distinguish two adjacent voxels. Second, k-space is filled by stepping from a maximum negative phase-encoding gradient amplitude through zero to a maximum positive phase-encoding gradient amplitude in succeeding TR intervals.

A 180° phase shift provided by a maximum negative phase-encoding amplitude and a maximum positive phase-encoding amplitude is illustrated in Figure 18-15. Intuitively, it can be seen that the MRI reconstruction schemes deal with redundant data. Theoretically there is a mathematically defined difference between a negative phase-encoding gradient and a positive phase-encoding gradient of the same amplitude.

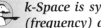 *k-Space is symmetrical about both the X (frequency) and Y (phase) axes.*

The spatial frequency lines acquired on either side of the zero amplitude phase-encoding

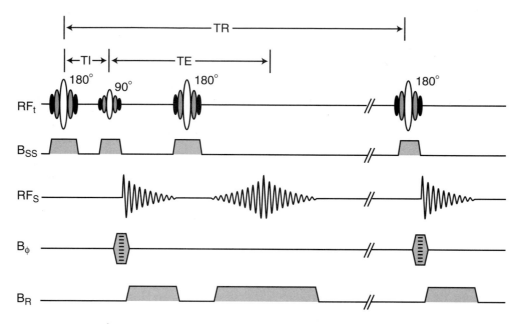

Figure 18-11 Inversion recovery spin echo pulse sequence.

gradient (G_Φ) are symmetrical. This mathematical relationship is called **Hermitian symmetry.**

During imaging, this symmetry can be destroyed in k-space by flow, RF phase shifts, and T2 relaxation while the signal is sampled. In the time domain, misadjusted quadrature signal detection, shifts of the sampling grid, and gradient eddy currents that cause the echo to shift during acquisition also cause the data to be non-Hermitian.

The entire k-space is usually measured in SE imaging to avoid artifacts within the image caused by any violation of the assumption of Hermitian symmetry. The redundant data improves the signal-to-noise ratio (SNR) at the cost of imaging time.

A number of approaches to fast imaging are designed so that half the data are calculated during image reconstruction by assuming Hermitian symmetry, rather than being acquired during signal detection. This technique is often termed *half Fourier imaging* (HFI). Using either half of k-space (Figures 18-16 and 18-17) and calculating the other half are sufficient to produce an MR image.

Such techniques have also been clinically exploited, as in rapid acquired spin echo (RASE), but have become less important for the clinical routine, even though they are slightly superior to SE for certain applications.

Usually there are even better alternatives for those applications (Chapters 19 and 20). With half Fourier acquired single shot turbo spin echo (HASTE), the HFI technique has another useful clinical application. As for the SE method, only half of the data are sampled, and the other half are then calculated. An additional eight lines are sampled for the phase correction to compensate for violations of Hermitian symmetry.

The lines of k-space to be measured are acquired from multiple SEs with a single excitation. Figure 18-18 is a clinical example of a T2 weighted (T2W) study acquired within 1 second with the HASTE approach. HASTE can

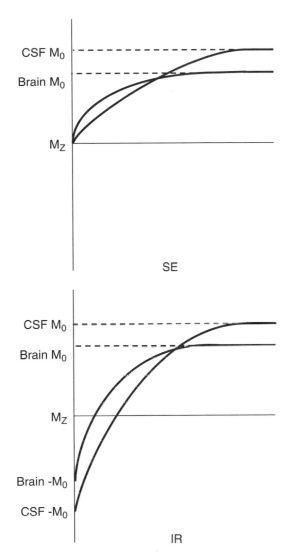

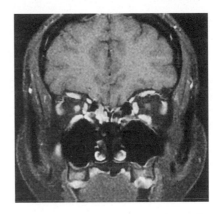

Figure 18-13 Fat suppression enhances the ability to detect right-sided optic neuritis by reducing the high fat signal from surrounding tissue. (Courtesy Robert Tien, Singapore.)

Figure 18-12 Longitudinal magnetization between tissues is greater with inversion recovery *(IR)* than with spin echo *(SE)*.

be combined with inversion recovery magnitude (HASTIRM) to null out fat (Figure 18-19).

Rapid Acquired Relaxation Enhanced Imaging

In 1986, Hennig suggested the use of multiple SEs with phase-encoding between each SE to measure k-space. Hennig named his pulse sequence rapid acquired relaxation enhanced (RARE) technique.

The RARE technique at the time was geared toward heavily T2W applications. The images were inferior in quality to SE images. They had blurring, rippling, and banding artifacts, which prevented widespread clinical acceptance.

In 1989, Mulkern and Wong were working on T2 measurements and needed a fast T2W localizer. They adapted Hennig's idea, recognizing the clinical potential of RARE. They reduced the heavy T2W and minimized the T2 decay-related artifacts. Their technique is known as *fast spin echo* (FSE), and a sample pulse sequence is shown in Figure 18-20. This method has been adapted and refined by many vendors and marketed with trade names, such as turbo spin echo (TSE), dual echo fast acquisition interleaved spin echo (DEFAISE), and contiguous slice fast spin echo (CSFSE).

These FSE pulse sequences use multiple 180° RF pulses to produce up to 16 SEs within a single TR interval. Half the SEs may be used to produce proton density weighted (PDW) images and half for T2W images. A typical pulse sequence uses a TR of 4000 ms and effective TEs of 30 and 110 ms to produce a 20-slice, double echo examination in less than 5 minutes.

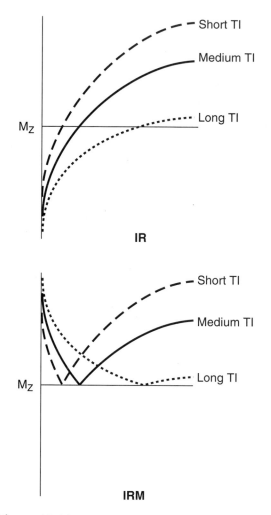

Figure 18-14 Inversion recovery imaging has a contrast range from $-M_0$ to M_0. Inversion recovery magnitude *(IRM)* considers only the absolute value of M_Z and has a contrast range from 0 to M_0.

 FSE imaging uses multiple SEs within a TR, with each SE obtained by a different B_Φ.

Implementing FSE requires hardware changes for faster RF pulses and shielded gradients to allow acquisition of one SE every 10 to 15 ms with multiple RF excitations. However, the required hardware changes are modest compared with those required for echo planar imaging (EPI) in which SEs are obtained every millisecond (Chapter 22).

Because multiple echoes are used to fill k-space, what echo time should be assigned to the image? Because of the importance of low spatial frequencies and those phase-encoding steps with low gradient amplitudes, the echo time at which those Fourier lines are sampled are the important ones. The contrast at that time will dominate the image contrast.

This time is called the **effective echo time** and is used as the echo time assigned to the image (Figure 18-21). Spin echo trains as long as 64 are successfully used, but a 4-echo train is normal. However, as the echo time is increased, the echoes become more heavily T2W, and artifacts can be generated.

The effective echo time is that SE obtained with the lowest amplitude B_Φ, usually the middle SE.

After a first enthusiastic clinical evaluation of this technique, there came a period of caution triggered by observation of differences in contrast between FSE and SE (e.g., bright fat) and by concerns of losing small objects in FSE imaging.

The effect from the signal relaxation during data sampling is similar to the effect observed when a reduced matrix size is used. Depending on the order of phase-encoding, the spin echo train length (ETL), and SE spacing, those spatial frequencies acquired during very late echoes with low signal contributions are underrepresented.

Acquiring high spatial frequencies with the early SEs causes an overrepresentation, and edge-enhancing artifacts may be observed. Acquiring the high spatial frequencies with late SEs causes underrepresentation, leading to ringing artifacts and blurring. Small objects may be lost because the spatial resolution is effectively decreased.

In FSE imaging, the signal for each subsequent measured line of k-space changes because of T2. This is unlike SE imaging in which the signal contribution is constant for each meas-

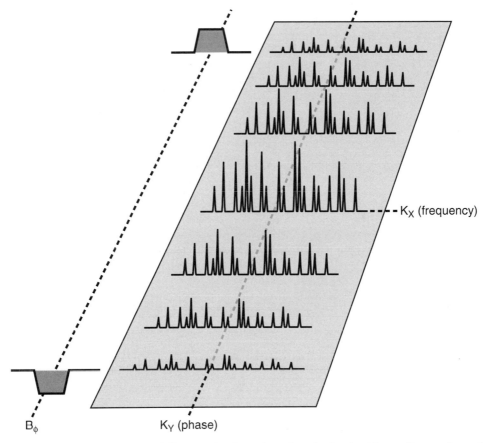

Figure 18-15 There is no difference in the spin echo obtained with gradients of equal amplitude but different polarity.

ured line. This condition is the cause of broadening of the point spread function and is the origin for the blurring, rippling, and banding artifacts sometimes observed in FSE imaging.

The biggest concern in the clinical use of FSE is the fear of not imaging small objects. The low spatial frequencies influence the contrast resolution. The high spatial frequencies influence edge definition and resolution of small objects.

If high spatial frequencies are with the late SEs, they will be underrepresented because of the low signal intensity caused by the T2 relaxation. As with any other imaging technique, pulse sequences and protocols have to be designed to prevent the loss of small objects or small lesions.

 With FSE, superior spatial resolution with better contrast resolution can be obtained in a reduced measurement time.

Besides the potential reduction in measurement time, FSE has expanded clinical capabilities that were otherwise too time-consuming, such as the selection of a TR beyond 3 seconds and the acquisition of 512 or even 1024 matrices. TIs of several seconds have been applied to null out the signal from fluid in FLAIR or IRM methods to study periventricular lesions (Figure 18-22).

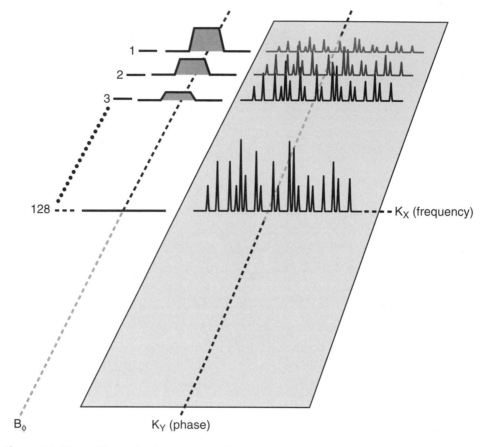

Figure 18-16 Half Fourier imaging speeds image acquisition with little cost in signal-to-noise ratio.

The application of three-dimensional SE techniques has been developed. Using a higher spatial resolution than usually acquired with SE imaging minimizes the concern of losing small objects.

The argument is now quite the opposite; with FSE, better spatial resolution can be achieved in less time than with SE. The result is less motion artifact and reduced phase artifact from flowing blood.

Ordering of k-Space

The measured lines of greater importance to image contrast are those in which the low spatial frequencies are sampled. Low spatial

frequencies represent the coarse structure of the patient and determine the contrast of the image. Those lines of k-space are sampled with low amplitude phase-encoding gradient magnetic fields.

If multiple lines are acquired with more than one SE, the SE following the weakest phase-encoding gradient pulse is called the *zero order spin echo*. The sampled line for this zero order SE fills the zero order in k-space and defines the effective echo time. Without changing the basic pulse sequence, the weighting of the achieved image is changed according to the effective echo time by just reordering the measurement of k-space.

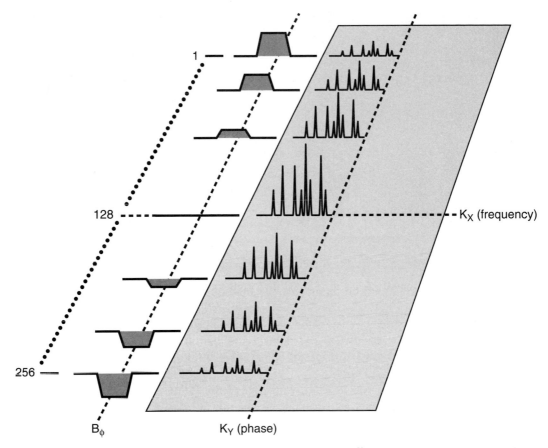

Figure 18-17 Half Fourier imaging can be done equally well with data from either half of k-space.

CONTRAST ENHANCEMENT WITH FAST SPIN ECHO

The differences between the contrast achieved with FSE and the contrast observed in SE imaging are most noticeable in fat (Figure 18-23), in delineation between gray and white matter, and in a reduced sensitivity to magnetic susceptibility gradients with FSE. The better delineation of gray and white matter can be explained as magnetization transfer saturation (MTS) phenomenon (see Chapter 19).

First, let us consider the major relaxation mechanism of protons in tissue. This is dipolar coupling. However, dipolar coupling between protons in water molecules does not happen readily because these molecules are tumbling about and rarely interact.

Also, the free water protons have no other spins to pass their excess energy to. Thus the T1 of pure water can be long, up to several seconds. However, those water molecules that become attached to a macromolecule, bound water, can pass their energy to the protons within the macromolecule because of their fixed geometrical relationship. This is the dipole-dipole interaction, and it has a range of several hundreds of micrometers.

Now, if the bound water protons come into the vicinity of the free water protons, the free water protons have a greater likelihood of giving

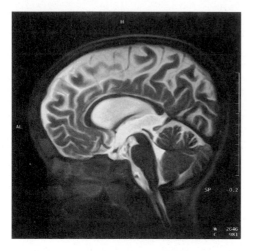

Figure 18-18   A HASTE image, which is always T2 weighted, showing a hydrocephalus (one excitation, 10.9 ms echo spacing, 87 ms effective echo time). (Courtesy William Faulkner, Chattanooga, TN.)

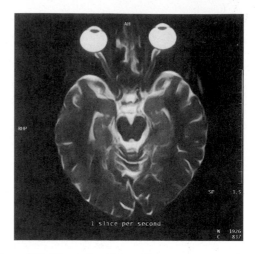

Figure 18-19   A HASTIRM (i.e., HASTE combined with IRM) to null the fat signal (150 ms inversion time before starting the HASTE sequence). (Courtesy William Faulkner, Chattanooga, TN.)

their energy up to the bound water protons. This is due to these protons being fixed to a slowly tumbling macromolecule, and thus they stay in the neighborhood a bit longer than other free water protons.

The bound water protons now act as a conduit for the energy to be transferred from the free water protons through the bound water protons to the protons in the macromolecules. The bound water acts like an energy pipe, and

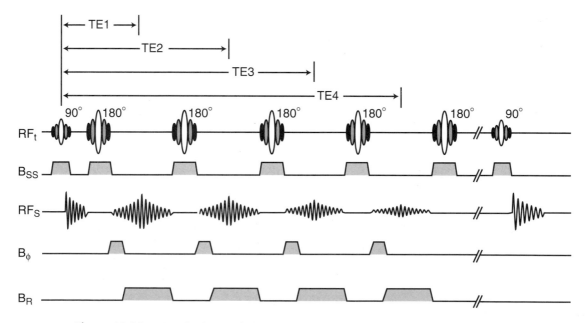

Figure 18-20   Signal relaxation during sampling of fast spin echo pulse sequence.

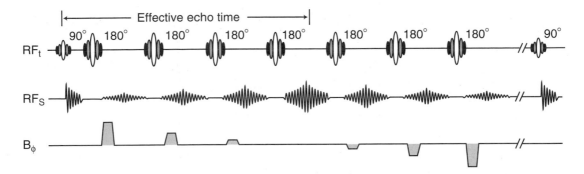

Figure 18-21 Determination of effective echo time during fast spin echo imaging. The maximum signal occurs near the center of k-space (maximum contrast resolution).

the macromolecules act as an energy sink. More important, the net result of this improved energy transfer mechanism is the decrease of T1 from what it would be if there were no macromolecules present.

When an off-resonance MTS RF pulse is applied to the bound water, the bound water protons receive all the energy they can handle. These protons are now saturated and will not be able to pass off any of the energy from the free water protons until they get rid of the energy from the MTS RF pulse. This blocking

of the energy transfer pathway effectively increases T1 for tissues that have a large concentration of macromolecules and makes them appear darker on the T1W image.

 Blood is not affected by MTS, and therefore this process improves contrast on MR angiograms.

In FSE, multiple 180° RF pulses are used for refocusing the spins into an SE. The RF pulse for one slice is off resonance for the remaining slices, causing a saturation of the short T2 components.

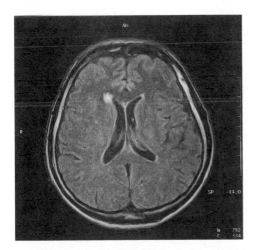

Figure 18-22 A periventricular lesion is seen on this FSEIRM (fast spin echo inversion recovery magnitude) image (T1, 2200 ms; repetition time, 9000 ms; effective echo time, 150 ms). (Courtesy R. Nick Bryan, Philadelphia, PA.)

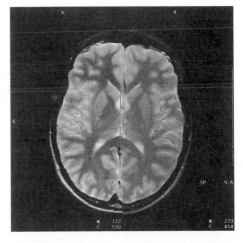

Figure 18-23 *Left side,* fast spin echo. *Right side,* conventional spin echo. Notice the hyperintense subcutaneous fat in the lower left of the image. (Courtesy R. Nick Bryan, Philadelphia, PA.)

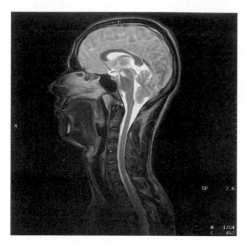

Figure 18-24   T2W FSE study of the cervical spine (TR, 3250 ms; effective echo time, 112 ms). (Courtesy Pedro Diaz-Marchan, Houston, TX.)

By means of magnetization transfer, this leads to increased saturation of the free water.

This saturation causes a further improvement in contrast and is, to a certain degree, responsible for the better contrast between gray and white matter in FSE imaging. The resulting FSE contrast is true T2 contrast, rather than the T2* contrast associated with GRE imaging (see Chapter 20).

Stimulated Echoes

Another significant difference between FSE and SE is the use of **stimulated echoes.** The effect of a 180° refocusing RF pulse is not only to refocus. There is also a component of net magnetization that is unaffected, and thus an additional echo is also created. The latter has its origin within the side lobes of the slice profile where the RF pulse is less than 180°.

In SE, these so-called stimulated echoes are eliminated with a gradient spoiler or an RF spoiler. In FSE, these stimulated echoes are used and contribute up to 15% to the overall signal.

Gradient Motion Rephasing

In addition to increased signal contribution, these stimulated echoes make the pulse sequence design a bit more complicated when

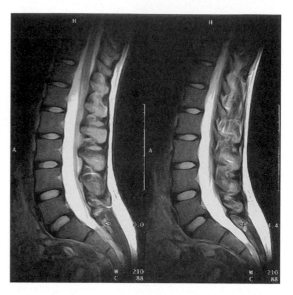

Figure 18-25   T2 weighted fast spin echo study of the lumbar spine acquired in 2 minutes (repetition time, 4000 ms; effective echo time, 120 ms). (Courtesy Pedro Diaz-Marchan, Houston, TX.)

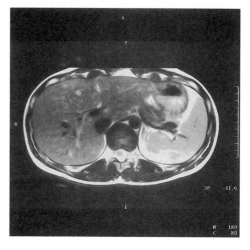

Figure 18-26   T2 weighted fast spin echo of the liver acquired in only 18 seconds (repetition time, 1240 ms; effective echo time, 120 ms). (Courtesy Hani Haykal, Houston, TX.)

it comes to implementing gradient motion rephasing (GMR). The gradient magnetic field timing has to be arranged considering not only primary SEs but now also the secondary or stimulated echoes.

J-coupling

The term *J-coupling* helps explain the relatively bright fat observed in T2W FSE imaging (see Chapter 9). For a complicated structure like fat, there is a coupling mechanism between spins that forces them to more slowly dephase despite the 180° refocusing RF pulse. This dephasing superimposed on the T2 relaxation results in the additional signal loss seen in SE imaging.

For a rapid sequence of 180° refocusing RF pulses, it can be shown that this J-coupling pattern is broken. The missing J-coupling dephasing means relatively more signal and is partially responsible for the bright fat on FSE imaging.

Clinical Applications of Fast Spin Echo

Fast spin echo seems to replace SE in all major applications. For most examinations, the time saved with the use of multiple echoes per TR is less often used to reduce measurement time than to increase spatial resolution. Increasing matrix size can be used to improve the spatial resolution.

With the use of a rectangular field of view in conjunction with FSE techniques, imaging of the spine is done faster with a significantly increased spatial resolution compared with SE imaging techniques. Figure 18-24 shows a T1W cervical spine study acquired in 3 minutes, 25 seconds, with a 512 matrix.

For the lumbar spine study shown in Figure 18-25, the time savings of the FSE technique is even more obvious. A T2W, 512 matrix image is obtained in 1 minute, 56 seconds.

For abdominal applications, T2W measurements can now be acquired in a breathhold, as shown in the 512-matrix image in Figure 18-26. FSE techniques are successfully applied to pelvic and orthopedic studies as well.

CHALLENGE QUESTIONS

1. For two-dimensional Fourier transform (2DFT) MRI, which gradient coil is energized to produce a given slice?
2. What are some advantages to FSE imaging over SE imaging?
3. What is the purpose of the 180° RF refocusing pulse in SE imaging?
4. Describe the difference in the pulse sequence between SE and FSE.
5. What does the second FT refer to in 2DFT MRI?
6. What is GMR?
7. What do STIR and ABSIR relate to?
8. What is a stimulated echo?
9. What is meant by Hermitian symmetry?
10. What is effective echo time?

Chemical Shift and Magnetization Transfer

The gyromagnetic ratio for hydrogen is 42 MHz/T. Therefore, in a 1-T B_0 field, hydrogen nuclei precess with a resonant frequency of 42 MHz. Table 19-1 summarizes hydrogen proton resonant frequency at several other B_0 values.

For a magnetic resonance imaging (MRI) signal to be obtained from tissue, the transmitted radiofrequency (RF_t) must be at the prescribed resonant frequency, say 42 MHz for a 1-T MRI system, to excite the proton spins. However, this situation applies only to proton spins in water, so-called free water.

Although water makes up approximately 80% of all tissue molecules, hydrogen is only approximately 60% of all tissue atoms. Nevertheless, the hydrogen in water predominates and is the principal source of the magnetic resonance (MR) signal.

 Sixty percent of the atoms of human tissue are hydrogen atoms.

However, proton spins in other tissue atoms also contribute to the MR signal if they are excited at the proper resonant frequency. Many schemes have been proposed for compartmentalizing body tissue for the purpose of MRI. The three-compartment model (Figure 19-1) is the simplest and all that is necessary for the discussion of magnetization transfer (MT)— water protons, fat protons, and macromolecular protons. Before proceeding to MT, consider again chemical shift because they are related.

CHEMICAL SHIFT

A revisit to the discussion of the parts per million (ppm) scale in Chapter 9 will show that

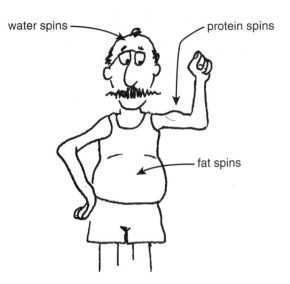

Figure 19-1 The three-compartment model of proton spins in the patient.

ppm is a relative value compared with the standard molecule tetramethylsilane (TMS). TMS is assigned an arbitrary value of 0 on the ppm scale. Water protons are shifted downfield 4.7 ppm and those of fat, 1.2 ppm. This is shown in the spectrum of Figure 19-2.

In a 1-T B_0 field, water protons will resonate at 4.7 Hz lower than TMS. Fat, protons have a resonant frequency 1.2 Hz below that of TMS in a 1-T B_0 field.

All hydrogen in water is bound to oxygen in the same manner. Therefore the water peak is narrow and intense. Hydrogen in fat is bound in many different ways, and this causes the fat peak to be broader and less intense. It is actually the result of many individual spectral lines, each representing a different chemical bond.

TABLE 19-1	Resonant Frequency for Hydrogen Protons as a Function of Magnetic Field Strength B_0						
B_0	0.2 T	0.35 T	0.5 T	1.0 T	1.5 T	3.0 T	4.0 T
Resonant frequency	8 MHz	15 MHz	21 MHz	42 MHz	63 MHz	126 MHz	168 MHz

The resonant frequency for fat differs from that for water because of very small differences in the local magnetic field. Both molecules may reside in an equal B_0 field, but the local magnetic field is slightly different and determined by the configuration of the rest of the bound molecule. Hydrogen spins and other nuclear spins in the same molecule cause this disturbance of the local magnetic field.

 Free water protons and fat protons have a resonance frequency separation of 3.5 ppm.

Because fat and water proton spins are at 4.7 and 1.2 ppm, respectively, their resonant frequency separation is (4.7 − 1.2 = 3.5) 3.5 ppm. At 0.5 T, the frequency difference is small. However, at 1.5 T and higher, the frequency difference can result in a significant artifact.

Fat/Water Chemical Shift
at 0.5 T: 3.5 ppm × 0.5 T × 42 MHz/T
= 73.5 Hz
at 1.5 T: 3.5 ppm × 1.5 T × 42 MHz/T
= 220.5 Hz
at 3.0 T: 3.5 ppm × 3 T × 42 MHz/T
= 441 Hz

Consider the water-filled cyst in the fat glob of the patient in Figure 19-3. The direction of the chemical shift is always along the direction of the frequency-encoded read gradient magnetic field, B_R. The amplitude of the shift is proportional to the external magnetic field, B_0. The appearance of the chemical shift as an artifact is determined by the receiver sampling bandwidth.

For a 256 × 256 image matrix, there will be 256 MR signals acquired with 256 different phase-encoding gradient magnetic fields, B_Φ. Each signal will be sampled and encoded to 256 pixels along the frequency axis. In k-space, the frequency axis is K_Y.

 Receiver bandwidth is the frequency at which an MR signal is sampled.

If the receiver sampling bandwidth is, for instance, 8 kHz, the signal will be sampled as shown in Figure 19-4, and at 1.5 T the pixel shift is approximately 7. Increasing the sampling bandwidth to 32 kHz increases the number of samples and reduces the chemical shift to less than 2 pixels.

Sampling Bandwidth/Pixel Shift
$\dfrac{8\ \text{kHz}}{56\ \text{Pixels}}$ = 31 Hz/pixel
= 2 pixel @ 0.5 T, $\left[\dfrac{73.5}{31}\right]$
= 7 pixel @ 1.5 T, $\left[\dfrac{220}{31}\right]$
$\dfrac{16\ \text{kHz}}{256\ \text{pixels}}$ = 63 Hz/pixel
= 1 pixel @ 0.5 T, $\left[\dfrac{73.5}{63}\right]$
= 3 pixel @ 1.5 T, $\left[\dfrac{220}{63}\right]$
$\dfrac{32\ \text{kHz}}{256\ \text{pixels}}$ = 125 Hz/pixel
= 0.5 pixel @ 0.5 T, $\left[\dfrac{73.5}{125}\right]$
= 2 pixel @ 1.5 T, $\left[\dfrac{22.0}{125}\right]$

MAGNETIZIATION TRANSFER

The proton MR spectrum of Figure 19-2 is not exactly complete. In addition to the resonance peaks of water protons and fat protons, there is a broad background of spins from protons in macromolecules and water bound to macromolecules (Figure 19-5).

Fat and water protons exhibit narrow resonant peaks and relatively long T2, on the order of tens of milliseconds. Macromolecular protons and their associated bound water protons

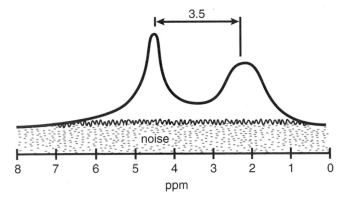

Figure 19-2 The proton magnetic resonance spectrum, showing the separation of 3.5 ppm between fat and water.

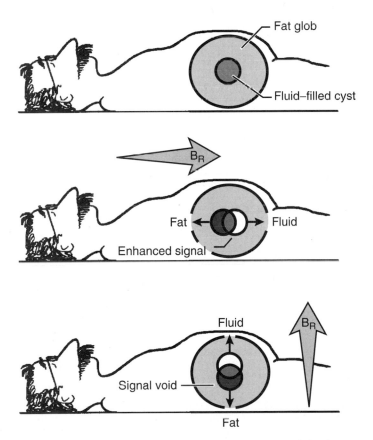

Figure 19-3 The chemical shift artifact appears in the direction of the frequency-encoded read gradient magnetic field, B_R.

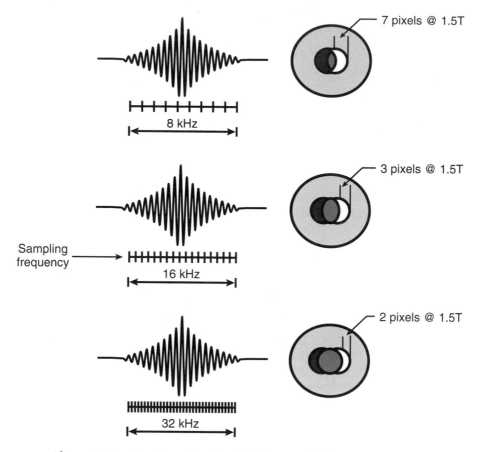

Figure 19-4   Signal sampling bandwidth controls chemical shift artifact.

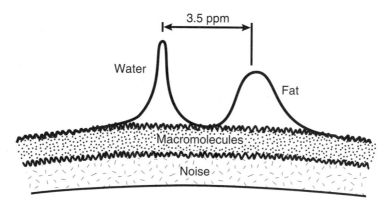

Figure 19-5   The broad spectrum of magnetic resonant frequencies of protons bound to macromolecular reduces contrast by transfer of magnetization to water protons.

exhibit a wide spectrum of resonant frequencies and a very short T2, less than one millisecond.

These characteristics of resonance and T2 result in a transfer of magnetization from free water through bound water to macromolecular protons, resulting in reduction in image contrast. Two methods are used to enhance image contrast by accentuating the signal from water protons.

The use of inversion recovery to saturate fat protons and suppress their signal was discussed in the previous chapter. A 180° RF inversion pulse is followed by a 90° pulse applied at an inversion time (TI), which just matches the time when fat longitudinal magnetization is relaxing through zero from $-M_Z$ to $+M_Z$ (Figure 19-6).

The fat saturation pulse sequence removes those bright tissues from the image and therefore improves the contrast of remaining tissue. However, more can be done by transferring the

magnetization from macromolecular protons and associated bound water protons.

The signal from water protons is relatively long, relatively intense, and of narrow frequency range. The signal from macromolecular protons and bound water protons is very short and of low intensity and wide frequency range. However, it is a signal that can obscure the contrast of free water protons.

The signal from free protons can be increased by saturating the bound spins with an RF pulse offset from the water resonance by a few kilohertz (Figure 19-7). This effectively saturates the magnetization of bound water protons so that they no long act as a conduit to transfer energy from free to bound state. The result is better contrast for fat/water protons.

The MT saturation pulse is followed by any number of routine imaging pulse sequences. Figure 19-8 is an example of MT gradient echo

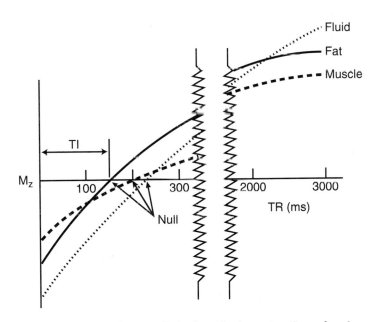

Figure 19-6 The signal from fat is nulled when the inversion time of an inversion recovery pulse sequence occurs at the time fat $M_Z = 0$.

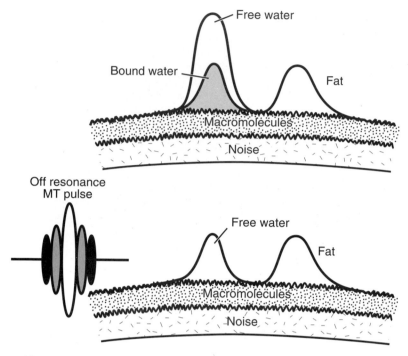

Figure 19-7 With the application of a broadband RF pulse centered off the water/proton peak, the macromolecular protons become saturated and magnetization is transferred to water.

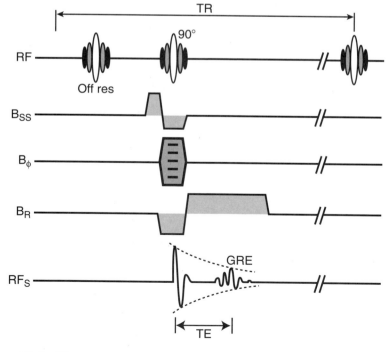

Figure 19-8 The magnetization transfer pulse is an off resonance pulse that precedes a normal imaging pulse sequence, such as the gradient echo shown here.

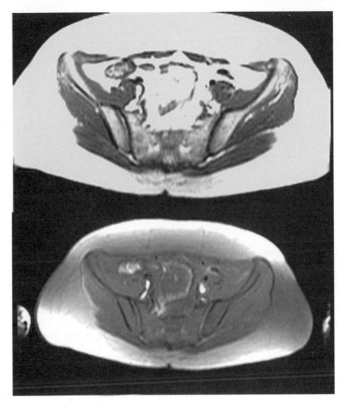

Figure 19-9 An example of incomplete fat saturation due to magnetic field inhomogeneity. (Courtesy Wlad Sobol, Birmingham, AL.)

imaging. The mechanism of MT is not completely understood, but it involves the saturation and therefore suppression of signal from macromolecular and then bound water. Incomplete fat saturation is demonstrated in Figure 19-9.

MT techniques are particularly helpful in magnetic resonance angiography (MRA) and contrast enhanced imaging. During MRA, MT improves vessel contrast by suppressing surrounding tissue. Gadolinium contrast imaging is similarly enhanced by suppressing the bound water signal, which does not bind to gadolinium as free water does.

CHALLENGE QUESTIONS

1. What happens if the RF pulse programmer is tuned to 70 MHz in a 1.5-T MRI system?

2. New imaging systems are being installed with a $B_0 = 3$ T. What is the operating frequency for such an MRI system?
3. Why is hydrogen used for MRI?
4. What is magnetization transfer (MT)?
5. Which has lower resonant frequency: hydrogen in fat or hydrogen in water?
6. Relative to mobile water protons, at what frequency do macromolecular protons and bound water protons resonate?
7. What is the general relationship between receiver bandwidth and the chemical shift artifact?
8. What is the chemical shift between fat and water for a 512-image matrix sampled with a 16-kHz receiver?
9. Along which gradient magnetic field—B_{ss}, B_Φ, or B_R—would a chemical shift artifact appear?
10. What is meant by fat saturation?

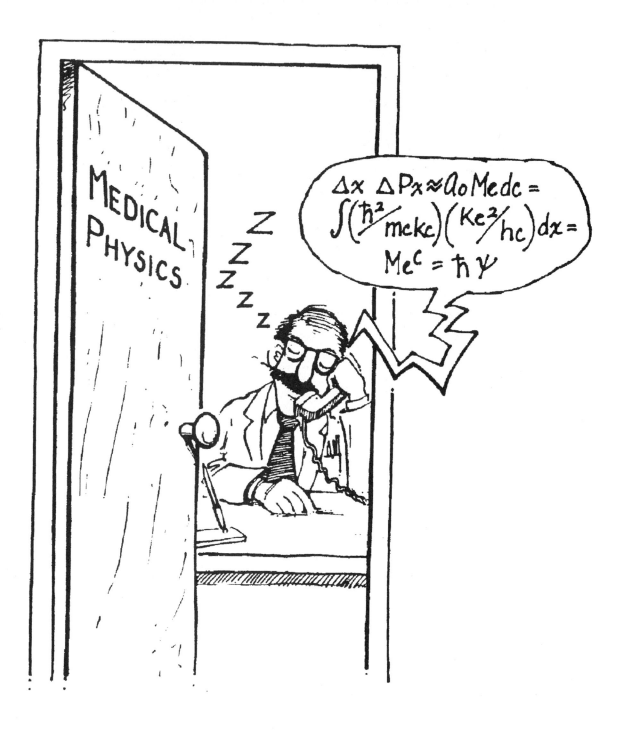

Chapter 20

Gradient Echo Imaging

OBJECTIVES

At the completion of this chapter, the student should be able to do the following:

1. Distinguish between a spin echo and a gradient echo.
2. Explain how a gradient echo is formed using a bipolar read gradient.
3. Identify a steady state pulse sequence.
4. Explain the meaning of a stimulated echo.
5. Define Ernst angle.
6. Discuss the contrast weighting of FLASH and FISP.

OUTLINE

In 1984, the desire for faster imaging led to the introduction of a group of pulse sequences. These pulse sequences lack the 180° radiofrequency (RF) refocusing pulse used in spin echo (SE) imaging.

The elimination of the 180° RF pulse allows the use of a shorter repetition time (TR) than is possible with SE imaging. This results in a decrease in the available longitudinal magnetization (M_Z), leading to a lower signal-to-noise ratio (SNR) and less contrast than if TR were shortened while the flip angle remained at 90°.

The solution to this problem was extracted from nuclear magnetic resonance (NMR) spectroscopy in which the flip angle is not fixed at 90°. Rather, it is optimized for the TR of the measurement and the spin-lattice relaxation time (T1) of the sample. The use of excitation flip angles less than 90°, the use of an α pulse, and the omission of the 180° RF refocusing pulse have allowed adequate SNRs within shorter sampling times.

 In gradient echoes (GREs), spins are refocused with a gradient magnetic field, rather than a 180° RF pulse.

THE GRADIENT ECHO

Figure 20-1 shows the basic pulse sequence for GRE imaging. Immediately after a low flip angle

excitation, α pulse, in the presence of a slice select gradient magnetic field (B_{SS}), a free induction decay (FID) is generated. The negative lobe of B_R is a rephasing lobe. Spins are in phase and precessing at the same frequency (Figure 20-2).

As in SE imaging, the phase-encoding gradient magnetic field (B_Φ) is energized momentarily to produce a difference in phase along the Y-axis. The spins in any column along the Y-axis precess at the same frequency, but now a difference in phase occurs (Figure 20-3). Still, each spin relaxes with equal T2* relaxation time.

If a frequency-encoding read gradient magnetic field (B_R) is energized simultaneously with or after the phase-encoding gradient magnetic field B_Φ, the spins dephase with T2* relaxation time (Figure 20-4).

The read gradient magnetic field, B_R, causes a range of resonance frequencies during data acquisition. This range in frequencies also causes dephasing, which needs to be considered and compensated. Providing B_R with opposite polarity and half the duration of that same gradient during the data acquisition causes an accelerated dephasing; this is followed by

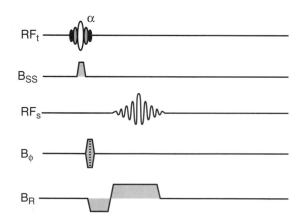

Figure 20-1 The basic pulse sequence for gradient echo imaging.

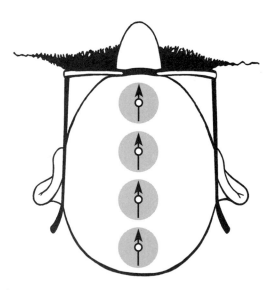

Figure 20-2 Following an α pulse all spins precess at the same frequency with the same phase and dephase with the same T2*.

rephasing and the generation of a gradient-refocused echo, which is known as a gradient echo or GRE (Figure 20-5).

Another view of this method of echo formation is shown in Figure 20-6. The GRE is shown here as forming within the FID. This is the principal reason GRE can be so fast.

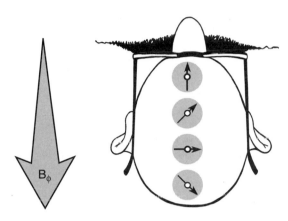

Figure 20-3 When a pulsed phase-encoding gradient magnetic field is applied for an instant to the spins of Figure 20-2, a phase change occurs.

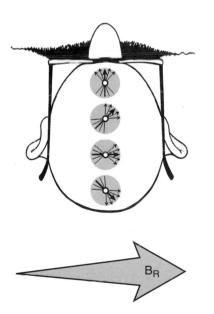

Figure 20-4 When a frequency-encoding gradient magnetic field is applied to the spins of Figure 20-3, T2* relaxation is accelerated.

T2 VERSUS T2*

The GRE signal is generated from an FID when the dephasing gradient is applied early in the FID and immediately reversed. The GRE forms within the time of the FID, and the amplitude depends on T2*.

When an SE is used to generate a GRE, the refocusing B_R can be switched during the first half of the SE (Figure 20-7, *A*) or after the center of the SE (Figure 20-7, *B*). In either case, the amplitude of the GRE depends on T2*. Radiologists rarely use this technique because it requires more time and more intense RF.

In addition to the gradient magnetic fields that are energized in conjunction with a selective excitation α pulse for the purpose of spatial encoding, patient- or system-related factors cause spin dephasing, which makes T2* still shorter. Inhomogeneity of the primary static magnetic field (B_0) and the magnetic susceptibility differences among tissues are typical sources for such spin dephasing.

The influence of B_0 inhomogeneity is further described in Figure 20-8. The voxel in Figure 20-8, *A*, contains five spins aligned and in phase to produce transverse magnetization, M_{XY}, precessing with frequency ω. These spins dephase with time because of T2 relaxation.

In Figure 20-8, *B*, the B_0 does not have uniform intensity (magnetic field inhomogeneity) as indicated by the small arrow. The result is accelerated relaxation (dephasing), which is T2* relaxation.

Even faster relaxation will result if a gradient magnetic field is applied to the voxel. In Figure 20-9, *A*, the application of B_R causes the spins that were dephasing with T2* relaxation time to dephase even more rapidly. If the polarity of B_R is reversed, as in Figure 20-9, *B*, the accelerated dephasing is reversed and the spins rephase to form a GRE. The amplitude of this GRE is that of the FID at that time of relaxation.

Because they usually remain at the same location and are constant over time, these dephasing mechanisms are refocused with the

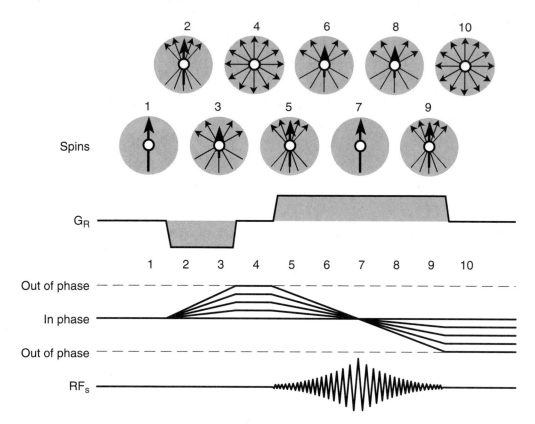

Figure 20-5 A bipolar read gradient magnetic field, B_R, instead of a 180° radiofrequency *(RF)* pulse, produces the gradient echo.

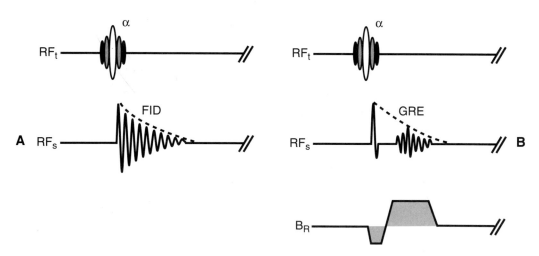

Figure 20-6 **A,** When B_R is energized during a free induction decay, spins dephase more rapidly. **B,** Reversing the polarity of B_R causes the spins to rephase, forming a gradient echo *(GRE)*.

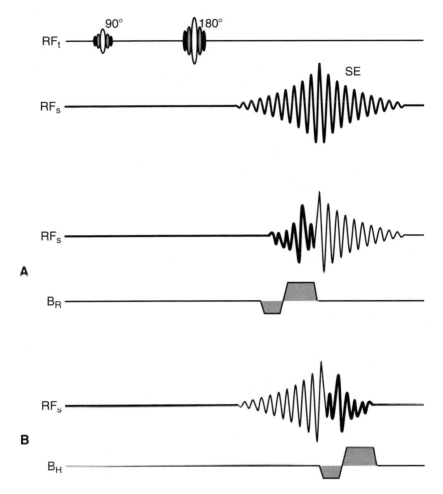

Figure 20-7   A gradient echo can be formed either early or late within a spin echo *(SE)*.

180° RF pulse used in SE imaging. The amplitude of the signal intensity in SE imaging depends on T2, not T2* (Figure 20-10, *A*).

With GRE imaging, the additional dephasing mechanisms contribute to the image contrast and the apparent spin-spin relaxation time is dominated by T2*, rather than T2 (Figure 20-10, *B*). Figure 20-11 shows the dephasing effects of magnetic susceptibility gradients at the base of the skull.

Steady State

One of the first groups to develop GRE imaging called its technique *fast low angle shot*

(FLASH). Other acronyms such as GRASS, FAST, and ROAST also surfaced.

FLASH uses a steady state for the longitudinal component of the macroscopic magnetization, M_z (Figure 20-12). Three repetitions from a long train of low flip angle α pulses are shown in Figure 20-13. Each α pulse generates an FID, as well as SEs. The SEs occur because of the rephasing of spins from the previous α pulses. The total signal, RFs, is the sum of the FID and the SE.

The further away from the fully relaxed state M_z is, the larger the relaxation. With every small flip angle excitation, the M_z

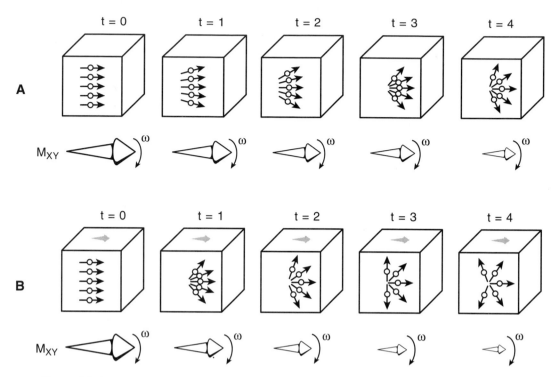

Figure 20-8 **A,** Spins randomly dephase because of T2 relaxation. **B,** Dephasing is more rapid in the presence of a gradient magnetic field as a result of reversible magnetic field inhomogeneities.

shrinks to the point at which the amount of M_Z recovered because of longitudinal relaxation equals the amount of M_Z reduced because of the low flip angle excitation.

 Steady state is the condition of constant longitudinal magnetization after repeated α pulses.

In other words, if the decrease in M_Z because of the excitation is larger than the amount recovered during the TR, the M_Z becomes smaller. A point is reached at which the reduction of magnetization caused by the excitation equals the same amount as the recovery during TR. That condition is **steady state** (Figure 20-14).

If the longitudinal magnetization is far from its fully relaxed state of equilibrium, the absolute recovery is relatively high. This is because exponential relaxation implies that a constant fraction of the remaining difference is recovered in a given time increment. This situation is likely to occur for the steady state of a large flip angle excitation or with short TRs. A decrease in longitudinal magnetization caused by the large flip angle excitation can only reach equilibrium with an appropriate recovery during the time between excitations (TR).

If the longitudinal magnetization is close to equilibrium, the absolute recovery is relatively low. This situation often occurs with the steady state of a low flip angle excitation or with relatively long TRs.

Low Flip Angle

For NMR applications with a short TR, a 90° excitation may not necessarily provide the strongest magnetic resonance (MR) signal. For a low flip angle, only the component of the M_Z

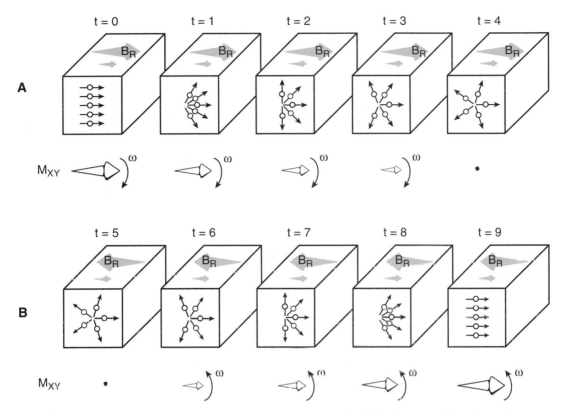

Figure 20-9 **A,** In the presence of a gradient magnetic field, dephasing of the free induction decay increases more rapidly and results in faster reduction in M_{XY}. **B,** Reversing the gradient magnetic field focuses the spins to a weaker signal intensity.

that is projected onto the XY plane produces a signal.

Consider the vector diagram in Figure 20-15. After an RF pulse of 20°, the M_Z decreases only 6% (Cos 20° = 0.94), whereas transverse magnetization, M_{XY}, which is the source of the MR signal, increases to 34% of M_0 (Sin 20° = 0.34).

Increasing the flip angle of the α excitation RF pulse removes the M_Z further from equilibrium while increasing M_{XY}. Table 20-1 shows these changing values for various flip angles. With flip angles less than 60°, more than half of the longitudinal magnetization remains.

Assume that M_{XY} is dephased or **spoiled** before each α pulse in a steady state echo train. For extremely short TRs, low flip angles result in greater signal intensity than those obtained

TABLE 20-1	Relative Longtitudinal and Transverse Magnetization as a Function of Flip Angle Immediately after Radiofrequency Pulse	
Flip Angle (degrees)	**Percent M_Z**	**Percent M_{XY}**
0	100	0
10	98	17
20	94	34
40	77	64
60	50	87
90	0	100

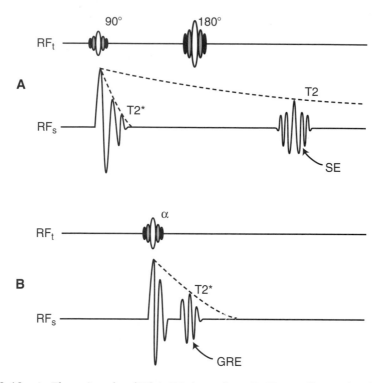

Figure 20-10 **A,** The spin echo *(SE)* is T2 dependent. **B,** The gradient echo *(GRE)* is T2* dependent.

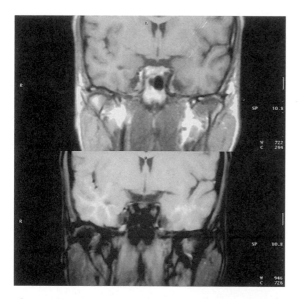

Figure 20-11 Differences in magnetic susceptibility among tissues at the base of the skull result in the dephasing effects shown. (Courtesy Susan Weathers, Houston, TX.)

after the 90° RF pulse of SE with the same short TR (Figure 20-16). At the TR, where M_Z for an α pulse crosses that for a 90° RF pulse, M_Z is almost at equilibrium for the α pulse while it is still increasing for the 90° RF pulse.

Ernst Angle

Depending on TR and the longitudinal relaxation time of tissue (T1), the most intense MR signal is produced with a specific flip angle, the Ernst angle, which is less than 90°. For a given T1 relaxation time, the MR signal might be higher with the use a flip angle lower than 90° (Figure 20-17).

The same signal can also be achieved with a lower flip angle and shorter TRs. For longer TRs, the use of a low flip angle turns into a disadvantage because the available M_Z is underused. For a given TR and for a specific T1 relaxation time, the Ernst angle is always the optimal flip angle in which a maximum signal can be achieved (Figure 20-18).

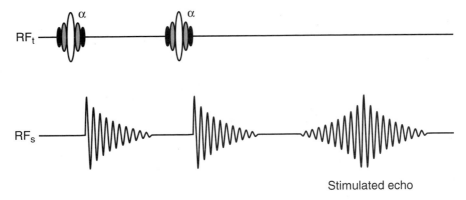

Figure 20-12 A stimulated echo is produced by refocusing the free induction decay.

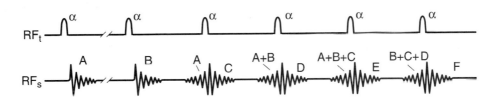

Figure 20-13 Once the steady state is established, stimulated echoes are refocused from several preceding free induction decays. The result is strongly influenced by spin-spin relaxation.

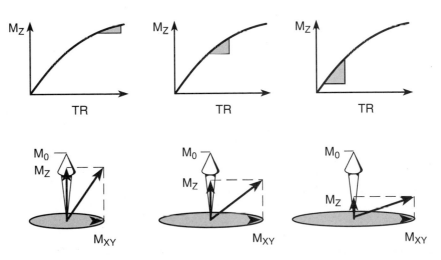

Figure 20-14 A steady state is established.

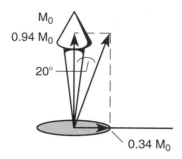

Figure 20-15 This vector diagram shows how a small α pulse can produce relatively large M_{XY}.

 The shorter the TR, the smaller the flip angle necessary to achieve maximum signal intensity.

The optimum flip angle is a compromise between projecting enough magnetization onto the XY plane to induce sufficient signal and leaving enough in the longitudinal direction to use for the next excitation. This approach provides a different contrast than that observed in SE imaging.

FLASH VERSUS FISP

With FLASH, gradient magnetic field spoiling (or RF spoiling) is generally used to destroy the phase coherence of M_{XY} (Figure 20-19). This approach is identical to the technique used in SE imaging to avoid stimulated echo-related artifacts. With this spoiling, only the M_Z and its recovered portion become involved in the next measurement.

There is another group of GRE pulse sequences that operates with a steady state for the M_Z and the M_{XY}. This group is called *fast imaging with steady state precession* (FISP) or *steady state coherent* (SSC) sequences. In FISP or SSC sequences, the aim is to establish not only a steady state in the longitudinal direction but also a steady state within the transverse plane (Figure 20-20).

Rather than spoiling the transverse magnetization that has been dephased for the purpose of spatial encoding, the magnetization is rephased after data acquisition. This is accomplished by designing the gradient waveform so that the areas of positive and negative amplitude cancel and the waveform is balanced. Because this is repeated for each measured line of k-space, it is expected that a steady state also develops in the transverse plane.

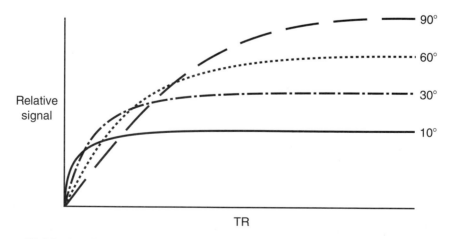

Figure 20-16 For tissue with a given T1 relaxation time, signal intensity is higher with a flip angle that is less than 90° and has a short repetition time *(TR)*.

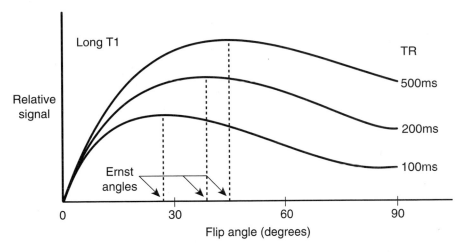

Figure 20-17 The Ernst angle is the flip angle that produces the strongest signal at a given repetition time *(TR)*.

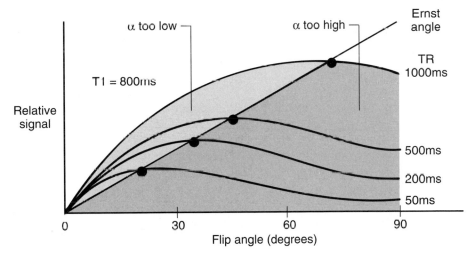

Figure 20-18 The Ernst angle is a function of repetition time *(TR)* and T1.

 A pulse sequence with a gradient balance in all three directions is referred to as a true FISP.

Balancing in the read direction of phase-encoding alone, with the standard variation of FISP, leads to an integration of the steady state free precession (SSFP) signal over a so-called resonant offset. This is also called *resonant offset acquisition into steady state* (ROAST). A true FISP, including gradient motion rephasing (GMR), is also known as *constructive interference of steady state* (CISS).

A difference in image appearance between FLASH and FISP occurs only if certain conditions are fulfilled. First, only tissues with a long T2* show an enhanced signal. For short T2*, the dephasing becomes too rapid to build

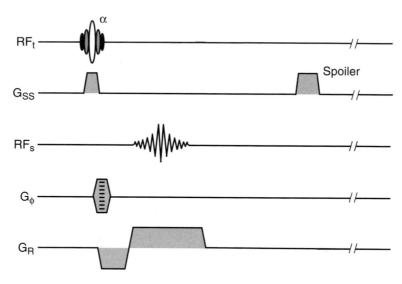

Figure 20-19   A gradient magnetic field spoiler destroys the phase coherence of M_{XY}.

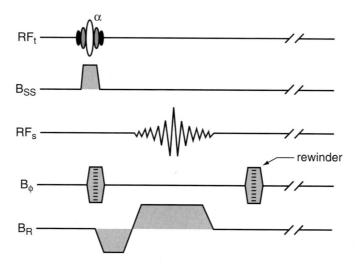

Figure 20-20   Some GRE sequences, such as FISP and SSC, establish the steady state in both M_Z and M_{XY}.

up a steady state of the transverse component. Second, the transverse component is nurtured according to the projection of the longitudinal component.

The larger the flip angle, the bigger the contribution to the transverse steady state.

Because the steady state in the transverse plane, M_{XY}, must be developed and maintained over several repetitions, T2* dephasing tends to destroy this coherence. Consequently, the shorter the TR, the better the image contrast.

Finally, the contribution to the transverse steady state should appear at the same phase for a constructive interference. Any motion of the patient that changes the phase history does not provide the necessary phase coherence, and the transverse steady state is not established. FISP, GRASS, FFE, and FAST are trade names for such SSFP sequences.

CONTRAST-ENHANCED TECHNIQUES

Once the steady state is reached after two or three α pulses, signal intensity occurs because of both the FID and the SE (Figure 20-21). A GRE obtained from this signal at echo time (TE) is generated with the sum signal of both the FID and the SE. Such a GRE mixes contrast dependent on proton density (PD), T1, and T2 as determined by the values of TR, TE, and α.

Contrast manipulation in GRE imaging is accomplished by precisely timing the read gradient magnetic field, B_R.

If the phase of the α pulse reverses or cycles properly, the SE component of the signal can be suppressed (Figure 20-22). The GRE formed

under this condition only reflects the FID and exhibits T1 weighted contrast.

If the refocusing gradient is energized before the α pulse (Figure 20-23), the result is the same as removing the FID. With this the GRE is formed from only the steady state SE and results in a T2 weighted image. Table 20-2 summarizes the relationship between image contrast and the type of signal used to generate the image.

Precession of steady state imaging fast (PSIF) is an SSFP sequence that produces an RF SE, rather than a GRE. PSIF is not a GRE sequence. The name, PSIF, shows that it is a time-reversed FISP. The data are first acquired, then comes the phase-encoding, and finally the excitation (Figure 20-24).

Although PSIF looks like a violation of causality, it is not. The signal collected with a PSIF technique has been prepared in the previous excitation. Because the echo is created in the previous excitation, the effective echo time is approximately twice the TR. That explains the heavy T2 weighted results.

This technique can be used to study the inner ear (Figure 20-25). A double echo sequence in which both the FISP echo and the

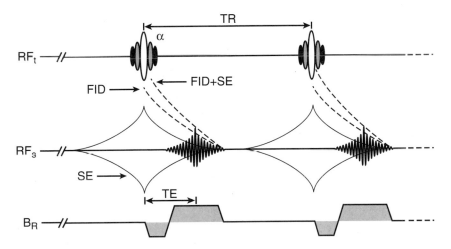

Figure 20-21 In the steady state, signal intensity occurs because of both the free induction decay *(FID)* and the spin echo *(SE)*.

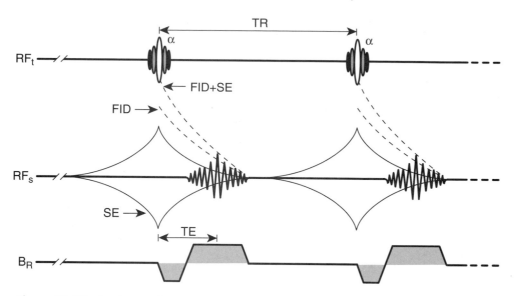

Figure 20-22 In the steady state, suppressing the spin echo *(SE)* component of the signal results in T1 weighted contrast.

PSIF echo are acquired is called *fast-acquired double echo* (FADE).

Adding the FISP echo and the PSIF echo increases the T2 weighting of the basic FISP

image. This approach allows a better delineation of fluid, fat, and cartilage (Figure 20-26), making it promising in orthopedic work. This is called *double echo steady state* (DESS).

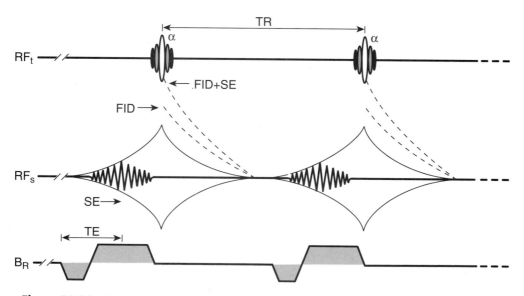

Figure 20-23 In the steady state, suppressing the free induction decay *(FID)* component of the signal results in T2 weighted contrast.

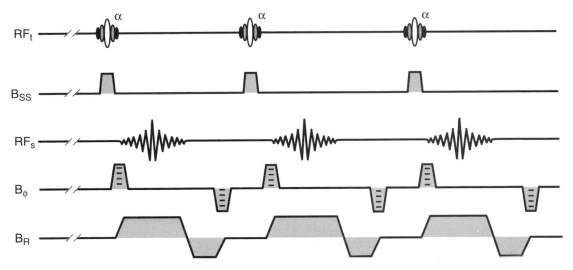

Figure 20-24 The PSIF pulse sequence.

TABLE 20-2	Image Contrast Weighting According to Gradient Echo Signal Used

GRE Signal	Weighting Image Contrast
FID × SE	Mixed
FID	T1W
SE	T2W

FID, Free induction decay; *GRE,* gradient echo; *SE,* spin echo; *T1W,* T1 weighted; *T2W,* T2 weighted.

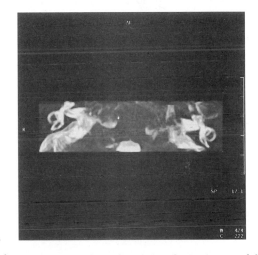

Figure 20-25 A three-dimensional PSIF image of the inner ear (TR = 17 ms, effective TE = 30 ms). (Courtesy Susan Weathers, Houston, TX.)

On the basis of the GRE method, new clinical applications have surfaced and are well established. Some examples include applications in orthopedics (Figure 20-27) and dynamic studies of the heart with the use of breathhold imaging techniques (Figure 20-28).

Whenever a GRE application uses a flip angle between 30° and 70°, it is probably an Ernst angle approach. The Ernst angle is also determined for time-of-flight (TOF) angiography in which both relaxation of blood and tissue replacement need to be considered. The same criterion, maximizing signal strength by choosing the optimum flip angle, is also used in ultrafast GRE imaging.

The absolute relaxation is lower when most of the net magnetization lies along the Z-axis. Although that relaxation is a function of the longitudinal relaxation time, T1, for that tissue, the differences in absolute relaxation of net magnetization are small for even great differences in T1. If only a small part of the available

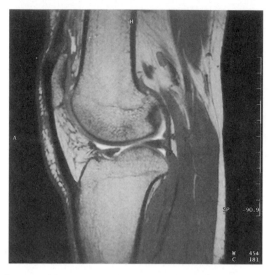

Figure 20-26 A three-dimensional DESS image of the knee showing destruction of cartilage (TR = 28 ms, effective TE = 52 ms). (Courtesy Tom Hedrick, Houston, TX.)

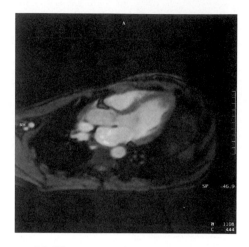

Figure 20-28 A two-dimensional image in a dynamic study of a long axis view of the heart showing the aortic outflow tract and the mitral valve (TR = 40 ms, TE = 7 ms, α = 30°, 6 min). (Courtesy Tom Hedrick, Houston, TX.)

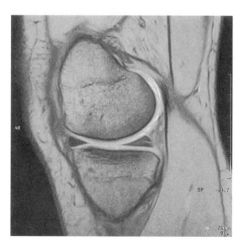

Figure 20-27 A two-dimensional example of a meniscal tear (TR = 560 ms, TE = 10 ms, α = 60°, 7 min). (Courtesy Tom Hedrick, Houston, TX.)

net magnetization is projected onto the XY plane, while most magnetization remains in the longitudinal direction, then only a slight disturbance from equilibrium occurs and the absolute relaxation is small.

Such a recovery rate is almost independent of the T1. Using an extremely low flip angle

(i.e., 5° to 15°) establishes a situation in which the MR signal strength is almost constant, even with shorter TR times and tissues with significant differences in T1 relaxation times.

CHALLENGE QUESTIONS

1. What is the principal advantage to GRE imaging?
2. What are the general characteristics of Ernst angle imaging?
3. What mechanism is used to rephase spins during GRE imaging?
4. What characterizes SSFP imaging?
5. Why is the read gradient magnetic field, B_R, bipolar in GRE imaging?
6. Graphically illustrate the difference between T2 and T2*.
7. What principally determines the value of T2*?
8. What is the difference between FLASH and FISP?
9. What is the Ernst angle?
10. How does signal intensity vary with flip angle from 5° to 90°?

Chapter 21

Faster Imaging Techniques

OBJECTIVES

At the completion of this chapter, the student should be able to do the following:

1. Identify the pulse sequence characteristic of turbo imaging.
2. Explain the use of a preparation pulse in fast imaging.
3. Describe sequential filling of k-space and its application.
4. Define isotropic imaging and the application of MPRAGE technique.
5. Draw a GRASE pulse sequence.

OUTLINE

TURBO IMAGING
GRADIENT AND SPIN ECHO IMAGING

Speeding up image acquisition by reducing the repetition time (TR) and flip angle, α, causes a loss of contrast in gradient echo (GRE) images. Those parameters, which are usually available to improve contrast, are constrained by speed and signal-to-noise requirements

Improved T1 weighted (T1W) contrast can be obtained in a fashion similar to that used in spin echo (SE) imaging with the inversion recovery (IR) technique. Recall that in IR SE, the inversion of spins occurs before each sampled line of k-space.

TURBO IMAGING

These methods often have names with a *turbo, snapshot, insta,* or *hyper* prefix. GREs are acquired after several α pulses prepared by an inversion pulse (Figure 21-1). For each line of k-space, a different spatial frequency in the direction of phase-encoding is sampled with each phase-encoding step.

 Low spatial frequencies, which contain the patient's coarse structure, follow weak phase-encoding gradients.

Low spatial frequencies are more important to image contrast than high frequencies, which primarily contribute to edge enhancement and spatial resolution. Understanding this spatial frequency weighting is the key to understanding both the image contrast behaviors of faster imaging and the way that a static image can be obtained from a moving object.

 High spatial frequencies, which contain the patient's fine structure, follow strong phase-encoding gradients.

TurboFLASH, snapshotFLASH, snapshotGRASS, and others are all similar imaging techniques that were introduced at different times by different groups who worked with different equipment. In this discussion, these techniques are identified as "turbo" because that is the term most adopted.

The common approach to turbo imaging is a 180° inversion pulse at the beginning of the sequence to generate T1W contrast. Other spin preparation methods have been introduced to provide T2 weighted (T2W) contrast or flow-diffusion weighting. With this technique, the data are acquired while the tissue relaxes.

Each line of k-space deals with a different amount of longitudinal magnetization (M_Z). In other words, each line has a slightly different T1W. The lines of k-space acquired with low

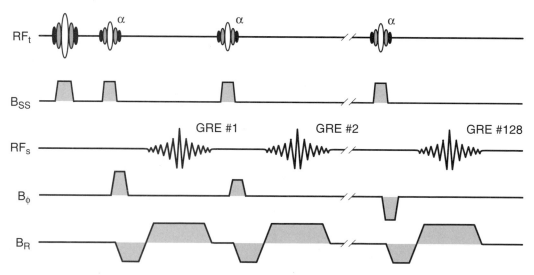

Figure 21-1 Data acquisition for turboFLASH imaging techniques.

amplitude phase-encoding gradients that sample the lower spatial frequencies are important for image contrast.

For certain clinical applications, these turbo techniques challenge the established GRE technique. Although the GRE technique provides an image within 10 seconds, turbo pulse sequences are 10 times faster and provide an image within 1 second.

One-second images bring to mind new clinical applications; however, the simultaneous multislice GRE technique is almost as fast as the sequential multislice turbo approach in abdominal imaging within a breathhold. Nevertheless, because the turbo technique results in an image one slice at the time, there is a noticeable reduction in motion artifacts.

When compared with GRE, turbo imaging has additional degrees of freedom to control the contrast within the image. In Figure 21-2 a breathhold liver study acquired with a GRE technique is compared with one acquired with the turboFLASH technique.

These turbo imaging techniques significantly increase the diagnostic capabilities of magnetic resonance imaging (MRI) in applications like the imaging of the first pass of con-

trast agents, such as Gd-DTPA (gadolinium-diethylene-triamine-pentaacetic acid). Studying the temporal course of Gd-DTPA distribution within liver and breast lesions or for brain perfusion studies results in a better temporal resolution and sometimes a better signal-to-noise ratio (SNR) than GRE imaging.

When the available magnetization changes over time, as in the turbo methods, another imaging parameter becomes an issue: the scheme of filling k-space. The order in which k-space was filled in SE or GRE imaging was unimportant because the acquisition began after reaching a steady state. Each line of k-space dealt with the same amount of M_Z.

 The order in which k-space is filled during turbo imaging adjusts image contrast.

With turbo imaging, this condition is no longer fulfilled. The k-space–ordering scheme becomes an adjustable parameter to achieve the desired contrast. Figure 21-3, *A*, shows that k-space is being filled sequentially from the smallest phase-encoding gradient to the largest. In Figure 21-3, *B*, the filling of k-space is ordered by particular selection of the amplitude of the

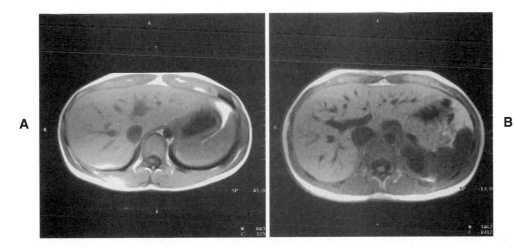

Figure 21-2 **A,** Breathhold liver image gradient echo. **B,** Breathhold liver image with turboFLASH.

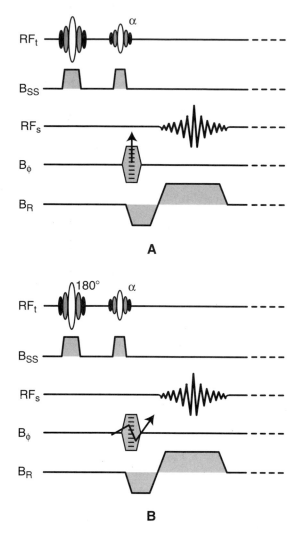

Figure 21-3 **A,** The k-space is normally filled sequentially from the lowest line up. **B,** The filling of k-spaces is selectable in turbo imaging to adjust contrast.

phase-encoding gradient. This tool is valuable because the course for the relaxation of M_Z is altered depending on the flip angle used throughout the signal acquisition.

Another degree of freedom for adjusting contrast occurs by changing the flip angle of the radiofrequency (RF) excitation pulse from one Fourier line to another. An RF pulse of a given angle excites the same fraction of the Z-axis magnetization regardless of the degree of

relaxation. Thus the early Fourier lines would be measured from stronger transverse magnetization (M_{XY}) than later lines when the flip angle increases for the later Fourier lines.

It is possible to use a larger fraction of the Z-axis magnetization, thereby keeping the magnitude of M_{XY} constant from line to line of k-space. This makes it possible to reduce the blurring effects observed for large differences in signal response from one Fourier line to another.

Consider a turbo technique applied to the heart with 64 phase-encoding steps and a 10-ms TR. This would result in an imaging time of 640 ms. Such an imaging time is probably still too long to freeze heart motion, but this deficiency can be partially corrected by segmentation (Figure 21-4).

In SE and GRE imaging, this problem is solved by triggering the acquisition for each Fourier line to correspond with a fixed time in the cardiac cycle. In segmented faster imaging, a certain number of Fourier lines are acquired (e.g., 7 lines) so that a 133×256 matrix can be filled within 19 heartbeats.

Such a technique allows dynamic imaging of the heart with breathholding to reduce respiratory motion. Figure 21-5, *A*, is a segmented fast low angle shot (FLASH) with five lines per segment acquired in 1 min, 12 s. Figure 21-5, *B*, was obtained in 16 heartbeats (one breathhold) with nine Fourier lines per segment.

Mugler at the University of Virginia is credited with introducing the three-dimensional (3D) version of turbo techniques, called the *magnetization prepared rapid gradient echo* (MPRAGE) *technique.* In two-dimensional (2D) turbo imaging, the net magnetization is prepared before acquiring all the Fourier lines. To simply apply this approach to a 3D acquisition scheme is not advised because more excitations alter the course of the relaxation and destroy the initial preparation.

The solution is the use of turbo techniques for all in-depth phase-encoding steps. A recovery period is allowed before proceeding to the next in-plane, phase-encoding step, which begins again with the inversion to prepare M_Z

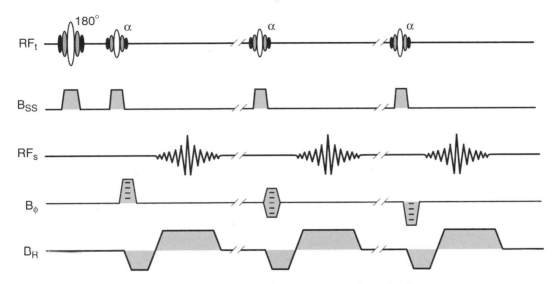

Figure 21-4 The concept of segmentation of Fourier lines.

(Figure 21-6). The amount of M_Z is the same for each step for in-plane phase-encoding. For the depth-encoding loop, the signal acquisition is done along the relaxation path. This accounts for the difference in contrast between turbo and MPRAGE techniques.

Using a varying flip angle reduces artifacts further. Spatial frequency filtering causes reduction by shaping the signal's approach to steady state. Acquiring data while M_Z relaxes applies a spatial frequency filter to the ideal spatial frequency spectrum.

 Spatial frequency filtering changes apparent spatial resolution and contrast resolution.

The term **filter** in this context comes from electrical engineering in which the relative strengths

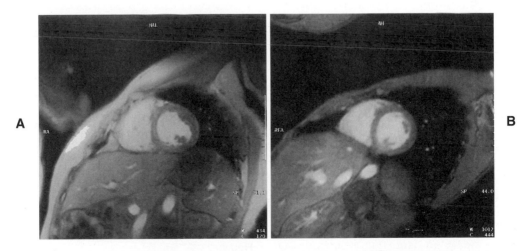

Figure 21-5 Short axis views of the heart acquired with varying degrees of segmentation.

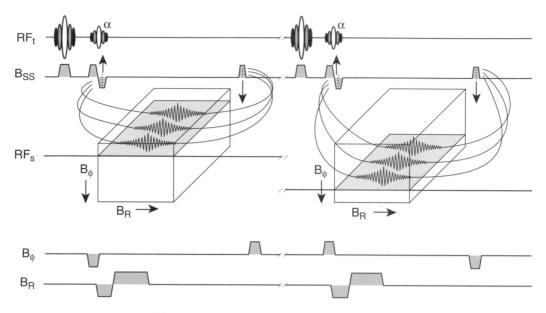

Figure 21-6 The MPRAGE pulse sequence.

of high and low spatial frequencies are modified. When high spatial frequencies are amplified, edge sharpness increases. When low spatial frequencies are amplified, blurring increases and apparent contrast resolution improves.

The same thing happens when measuring the high or low spatial frequencies. When the Z-axis magnetization is nearly relaxed, an emphasis of the high or low spatial frequencies produces an edge sharpness or blurring, respectively. As a result, the original object is inaccurately represented.

This spatial frequency filter is likely to produce image artifacts that appear as blurring, ringing, and edge enhancement. With variation of the excitation angle from one depth-encoding step to the next, it is possible to achieve a signal course where this spatial frequency filter effect is eliminated, resulting in fewer such artifacts. Figure 21-7 represents a T1W study of the head in which the entire head is imaged in approximately 7 minutes with an isotropic resolution of 1.25 mm.

GRADIENT AND SPIN ECHO IMAGING

Feinberg and Oshio introduced the combination of fast spin echo (FSE) and GRE, which they called gradient and spin echo (GRASE)

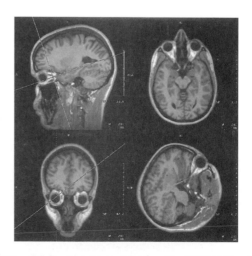

Figure 21-7 Image acquired with MPRAGE with isometric resolution of 1.25 mm and no gaps.

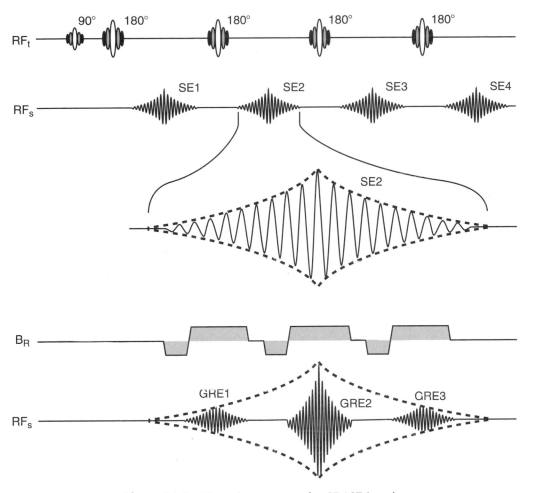

Figure 21-8 The pulse sequence for GRASE imaging

imaging. Rather than only one echo being sampled between 180° refocusing pulses, three GREs are acquired (Figure 21-8). The principal advantage of this technique is a significantly shorter echo train, which leads to more slices per TR and a lower RF power deposition.

Because the J-coupling pattern remains intact, this sequence also provides a fat intensity similar to SE techniques. The GRASE technique has a higher sensitivity to magnetic susceptibility, which is typical for GRE imaging techniques.

CHALLENGE QUESTIONS

1. What is TURBO imaging?
2. What does GRASE identify?
3. How does TURBO imaging differ from SE or GRE imaging in regard to the filling of k-space?
4. Which of the following pulse sequences results in more patient RF exposure: SE, IR, GRE, FSE, or GRASE?
5. Why is ordering of k-space so important for TURBO imaging?
6. What is meant by the term *high pass filter*?

7. What is meant by segmental imaging in cardiac studies?

8. Diagram the RF pulse sequence and signal acquisition sequence for a TURBO FLASH imaging technique.

9. What does the symbol B_Φ with the step indication mean?

10. What is isotropic imaging?

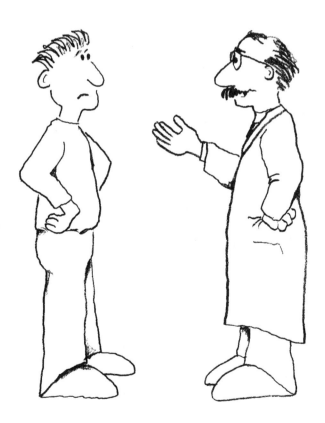

"I assure you... your magnetic personality
won't affect our MRI."

Chapter 22

Echo Planar Imaging

OBJECTIVES

At the completion of this chapter, the student should be able to do the following:

1. Diagram an echo planar imaging pulse sequence.
2. Describe the multiple ways that k-space is filled during echo planar imaging.
3. Identify the enhanced hardware requirements for echo planar imaging.
4. Report on several clinical situations that are particularly suited to echo planar imaging.

OUTLINE

ECHO PLANAR IMAGING
HARDWARE REQUIREMENTS

Echo planar imaging (EPI) is a method for extremely fast formation of the magnetic resonance (MR) image. Some of its commercial implementations have trade names that imply instantaneous image acquisition. Although that may be a slight exaggeration, imaging times of 50 ms to produce images of moderate quality are realistic.

ECHO PLANAR IMAGING

In 1977 Mansfield first introduced the concept of EPI. The distinguishing characteristic of EPI is the filling of k-space after a single radiofrequency (RF) excitation. Each line of k-space does not require separate spin excitation as in spin echo (SE) or gradient echo (GRE) imaging.

The entire k-space can be sampled and filled by measuring either the envelope of free induction decay (FID) or that of an SE. In either case, the entire image is acquired in a single RF excitation and therefore one repetition time (TR).

 The fundamental idea of EPI is to fill k-space with the magnetization produced by a single RF pulse.

SE and GRE techniques measure only a portion of k-space in each TR interval. That portion is typically one Fourier line of k-space. Thus T1 is a consideration because it is necessary to allow longitudinal magnetization to recover before the next portion of k-space can be measured.

EPI avoids this problem by measuring all of k-space in one pass. However, because this one pass may be rather long, spin-spin relaxation (T2) during signal sampling becomes an issue. The raw data measurements must be made rapidly to measure all of k-space before the transverse magnetization M_{XY} is substantially altered in magnitude by T2* relaxation.

Thus the magnetic resonance imaging (MRI) system must be capable of extremely fast and high-amplitude gradient switching and rapid data acquisition. Manufacturers have solved these engineering and hardware requirements.

A single RF excitation α pulse is followed by a 180° RF refocusing pulse. The MR signal read phase contains a train of GREs produced by rapidly switching the read gradient magnetic field (B_R) (Figure 22-1).

After a single excitation, the read gradient is switched from one polarity to another, generating a GRE each time. Phase-encoding is done with a small constant gradient throughout the acquisition. This way, each echo has a different phase-encoding and can be used to fill k-space. Acquisition times are about 10 times faster than those for the turbo imaging techniques described in Chapter 21.

The train of echoes obtained in EPI is produced by switching the gradient magnetic field and sampling the signal in the envelope of the SE. EPI GREs are produced with modifications of the scheme shown in Figure 22-1 and are termed *BEST* and *FLEET* by various vendors.

The original echo planar method proposed by Mansfield was complicated by limitations of his hardware. A more recent version, blipped echo planar, makes a better introduction to how EPI works.

Figure 22-2 shows the pulse sequence diagram of a blipped echo planar image. Figure 22-3 shows the path through k-space that is traversed in sampling the GRE signals.

There is only one RF pulse. The phase-encoding gradient waveform consists of a string of short, relatively weak "blips" (hence, the name of the sequence). Between each blip, the frequency-encoding gradient waveform is turned on rapidly to a maximum value and then turned off just before the next blip. Signals are acquired between the blips.

The frequency-encoding read gradient magnetic field, B_R, alternates between positive and negative amplitude. This is the reason the path in the k-space goes back and forth. The phase-encoding gradient pulse moves the path to the left edge of the k-space at the same time the frequency-encoding gradient pulse moves the path to the bottom.

The acquisition of data starts during the B_R pulse, which moves the path from left to right.

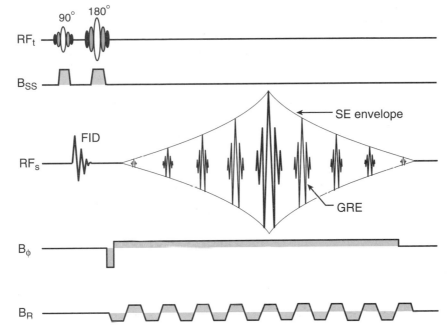

Figure 22-1 The basic pulse sequence for echo planar imaging.

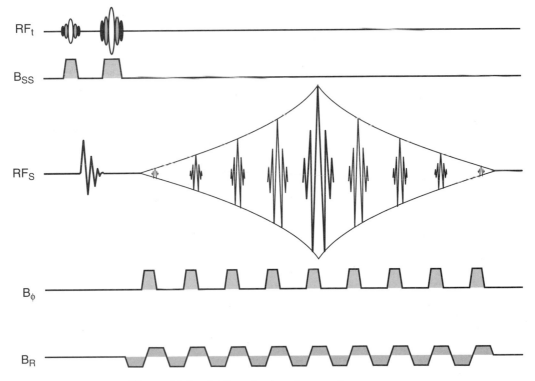

Figure 22-2 A blipped echo planar pulse sequence.

The blip pulse shifts the path up one row. Then another B_R pulse, which is of the opposite amplitude, moves the path from right to left. The phase-encoding gradient blips shift the path to different rows, and the frequency-encoding gradient pulses sweep the path along a row.

Figure 22-4 shows images of the same slice from the same patient. The SE image (Figure 22-4, *A*) was acquired in 7 min, 8 s. The echo planar image (Figure 22-4, *B*) was acquired in 120 ms. There is still only one RF pulse used for excitation with EPI.

The transverse magnetization is prepared by the 90° and 180° RF pulses, and then the regular blipped echo planar gradient waveforms follow. T1 weighted (T1W) sequences can be constructed in a similar fashion by placing RF pulses that implement a partial saturation or an inversion recovery (IR) contrast weighting in front of the echo planar acquisition.

HARDWARE REQUIREMENTS

The hardware requirements of EPI include switching the frequency-encoding gradient and receiving the MR signals rapidly and nearly continuously. These hardware requirements were the original impetus for the development of shielded gradient coils; the eddy currents induced in unshielded gradient coils destroy the EPI signal, even if they are sufficiently small to allow routine SE and GRE imaging.

Exceedingly fast, high-intensity gradient magnetic fields are required for EPI. Rise and fall times of approximately 100 µs are required.

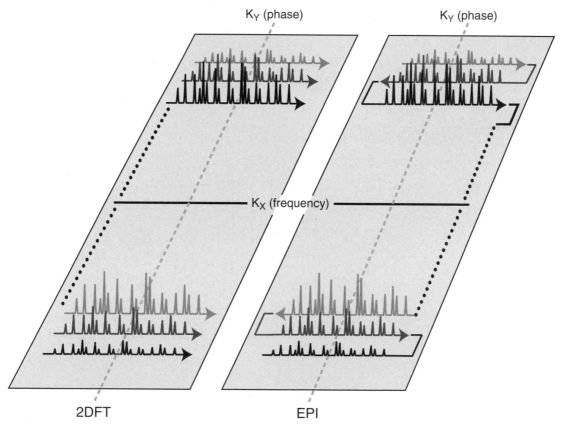

Figure 22-3 The path through the k-space traversed in blipped echo planar imaging.

Gradient magnetic fields exceeding 25 mT/m are necessary.

The attractions of EPI have encouraged engineering to overcome these technical obstacles. The use of a single excitation RF pulse means that the echo planar image reflects a brief interval of time.

 Echo planar images can be obtained at radiographic speed, approximately 50 ms.

SE and GRE techniques must image dynamic processes by synchronizing to the physiological cycle, as in cardiac imaging. It is assumed that the variations from cycle to cycle are minimal to measure each line of k-space at the same phase of a physiological cycle.

EPI excites the spins once and then rapidly acquires all the data needed for the image. In its faster implementations, EPI has temporal resolution equivalent to ultrasound and electron beam computed tomography (EBCT). Thus it is possible to image patients with cardiac arrhythmias and to look at fast processes in the brain, such as oxygen use and contrast

agent dynamics. EPI is also used for dynamic imaging of the viscera and the human fetus.

EPI requires special MRI hardware and data-handling capacity. However, a number of methods similar to echo planar that do not require such exotic hardware have been proposed and investigated. The gradient and spin echo (GRASE) method mentioned in Chapter 21 is an example of a hybrid of fast spin echo (FSE) and EPI. Between each pair of 180° RF pulses, not just one SE but several GREs are formed. Those GREs are the same as the echoes generated by the echo planar approach.

There are a number of methods for filling k-space in patterns such as spirals, square spirals, and rosettes. These methods map the entire k-space with the magnetization from a single RF pulse, although some of the implementations of these ideas segment the acquisition and use a few RF pulses to cover all of k-space.

Image contrast can be readily manipulated in EPI to accentuate tissue differences of proton density (PD), T1, or T2. Spin preparation

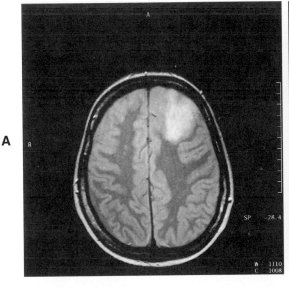
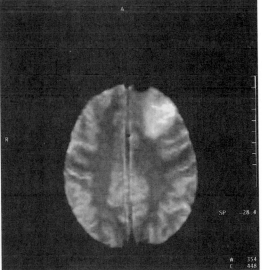

Figure 22-4 T2 weighted images acquired by **(A)** spin echo in 7 minutes, 8 seconds and **(B)** echo planar imaging in 120 ms.

for fat or water suppression, chemical shift imaging, T1W with an inversion pulse, and flow encoding are possible.

 The principal advantage to EPI is the ability to freeze motion.

With EPI times of 50 to 100 ms, even cardiac motion, up to 10 cm/s, is reduced as in a radiographic image. Indeed, EPI represents cineradiography-like MRI.

A concern about the use of this technique has been the physiological stimulation threshold. A rapidly changing magnetic field (dB/dt) or its correlated electric field (dE/dt) may result in nerve stimulation, leading to muscle contraction. Very powerful gradient magnetic fields are necessary to produce high-resolution images or ultrashort imaging times.

The required rapid switching of these gradients can produce magnetic field changes up to 100 T/s. This is above the reported neural stimulation threshold of approximately 60 T/s. Ventricular fibrillation has been induced at 250 T/s. Most currently developed EPI techniques are well below that stimulation threshold.

Another problem for practical EPI is the chemical shift artifact. It is necessary to use some sort of technique, such as fat saturation, to minimize the intensity of the fat signal and avoid unacceptable degradation of the echo planar image.

Typical applications for EPI are dynamic studies of heart motion, first-pass tracing of contrast agents, functional imaging, and fast imaging of moving structures. With diffusion and perfusion mapping, this technique shows potential to further increase the diagnostic capabilities of MRI.

CHALLENGE QUESTIONS

1. What is the fastest mode of MR image acquisition and how fast is it?
2. What are the principal applications for EPI?
3. Which of the following RF pulse sequences deposits the least energy in tissue for a given image: SE, IR, FSE, GRE, EPI, or GRASE?
4. Why is fat saturation technique often required for EPI?
5. How can an entire image be formed with a single SE signal?
6. What particular potential hazard is associated with EPI?
7. Which of the following nuclear magnetic resonance (NMR) parameters—PD, T1, or T2—is changing during signal acquisition in EPI?
8. Which prevails in EPI: PDW, T1W, or T2W?
9. What is a shielded gradient coil, and why is it important for EPI?
10. What principal hardware characteristics are required for EPI?

Part V

Applications

Chapter 23

Magnetic Resonance Angiography

OBJECTIVES

At the completion of this chapter, the student should be able to do the following:

1. Describe the flow-void phenomenon.
2. Discuss the origin of flow-related enhancement.
3. Distinguish between time of flight and phase contrast magnetic resonance angiography (MRA).
4. Draw both two-dimensional (2D) and three-dimensional (3D) pulse sequences for MRA.
5. Explain plug flow, laminar flow, turbulent flow, and pulsatile flow.

OUTLINE

Motion affects magnetic resonance imaging (MRI) both beneficially and detrimentally. It is possible to measure motion and to determine information, such as myocardial velocity and blood flow. Vessels can also appear displaced or disappear entirely. Important structures can be obscured by motion artifacts. Nevertheless, there is widespread acceptance of magnetic resonance angiography (MRA), in which flowing blood is visualized directly.

The effects of motion in MRI can be separated into magnitude effects and phase-shift effects. Each of these produces artifacts and gives rise to methods of motion measurement and MRA. This chapter considers motion visualization and measurement.

 The four fluid motions of blood are plug flow, laminar flow, pulsatile flow, and turbulence.

The motion itself can be complicated. Fluid flow is often described as being **plug flow,** in which all of the fluid moves at the same speed (Figure 23-1, *A*). Fluid flow can also be described as fully developed **laminar flow,** in which the speed varies in a parabolic fashion across the lumen of the vessel. The speed is slowest at the walls of the vessel and fastest in the center (Figure 23-1, *B*). **Turbulence** is the random motion of blood in regions of discontinuity, such as stenosis or bifurcation.

Blood flow in the arteries is **pulsatile** with regular acceleration and deceleration (Figure 23-1, *C*). The velocity profile changes from pluglike (when the fluid is accelerated) to almost parabolic (when the force on the fluid is relatively constant).

In some vessels, such as the aortic root and the femoral arteries, the direction of flow can reverse briefly during part of the cardiac cycle. At specific points in the cardiac cycle, it is possible to have forward flow in some parts of the lumen and retrograde flow in others. Even some systemic veins have cyclic variations in flow caused by the respiratory cycle.

A plot of the velocity of blood flow as a function of distance from the center of the vessel is called a *velocity profile* (Figure 23-1, *A*, *B*, and *C*). The changing flow rate is shown in Figure 23-1, *D*, as a function of time for pulsatile flow.

There are two basic ways to display flowing blood and produce an MRA. During radiofrequency (RF) excitation, the inflow/outflow or "flight" of proton spins results in time of flight (TOF) effects. During signal sampling under the influence of the frequency-encoded read gradient magnetic field (B_R), spins moving in the direction of B_R experience a phase shift, resulting in phase contrast (PC) effects.

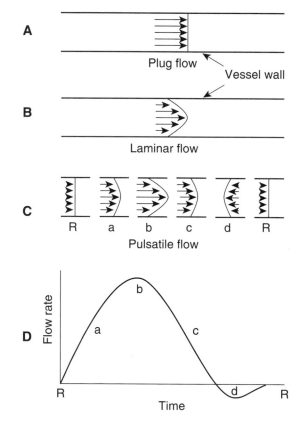

Figure 23-1 **A,** Plug flow occurs when the fluid throughout the vessel moves at the same velocity. **B,** Laminar flow is characterized by a parabolic distribution of velocities. Fluid near the vessel wall moves slowly while fluid near the center moves faster. **C,** In pulsatile flow, the periods of acceleration resemble plug flow, and the periods of constant flow resemble laminar flow. **D,** The blood flow rate changes with time.

Although physiological motions can be complex, only simple motion is considered in the following discussion of motion effects. This is one reason why there are a variety of MRA methods in regular use. Different methods are better in different regions of the body.

 Rapid blood flow results in dark blood; slow flow results in bright blood.

Depending on velocity, flowing blood can appear dark or bright. In general, for spin echo pulse sequences, rapidly flowing arterial blood creates a "flow-void" and appears dark. Slowly flowing venous blood usually appears bright.

Furthermore, the appearance of blood flow is very much a function of the pulse sequence, gradient magnetic field intensity, and slew rate. Additionally, flow-compensating gradient magnetic fields influence the visualization of flowing blood.

Three factors contribute to flow-void and signal loss during rapid blood flow: high velocity, turbulence, and dephasing. Similarly, three factors principally contribute to signal gain: flow-related enhancement, even-echo rephasing, and pseudogating.

MAGNITUDE EFFECTS

The discussions of equilibrium saturation in previous chapters assumed that the proton spins were stationary. When motion is perpendicular to the imaging slice, it is possible for spins that have experienced one or more RF pulses, and are therefore partially saturated, to be replaced by fresh spins.

The fresh spins may be at equilibrium (i.e., $M_Z = M_0$) because they have not yet experienced an RF pulse. Consequently, the fresh spins transported into the slice by motion can appear brighter than if they had remained stationary within the slice. Stationary spins would have been excited by recent RF pulses and thus are not at full equilibrium (Figure 23-2).

Spin-lattice relaxation (T1) is the process by which spins give up energy to the molecular environment to relax to equilibrium. The

replacement of partially saturated spins by fresh spins can be viewed as an acceleration of the T1 process. Of course, the fact that the new spins are different from the old spins must be ignored; however, that is the nature of MRI.

Turbulence

The identity of spins is inferred from their location. The lumen of a vessel actually contains a lot of different spins during the course of acquiring the data for a magnetic resonance (MR) image, yet they all appear to be the same in the image.

At regions of discontinuity in the vasculature, such as stenosis or bifurcation, flowing blood becomes turbulent (Figure 23-3). The result is exceptional intravoxel dephasing and loss of signal.

Flow-Void

Consider the situation present in spin echo imaging (Figure 23-4). To form a spin echo, blood must be subjected to both the 90° RF pulse and

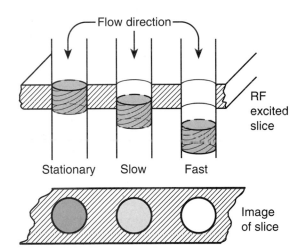

Figure 23-2 Stationary tissue is partially saturated by a regular radiofrequency *(RF)* excitation. Fluid flowing into the slice is at equilibrium and produces a stronger signal. The faster the flow, the greater the fraction of the slice thickness in which partially saturated blood is replaced by fresh blood during repetition time.

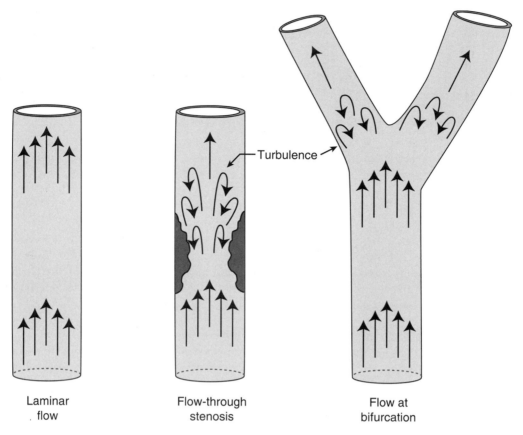

| Laminar flow | Flow-through stenosis | Flow at bifurcation |

Figure 23-3 Turbulent flow is disorderly flow that occurs in the region of a stenosis or downstream from a bifurcation.

the 180° RF pulse. Therefore stationary blood appears much like the surrounding tissue.

When blood moves slowly, many proton spins exit the imaging section and are not subjected to the 180° RF refocusing pulse. The result is reduced signal intensity.

When blood flow is very fast, the blood protons saturated by the 90° RF pulse leave the imaging section before the 180° RF refocusing pulse and no signal is emitted. The result is **flow-void.**

Flow-Related Enhancement

Contrary to flow-void with fast-moving blood is **flow-related enhancement (FRE),** associated with slow blood flow. During multislice

imaging, slow-moving blood entering the first slice (the entry slice) has a different spin property from the tissue slice.

Depending on the T1 of stationary tissue and the repetition time (TR) of the pulse sequence, the tissue will be in a state of partial saturation. The TR is too short or the T1 is too long, or both, for tissue spins to relax to equilibrium. With no flow, the stationary blood appears as the surrounding tissue (Figure 23-5).

Suppose the slice thickness is 10 mm and blood flow is 1 cm/s, typical for veins. Blood flowing into the slice is unsaturated at equilibrium, whereas that of surrounding tissue is partially saturated. Therefore the

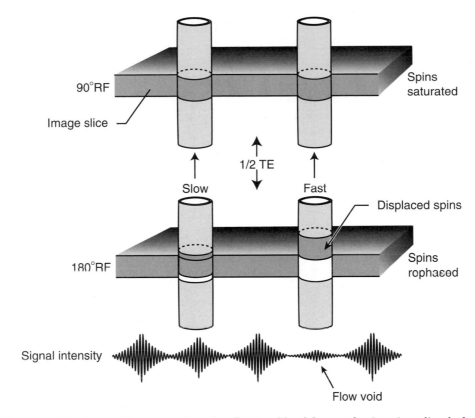

Figure 23-4 Flow-void occurs when fast-flowing blood leaves the imaging slice before receiving the 180° radiofrequency *(RF)* rephasing pulse.

inflowing blood will have higher magnetization available (M_Z) and will emit a stronger signal (FRE). The maximum FRE occurs when blood velocity is sufficient to just replace the blood in the imaging slice during TR.

 When blood velocity equals the slice thickness (mm) divided by TR (ms), FRE is maximum.

FRE is most visible on T1 weighted (T1W) images at short TR. The appearance of FRE in slices deep into the volume of multislice images reflects the parabolic shape of laminar flow and therefore may appear only in the center of the vessel lumen (Figure 23-6).

PHASE SHIFT EFFECTS

When an excited, stationary spin is in the presence of a gradient magnetic field, its precessional frequency depends on its position along that gradient magnetic field (Figure 23-7, *A*). Likewise, a spin that moves along the gradient has a precessional frequency that changes with its position along the gradient magnetic field (Figure 23-7, *B*).

The change in precessional frequency with motion along a gradient magnetic field can be directly observed, if the motion takes place while the B_R is energized. However, it is usually manifested as a phase shift that represents the total difference in precession between the

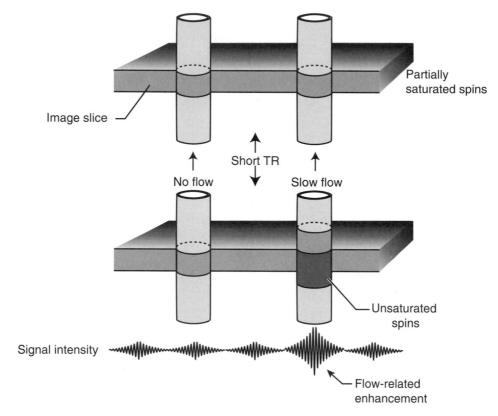

Figure 23-5 Flow-related enhancement occurs when blood flow is slow. Protons at equilibrium enter the slice, while protons in adjacent tissue are partially saturated. The unsaturated blood emits a higher intensity signal.

moving spins and stationary spins in the same voxel.

FLOW MEASUREMENT

It is possible to use a bipolar gradient pulse to sensitize the pulse sequence to motion so that the previously mentioned phase shift is linearly proportional to velocity (Figure 23-8). This is the basis of most flow-measuring methods in MRI. Table 23-1 relates the vendor acronyms used in marketing their respective flow compensation pulse sequences.

Flow compensation gradient magnetic fields are also called *motion artifact suppression technique* (MAST) and *gradient moment*

nulling (GMN). The term *moment* refers to zero order (stationary), first order (velocity), second order (acceleration), and third order (pulsatility motion). Gradient magnetic fields are tailored to null each order moment in flow-compensated imaging. Cardiac MRI (Chapter 26) requires multiple flow-compensating gradients.

During fast imaging with very short TR, every slice is an entry slice and FRE is prominent. Furthermore, because most vessels enter the imaging slice obliquely, the low-flip angle and short TR of fast imaging intensify FRE in all vessels.

The pulse sequence usually makes two measurements that have different sensitivities to motion along the motion-measuring direction.

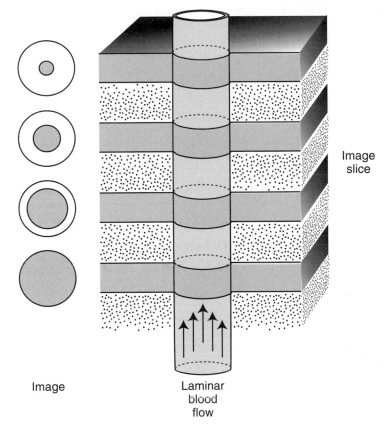

Image slice

Image

Laminar blood flow

Figure 23-6 Because of laminar blood flow, the flow-related enhancement takes on a varying appearance in multislice imaging.

The velocity is then determined from the difference in phase between these two measurements.

Dual measurements are necessary because there are other effects that produce phase shifts in an MR image. These include chemical shift differences and magnetic susceptibility differences.

These sources of phase shift give the same amount of phase shift in both motion-sensitive measurements, whereas motion gives rise to different amounts of phase shift in the two measurements. Thus the difference between the two measurements yields phase shifts that only arise from motion. This phase shift difference is directly related to velocity in the sensitive direction.

 Phase shifts can distinguish true from false lumens in aortic dissections.

Flow is usually measured by multiplying the velocity of each pixel by the area of the voxel that is perpendicular to the direction of motion sensitivity. This gives a reasonably accurate result in vivo, although the phase shift of the pixel represents a nonlinear averaging of the velocities present in the voxel. Improvements of the method and clinical flow packages are available on most imaging systems.

It is also possible to use intensity effects to measure flow. For example, one method of flow measurement is to apply a thin saturation pulse in a plane that is perpendicular to the

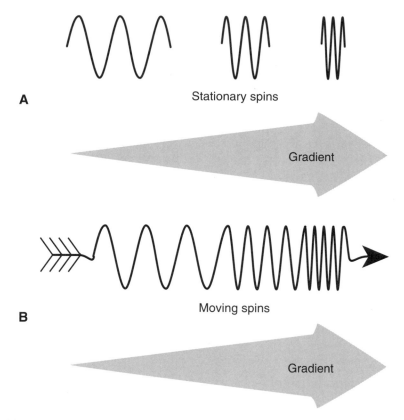

Figure 23-7   A, Stationary spins resonate at different frequencies depending on location along a gradient magnetic field. **B,** Spins moving along that gradient have a constantly changing resonant frequency. This is similar to the sound made by a trombone that is played while moving the slide.

imaging plane. This makes a dark line across the image. If a number of images are acquired at varying delays from this saturation pulse, the dark line moves in regions of moving tissue (e.g., flow in blood vessels).

The displacement of the line during the known delay between saturation and measurement can be divided by the delay time to give a velocity estimate. For example, this method has been used to detect and measure retrograde flow in the blood vessels serving the kidneys.

The two broad categories of motion artifacts are those related to intensity errors and those related to phase-shift errors (Chapter 28). The phase-shift errors are often detected as streaks

emanating from arteries of the heart chambers. These streaks are parallel to the phase-encoded direction of the two-dimensional Fourier transform (2DFT) image. Intensity errors can actually be beneficial, and they are exploited to produce MR angiograms.

MAGNETIC RESONANCE ANGIOGRAPHY

MRA is now routine because of the benign nature of MRI; therefore MRA is useful as a screening procedure for suspected vascular disease.

MRA is used extensively to examine the extracranial circulation of the neck, especially

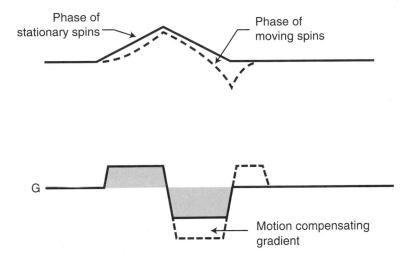

Figure 23-8 A bipolar gradient waveform consists of two pulses of equal area but opposite polarity. Thus it does not have a net effect on stationary spins. However, spins moving with a constant velocity gain less phase shift during the first pulse than they lose during the second. This results in a net phase shift proportional to velocity.

the carotid and vertebral arteries. It is also useful in examining the intracranial circulation, especially the circle of Willis.

Arteriovenous malformations and aneurysms are often examined by MRA. Although slow venous flow still poses technical challenges, MRA is used to examine all parts of the aorta, renal arteries, and peripheral circulation, including arteries and veins. MRA may be the only way to evaluate the circulation of patients who are allergic to iodinated x-ray contrast agents.

 Time of flight (TOF) and phase contrast (PC) are the two methods for MRA.

There are two ways to approach MRA: first analyze either the intensity or phase-shift mechanism for sensitivity to motion. Second, check to see whether the data acquisition is two-dimensional (2D) or three-dimensional (3D). Because these views are somewhat independent, the sensitivity mechanisms can be treated as fundamental, whereas the

TABLE 23-1	Flow Compensation Acronyms	
Vendor	**Name**	**Acronym**
General Electric	Flow compensation	FLOW COMP
Philips	Flow adjustable gradient waveform	FLAG
Hitachi	Motion artifact suppression technique	MAST
Siemens	Gradient moment rephasing	GMR
Toshiba	Flow compensation	FLOW COMP
	Flow artifact suppression technique	FAST

appropriateness of the data acquisition method (i.e., 2D or 3D) for each mechanism can be secondary.

Time of Flight Magnetic Resonance Angiography

The expression *time of flight* (TOF) has become popular to describe the intensity-based approach to MRA. Consider the effect of TR on the wash-in of fresh spins. The longer the TR, the larger the fraction of a vessel volume within the excited region (i.e., the 2D slice or the 3D volume) that contains fresh spins at equilibrium.

TOF attempts to capture this idea of spin replacement during the interval between RF stimulations of the excited region. It should not be confused with the different use of "TOF" in positron emission tomography (PET) image reconstruction.

In TOF MRA, the thickness of the excited region, the flip angle of the RF pulses, and the TR are optimized for the speed and direction of blood flow. This maximizes the contrast between the blood and the surrounding tissues.

The wash-in of fresh spins has partially enhanced the blood; a number of RF pulses within the interval of the past several T1s have partially saturated the surrounding tissues. TOF MRA works better for flow that is perpendicular to the smallest dimension of the excited region (e.g., perpendicular to the slice in a 2D acquisition) because it is easier to ensure that the fresh spins replenish the entire length of the vessel within the excited region. It works better for thinner excitation regions because it is easier to replenish the entire imaged length of the vessel.

TOF MRA is best with fast, gradient echo pulse sequences, which maximize signal from blood while minimizing tissue signal. Because of short TR, tissue is partially saturated and therefore exhibits low signal intensity. Because of short TR, FRE is maximized and vessels are bright.

 With 2D TOF, every slice is an entry slice and FRE is maximized.

TOF MRA also works better for faster flow, because more fresh spins are moved into the RF excited region. A potential problem arises from tortuous vessels that meander within the RF excited slice because it is more difficult to completely replenish the saturated blood with fresh blood.

Another problem arises in areas of disturbed flow, such as the carotid bulb, some aneurysms, or downstream of a constriction or bifurcation. In such cases, there may be a mixture of velocities and therefore a range of phase shifts within the voxel that reduces the brightness of blood in the region of disturbed flow by destructive interference. In essence, this is a reduced effective T2. Also, the higher orders of motion, such as acceleration present in these structures, lead to imperfect motion compensation.

Phase Contrast Magnetic Resonance Angiography

The other major type of MRA uses the phase-shift mechanism of flow sensitivity. PC MRA makes two measurements with different velocity sensitivities. The difference between the two measurements yields an image in which the phase shifts are proportional to velocity. For MRA purposes, pixels in the image that have significantly nonzero velocities belong within blood vessels and are shown as blood vessels.

Naturally, the considerations of TOF MRA are important in PC MRA, because a strong signal from flowing blood is important. However, it is possible to make PC MRA sensitive to relatively slow flow by changing the velocity sensitivity.

 PC MRA has the potential to combine structural MRA with functional velocity measurements.

The drawback to PC MRA is that it is only sensitive to motion in one direction, that of the motion-sensitizing gradient. Thus three measurements are needed to get isotropic motion sensitivity. This can be advantageous when the direction of blood flow is important; however, PC MRA can be a drawback when only the structure of the vascular tree is important and when TOF MRA provides adequate information in less time.

Two-Dimensional Magnetic Resonance Angiography

The early approaches to MRA were 2D, which remains a clinically significant approach for screening and quick MRA examinations. The 2D approach images a moderately thick slice so that there is high contrast between the vessels and surrounding tissues. This results in a projection image of the vessel against the background of the projected stationary tissues. This projection image is called maximum intensity projection (MIP).

The 2D approach works better with PC methods than with TOF methods because it is difficult to suppress the intensity of the stationary tissues in a thick slice at the same time that the vessels with flow in the plane of the slice are made as bright as possible (Figure 23-9).

PC can be acquired in 2D or 3D, just like TOF MRA. As with TOF MRA, PC MRA is faster in 2D and has better spatial resolution and signal-to-noise ratio (SNR) in 3D.

Three-Dimensional Magnetic Resonance Angiography

The highest quality MR angiograms are produced by 3D MRA. A 3D MRA adds spatial resolution in the third dimension, thereby making it possible to detect smaller vessels that would not stand out against the background in a 2D MRA. It also produces a 3D data set from which angiographic views of the vessels can be constructed from arbitrary directions.

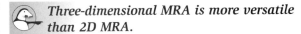 *Three-dimensional MRA is more versatile than 2D MRA.*

The price for this versatility is a longer acquisition time. As a result, some facilities make 2D MRAs for localization and a quick examination in case the patient becomes uncooperative, and then they proceed to 3D examinations that can yield more information (Figure 23-10).

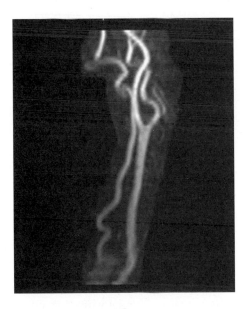 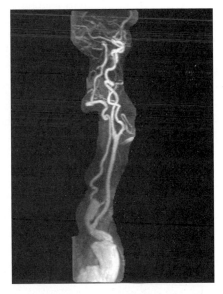

A **B**

Figure 23-9 Two-dimensional projection magnetic resonance angiography showing (**A**) carotid and (**B**) contrast-enhanced image of the same patient. (Courtesy Errol Candy, Dallas, TX.)

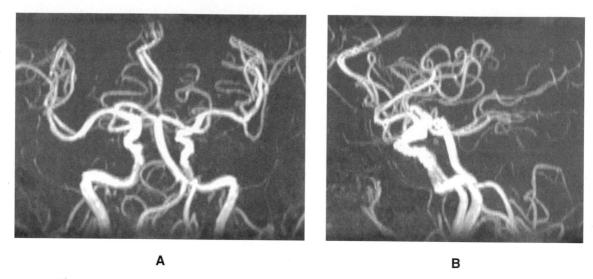

A   **B**

Figure 23-10   Three-dimensional maximum intensity projection, time of flight magnetic resonance angiography **(A)** midcoronal and **(B)** midsagittal views. (Courtesy Errol Candy, Dallas, TX.)

The angiographic view from a 3D data set requires a projection of the data. The most common algorithm is the MIP method (Figure 23-11). A ray line perpendicular to each pixel of the MIP image is projected through the 3D data set, and the value of the brightest pixel along the ray line is assigned to that pixel of the MIP image.

MIPs can be constructed from arbitrary points of view. It is possible to edit the 3D data set before the MIP so that only a subvolume is used for the MIP procedure. Thus it is possible to engage MIP for each carotid artery individually from a 3D data set of the neck.

The MIP algorithm produces MRAs that look natural. However, it is possible for small, lower intensity details to be overwhelmed by larger, brighter structures. Misleading depth information can also be produced, because the human visual system often expects bright objects to be closer than dim objects.

Among the solutions to this problem are depth-weighted MIP. Depth-weighted MIP attenuates the intensity of the brightest pixel along the ray line according to the distance between the pixel and the observer, rendering methods from computer graphics and stereoscopic presentation of the projections, which provide an improved depth perception and the appropriate relationships among structures in three dimensions (Figure 23-12).

Even with these improvements, MIP images contain many artifacts. MIP images are good for general visualization of a lesion. However, diagnosis and stereotactic surgery planning are made from the source images, not the MIPs.

Magnetic Resonance Angiography versus Digital Subtraction Angiography

MRA differs significantly from x-ray contrast angiography (i.e., digital subtraction angiography [DSA]). MRA depicts flowing blood; DSA shows the spaces into which iodinated contrast agents eventually make their way.

Thus MRA may not accurately depict the true lumen of a vessel because the flow is quite slow near the vessel wall. It is subject to signal dropout in regions of disturbed flow. MRA may not accurately demonstrate aneurysms or a thrombus. Experienced clinicians prudently

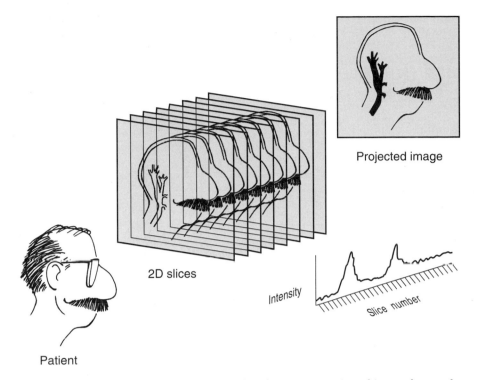

Projected image

2D slices

Intensity

Slice number

Patient

Figure 23-11 Maximum intensity projection (MIP) creates a projected image from a three-dimensional (3D) data set. Each pixel of the MIP image has the highest intensity of pixels along a ray projected through the 3D data set.

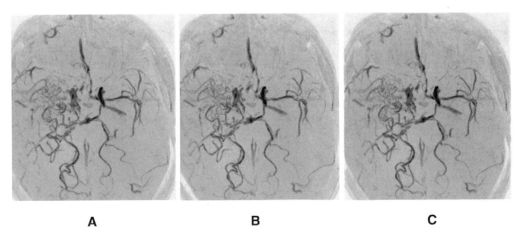

A   B   C

Figure 23-12 It is possible to create separate maximum intensity projection images for each eye so that the data set may be viewed stereoscopically. Images **A** and **B** can be viewed "wall-eyed" or with a stereoscopic viewer. Images **B** and **C** can be viewed "cross-eyed." (Courtesy Michael Mawad, Houston, TX.)

advise that raw MRA data be examined along with MIP images.

CHALLENGE QUESTIONS

1. What is the difference between laminar flow and plug flow?
2. Which is more accurate in depicting blood flow in abnormal vessels: MRA or DSA?
3. What are the two principal techniques used for MRA?
4. What change in the MRI pulse sequence is necessary to produce a three-dimensional Fourier transform (3DFT) MRA image?
5. What is the principal problem with attempting to image turbulent blood flow?
6. Which technique, 2DFT or 3DFT, produces better spatial resolution and/or contrast resolution in MRA?
7. If blood flow were 1 cm/s and the repetition time were 1000 ms, what slice thickness would produce the maximum flow-related enhancements?
8. What imaging parameters must be optimized for time-of-flight MRA?
9. What MRI pulse sequence maximizes flow-related enhancement?
10. Diagram the flow rate of blood in the aorta as a function of time during the cardiac cycle.

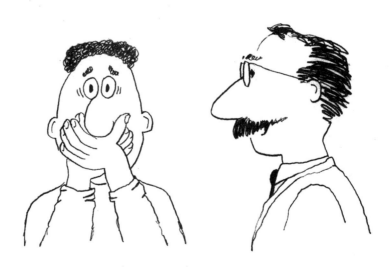

"When I told you to remove your earrings I meant all of your rings...including your tongue ring."

Chapter 24

Perfusion Imaging

The previous chapter described the imaging of large vessels with magnetic resonance (MR) techniques, magnetic resonance angiography (MRA). This chapter describes techniques for imaging blood microcirculation, **perfusion.** The following chapter describes magnetic resonance imaging (MRI) at an even lower anatomical level, **diffusion.**

 Both perfusion imaging and diffusion imaging are the bases for functional magnetic resonance imaging (fMRI).

Blood flows through the vascular tree into smaller and smaller vessels. Capillaries are the smallest vessels, and they are responsible for delivering oxygen and nutrients to tissues.

Imaging blood flow in capillaries is perfusion imaging.

Blood delivered to tissue, arterial blood, is oxygenated. Venous blood is removed from tissue through a similar capillary network as deoxygenated blood (Figure 24-1).

 Perfusion is the flow of blood through the capillary network.

The x-ray tube and a hot water radiator can serve to distinguish perfusion from diffusion. In an x-ray tube, the anode heat is dissipated by conduction to the rotor, convection from the housing, and radiation from the anode (Figure 24-2).

In a room-warming radiator, hot water is conducted through the coils of the radiator

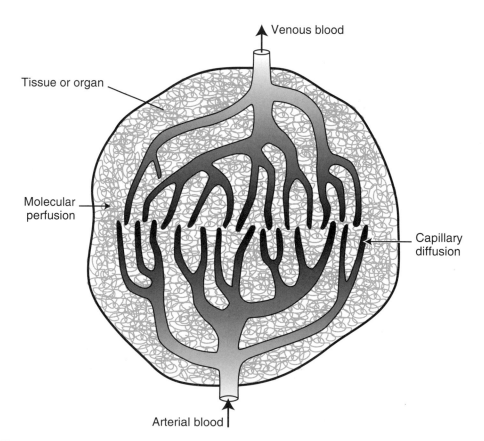

Figure 24-1 Blood entering tissue is oxygenated through oxyhemoglobin. Venous blood is deoxygenated through deoxyhemoglobin.

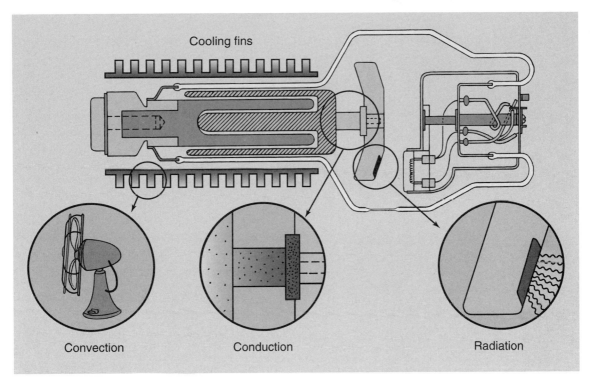

Figure 24-2 Heat from an x-ray tube anode is dissipated by radiation, conduction, and convection. Conduction and convection are analogous to perfusion and diffusion, respectively.

where heat is transferred to air molecules, which are convected through the room. In each of these examples conduction is analogous to perfusion; convection is analogous to diffusion.

There are two general approaches to perfusion imaging: the use of exogenous contrast agents and the use of endogenous contrast agents (Box 24-1).

EXOGENOUS MAGNETIC RESONANCE IMAGING

The use of exogenous contrast agents for studying brain perfusion has been practiced for some time with considerable success. Single photon emission computed tomography (SPECT) with ^{133}Xe, positron emission tomography (PET) with ^{15}O, and x-ray computed tomography (CT)

with an iodinated contrast agent provide the basic approach to what has become exceptionally effective MR perfusion imaging.

The use of any exogenous contrast material requires a bolus injection. The challenge is to acquire images during the first pass of the bolus of contrast material (Figure 24-3).

Box 24-1	*Two Approaches to Perfusion Imaging*

EXOGENOUS: The contrast agent originates outside of the organ or tissue.
ENDOGENOUS: The contrast agent is produced by manipulating the hydrogen spins within the organ or tissue.

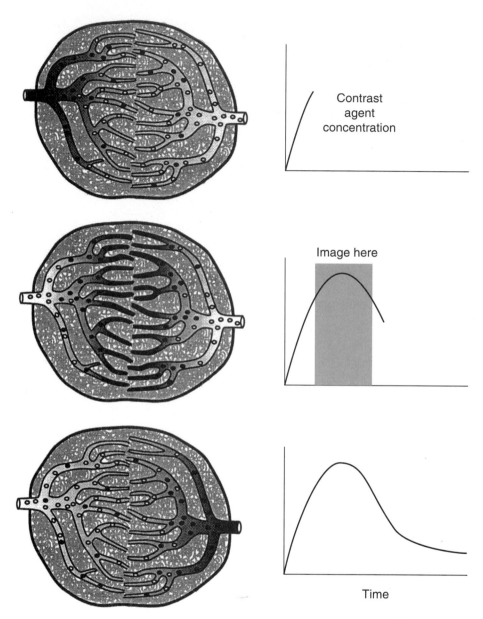

Figure 24-3 Imaging time is critical when a bolus of contrast material is injected.

MRI has a decided advantage over SPECT, PET, and CT in that no ionizing radiation is involved. Gadolinium chelates (Gd-DTPA) are most often used for MR perfusion imaging.

MR image appearance is very much affected by blood flow and bolus injection rate but, more important, by the radiofrequency (RF) pulse sequence. T1 weighted (T1W) pulse sequences show perfused tissue with increased signal intensity. T2* weighted (T2*W) pulse sequences result in reduced signal intensity (Figure 24-4).

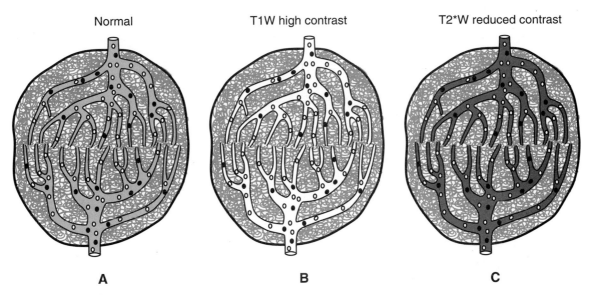

Normal T1W high contrast T2*W reduced contrast

A B C

Figure 24-4 **A,** Before bolus injection, there is little vascular contrast. **B,** After bolus injection T1 weighted *(T1W)* vasculature shows high signal while tissue parenchyma is unaffected. **C,** T2* weighted *(T2*W)* vasculature contrast is reduced because of susceptibility effects on tissue by the contrast medium.

The reversal in signal intensity is due to the paramagnetism of gadolinium. In the presence of an external magnetic field, B_0, paramagnetic materials increase the local magnetic field because of the magnetic susceptibility of tissue.

The magnetic susceptibility of tissue in the presence of a paramagnetic contrast agent causes an intravoxel gradient magnetic field, which effectively reduces T2*. The increase in local magnetization due to the paramagnetic contrast agent increases T1 relaxation.

The reduced signal from T2*W images and increased signal from T1W images can be sculptured with cleverly tailored RF and gradient magnetic field pulse sequences. These effects combine to produce the time-dependent signal for gray matter and white matter intensity shown in Figure 24-5.

The most common perfusion protocol used clinically today is T2* FID-EPI (free induction decay–echo planar imaging). It is used for tumor characterization, tumor recurrence, and stroke.

ENDOGENOUS MAGNETIC RESONANCE IMAGING

There are several disadvantages to the use of exogenous contrast agents. They add time and expense to any examination. If necessary, a considerable delay may be required before repeating the examination. Most important, the procedure is invasive.

The endogenous contrast agent that has stirred the most interest is blood. Arterial capillary blood carries oxygen fixed to the hemoglobin molecule. Venous capillary blood leaves tissue, having deposited its oxygen and picked up carbon dioxide.

 Arterial blood is oxyhemoglobin; venous blood is deoxyhemoglobin.

Oxyhemoglobin is diamagnetic and therefore does not influence blood magnetization or MR signal intensity. Deoxyhemoglobin is paramagnetic because it has four unpaired electrons and therefore behaves much like the gadolinium chelate contrast medium.

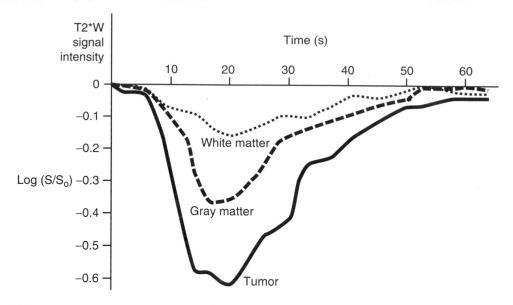

Figure 24-5 Intravoxel incoherent motion results in this time-related signal intensity pattern for brain tissue.

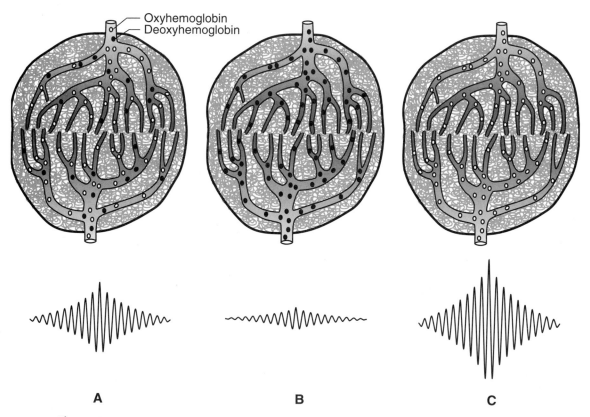

Figure 24-6 Blood oxygen level dependent imaging requires two images. **A,** Normal vasculature with mix of oxyhemoglobin and deoxyhemoglobin. **B,** Brain activity consumes oxygen, causing deoxyhemoglobin to form reducing signal. **C,** Replacement oxyhemoglobin results in increased signal.

🐢 *Deoxyhemoglobin shortens T2*.*

Neuroscientists have long understood that cerebral blood flow (CBF) increases in response to brain activity. Regardless of whether the brain activity is motor, as in tapping a finger, or visual, as in viewing a picture, or aural, as in speaking, each is accompanied by a hemodynamic response that increases, even to the point of oversupply, blood flow to the active region of the brain. This is the basis for fMRI.

The hemodynamic response is not instantaneous; it occurs over several seconds, which requires that MRI be done over a similar time period. Gradient echo imaging is acceptable, but echo planar imaging (EPI) is most successful.

The increased cerebral blood flow is imaged with fast pulse sequences tailored to deoxyhemoglobin and called *blood oxygen level dependent* (BOLD) imaging. BOLD imaging is shown schematically in Figure 24-6. With normal brain activity, there is a mix of oxyhemoglobin and deoxyhemoglobin (Figure 24-6, *A*). The hemodynamic demand from brain activity first causes deoxyhemoglobin to form (Figure 24-6, *B*), which reduces signal intensity because of accelerated T2* relaxation. Next, oxygenated inflowing blood displaces the deoxyhemoglobin and signal intensity increases (Figure 24-6, *C*).

BOLD images are obtained in paired acquisitions (Figure 24-7) and displayed in highlighted or subtraction mode. With the use of gradient echo pulse sequences with repetition time (TR), approximately several 100 ms, baseline images are acquired, and then the study is repeated during patient stimulation. Alternatively, with less than 100-ms EPI, baseline images and patient stimulation images can be cycled for increased temporal resolution because the cycling is less sensitive to patient motion (Figure-24-8).

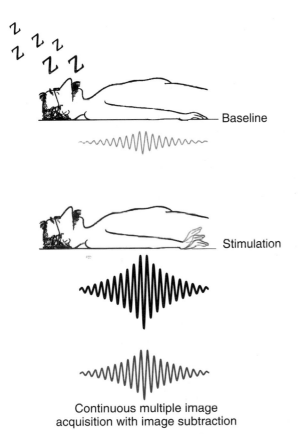

Continuous multiple image
acquisition with image subtraction

Figure 24-7 Functional magnetic resonance images are acquired as multiple repetitions of baseline—stimulated = highlighted image.

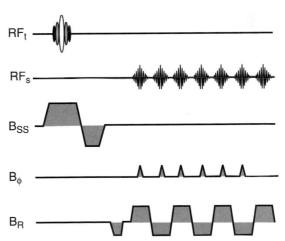

Figure 24-8 Exceptionally fast, less than 100 ms, functional magnetic resonance imaging is performed with echo planar imaging techniques to minimize the effects of patient motion.

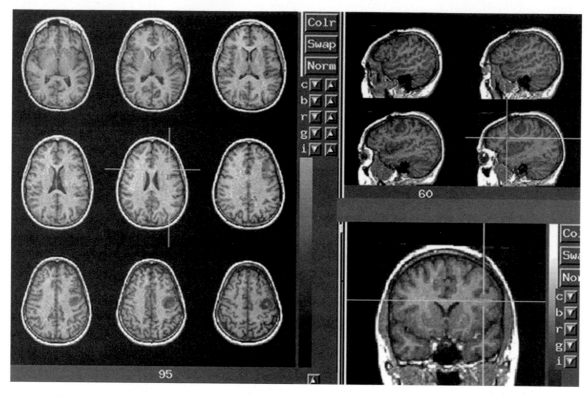

Figure 24-9 Representative functional magnetic resonance imaging showing areas of cortical activity in response to stimulation—finger tapping. (Courtesy Katey Meadors, Stillwater, OK.)

Once pairs of BOLD images have been acquired, highlighted or subtraction images are produced from the sets of baseline and stimulus images (Figure 24-9). Often color is used to dramatically indicate areas of cerebral stimulation.

The perfusion images in Figure 24-10 show delayed time to peak (TTP) in the right middle cerebral artery area. The cerebral blood volume (CBV) image shows normal regional CBV as flow equilibrates over time. Such "brain maps" are very effective perfusion studies for patients with a stroke. Such images are usually displayed in color.

CHALLENGE QUESTIONS

1. What is the difference between perfusion and diffusion?
2. What does BOLD stand for?
3. What type of MRI pulse sequences are used for fMRI?
4. Distinguish between exogenous and endogenous as the terms are applied to MRI contrast agents.
5. Which has shorter T2 relaxation time: oxyhemoglobin or deoxyhemoglobin?
6. SPECT and CT can produce excellent functional images. What is one significant advantage of fMRI over these other techniques
7. Describe the BOLD sequence for fMRI.
8. Why is fast imaging required for BOLD contrast fMRI?
9. What is the importance of imaging time for exogenous fMRI?
10. What is the effect of deoxyhemoglobin on proton density, T1 relaxation time, and T2 relaxation time?

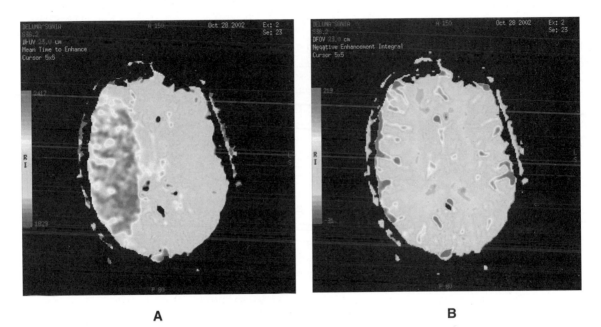

A **B**

Figure 24-10 **A,** Perfusion images of regional time to peak (TTP). **B,** Perfusion image of cerebral blood volume (CBV). (Courtesy Todd Frederick, Dallas, TX.)

Diffusion Imaging

Diffusion is one level closer to the cell than capillary perfusion. Diffusion is the random motion of molecules from a region of high concentration to one of low concentration.

TISSUE DIFFUSION

Diffusion is also termed *brownian motion* for Robert Brown, the English scientist who first identified this process as thermal or heat induced. At T = 0 K, absolute zero, there is no diffusion. As temperature increases, molecules in one medium vibrate, move, and diffuse into an adjoining medium more readily. The time required for molecules to diffuse from one medium to another is expressed by the diffusion coefficient, D.

Consider the situation shown in Figure 25-1. If one could isolate two different molecular species into compartments, with time, the mol-

ecules would mix. The rate at which such mixing occurs is best described by D.

If the diffusion is restricted, as occurs across a cell membrane, the diffusion distance is limited (Figure 25-2). These relationships are described mathematically by Fick's law and Einstein's equation, from which one can derive D. The diffusion coefficient has units of mm^2/s.

 Higher values of D represent faster rates of molecular diffusion.

The diffusion coefficient, D, has been measured for many body fluids. The reciprocal of D, a value termed *b* that depends only on gradient magnetic fields, is that which is computed for magnetic resonance (MR) images. Therefore the parameter b has units of s/mm^2.

The diffusion-imaging scheme is not unlike that for phase contrast (PC) magnetic reso-

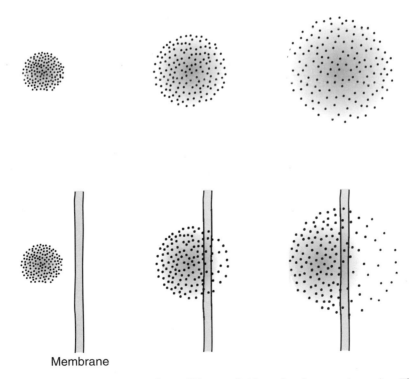

Membrane

Figure 25-1 Diffusion occurs when different fluid molecular species mix. The time required for complete mixing is a function of the diffusion coefficient, D.

nance angiography (MRA). The simplest pulse sequence is spin echo (Figure 25-3). The three gradient magnetic fields are produced for spatial localization. Additionally, one of the gradients is energized briefly on either side of the 180° radiofrequency (RF) refocusing pulse. This is called a **diffusion gradient**.

Now, consider the response of intravoxel spins due to diffusion during the period between the two diffusion gradient pulses (Figure 25-4). Spins moving randomly (diffusing) during application of the gradient have their transverse magnetization, M_{XY}, shifted in phase. At the time of the second diffusion gradient, this phase shift results in accelerated dephasing of the spin echo so that the intensity of the echo signal, S_0, is reduced to S as shown in Figure 25-5.

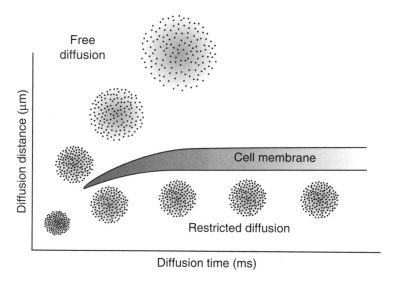

Figure 25-2 Diffusion is slower and limited when a barrier, such as a cell membrane, is present.

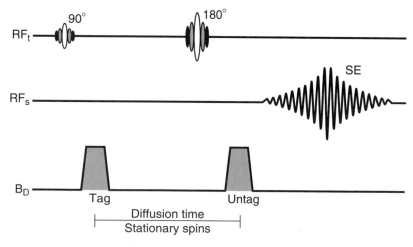

Figure 25-3 Spin echo diffusion imaging requires that a gradient magnetic field be pulsed briefly on either side of the 180° RF refocusing pulse.

The ratio of S/S_0 is called **signal attenuation** and given the symbol A. The value of A is a simple exponent in D and b.

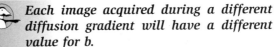

Signal Attenuation
$A = S/S_0 = e^{-bD}$

D is a property of the fluid, and b depends on the nature of the diffusion gradients (Figure 25-6). If there were no diffusion, the diffusion gradients would have no effect and a diffusion image would not be possible. The diffusion gradient may best be described as an indicator of membrane integrity.

PULSE SEQUENCES

For a diffusion image to be made, two or more signal acquisitions are required. Although previously described for spin echo imaging, nearly any pulse sequence can be used: steady state free precession (SSFP) stimulated echoes, gradient echoes (GREs), and echo planar imaging (EPI).

Subtraction of the two or more images results in a value for each pixel related to b. This value is calculated by regression analysis of each image to the exponential equation for signal attenuation given previously.

Each image acquired during a different diffusion gradient will have a different value for b.

The resulting diffusion image shows fast diffusion as bright and slow diffusion as dark. However, there are many confounding obstacles to successful diffusion imaging. Nevertheless, while the value of b differs with diffusion gradient intensity, the value of D is a constant tissue-related property.

The emergence of EPI has made rapid diffusion imaging possible. The improved gradient coil systems associated with EPI allow a more accurate determination of D. Gradient field strengths of 40 mT/m with slew rates of 60 T/m/s allow imaging of b factors to 500 s/mm². More intense gradient magnetic fields produce higher b-values or the same b-value at reduced time-to-echo (TE).

This cannot be done on slower, weaker MRI systems. One significant disadvantage of older systems is that the slow data acquisition allows for inadvertent motion.

Combining perfusion/diffusion images is illustrated in Figure 25-7, where there is a perfusion-diffusion mismatch. The small spots that are bright on the FLAIR and DWI images and dark on the ADC image represent dead tissue due to cytotoxic edema causing restricted

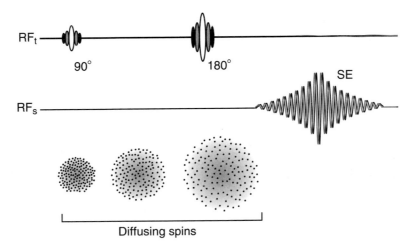

Figure 25-4 Spins diffusing during the time between the diffusion gradient magnetic fields experience a phase shift.

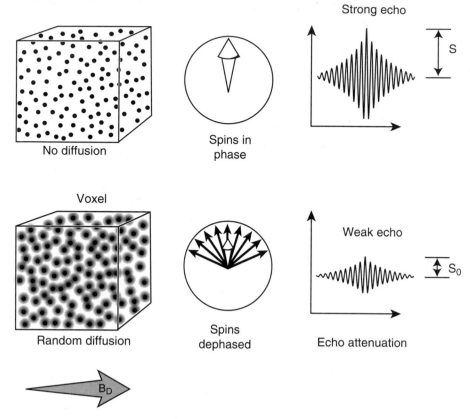

Figure 25-5 The quantity S/S_0 is the diffusion signal attenuation, A.

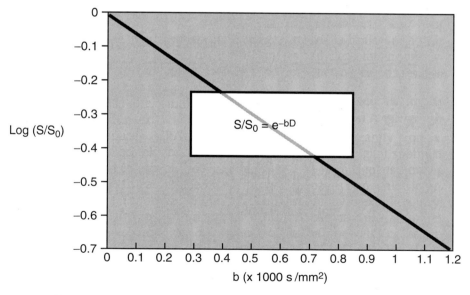

Figure 25-6 Diffusion signal attenuation as a function of b-values.

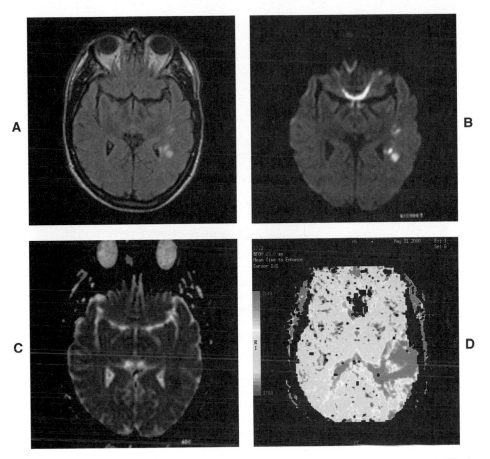

Figure 25-7 **A,** Fluid attenuated inversion recovery (FLAIR) transverse image. **B,** Diffusion weighted image (DWI) trace image with a b-value of 1000. **C,** Apparent diffusion coefficient (ADC) map of DWI image in **B. D,** Time to peak (TTP) perfusion map. (Courtesy Todd Frederick, Dallas, TX.)

diffusion and lengthened T2. The wedge-shaped area on the TTP perfusion image represents a larger area of delayed perfusion.

CHALLENGE QUESTIONS

1. What is a diffusion coefficient?
2. How is the diffusion coefficient measured?
3. Why do we use the b factor rather than the diffusion coefficient when evaluating diffusion imaging?
4. How does rapid perfusion appear, compared with slow perfusion?
5. How would the diffusion gradient be identified on an MRI pulse sequence diagram?
6. What is the ratio of S/S_0 called in diffusion imaging, and what is its meaning?
7. State the equation for signal attenuation and identify each parameter.
8. When the b factor is increased after increasing the amplitude of the diffusion gradient, what happens to signal attenuation?
9. What is brownian motion?
10. What are the two principal MRI pulse sequences used for diffusion imaging?

Chapter 26

Cardiac Magnetic Resonance Imaging

OBJECTIVES

At the completion of this chapter, the student should be able to do the following:

1. Identify the magnetic resonance imaging (MRI) system specifications necessary for cardiac MRI.
2. Describe the principal pulse sequences used for cardiac MRI.
3. Discuss the property of segmented k-space.
4. Identify the four principal imaging planes for cardiac anatomy.
5. Discuss the process of imaging myocardial perfusion.

OUTLINE

Heart disease is the number one cause of death in America for both men and women. Any improvement in early diagnosis would surely improve survival and quality of life.

Advances in magnetic resonance imaging (MRI) system hardware and pulse sequence development are resulting in significant advances in cardiac MRI, and it is now becoming an accepted method for a number of cardiac diseases. The types of tissue involved and the variation of motion in the heart make it tough on MRI. Nevertheless, cardiac MRI is helpful in evaluating both congenital and acquired heart disease.

There are three types of tissue in the heart: muscle of the myocardium, fat, and rapidly flowing blood. Each of these tissues has sufficiently different values of T1, T2, and proton density (PD) that cardiac imaging should be easy (Table 26-1).

However, motion gets in the way to complicate MRI. Movement of the diaphragm, the beating heart, and flowing blood result in very complex motion.

Flowing blood within the coronary arteries can be imaged with the techniques of magnetic resonance angiography (MRA). However, the gold standard remains x-ray coronary angiography because it has better spatial resolution and contrast resolution.

Myocardial perfusion can be imaged with the contrast agent gadopentetate dimeglumine (Gd-DTPA) or with the endogenous BOLD (blood oxygen level dependent) technique, although the BOLD technique is largely restricted to research.

Radioisotope imaging with thallium (^{210}Th) under stress remains the diagnostic test of choice for assessing myocardial ischemia, but MRI is likely to prevail in the near future because soft tissue attenuation artifact is not a problem. Furthermore, MRI can acquire multiple images with good spatial resolution in a heartbeat.

Wall motion imaging with spatially selective presaturation radiofrequency (RF) pulse techniques called **myocardial tagging** shows great promise for evaluation of myocardial ischemia. Wall position displacement as little as 1.0 mm can be detected, and wall motion abnormalities under stress occur before changes in the electrocardiograph (ECG) or development of chest pain.

 End expiration breathhold results in less motion artifact.

The main obstacle to adequate cardiac MRI is respiratory motion. With every breath, the heart moves up 3 cm vertically. Fortunately, breathhold images with good signal intensity and high resolution can be obtained with short breathholds of up to 16 seconds.

When attempting breathhold imaging, the technologist should carefully instruct the patient and direct the patient to practice. Breathholding at the end of inspiration results in considerable variability in heart positioning; breathholding at the end of expiration is preferred. Because not all patients can hold their breath, even for a short time, other methods have been developed to reduce artifacts caused by respiratory motion.

 Navigator echoes are fast, one-dimensional images used to monitor the position of the diaphragm.

The navigator echo is acquired immediately after each triggering of the ECG. If the diaphragm has moved more than a predefined distance, the signal is rejected and another signal is acquired at the same phase-encoding step.

TABLE 26-1	Approximate Values of MRI Parameters for Heart Tissue at 1.5 T		
Tissue	**T1**	**T2**	**PD**
Myocardium	760	40	0.8
Fat	290	50	0.9
Blood	700*	160*	0.9

*Very flow dependent.

Although navigator echoes allow good cardiac images to be obtained while the patient is breathing freely, a lot of signals are rejected. The total image time can take two to four times longer than it otherwise would.

IMAGING SYSTEM REQUIREMENTS

The rapid motion of heart tissue and the movement of blood place exceptional demands on the function of all components of the MRI system. Fast image acquisition requires precisely tuned electronics, robust gradient coils, and a high B_0 field intensity.

Several manufacturers have developed MRI systems specifically for cardiac MRI. These systems have short bore design, high B_0 field intensity, and strong, fast gradient coils.

 Minimum requirements for good cardiac MR imaging are 1.5 T, 15 mT/m, and 100 T/m/s.

Although most MRI systems advertise cardiac MRI capacity, several hardware features are necessary for good cardiac MRI. The following characteristics are essential if the full ability for cardiac MRI is to be achieved.

Static Magnetic Field. Although cardiac MRI can be done at B_0 as low as 0.2 T, 1.5 T is probably the minimum that should be used. The improved signal-to-noise ratio (SNR) at 1.5 T allows for faster imaging and high temporal resolution, even at high heart rates. The temporal resolution at lower field intensity is too low for state-of-the-art physiological evaluation.

Field of View (FOV) and RF Coils. A surface coil complement should be available. Dedicated phased-array cardiac coils, typically with four to six elements, allow for further improvements in SNR and contrast resolution. Also, in selected instances, they allow use of a small FOV (down to 10 cm) for detailed imaging, though there is reduced coverage because only selected elements of the array are used.

Gradient Coil Capacity. The gradient coils must be fast and intense. Switching times of not more than 200 µs are required. When energized, the coils must produce a gradient magnetic field of at least 15 mT/m but even higher is better for most applications.

 Slew rates of at least 100 T/m/s are desirable.

The fastest gradients now allow imaging with repetition time (TR) as low as 2 ms. With single-shot echo planar imaging (EPI) techniques, a 64 × 64 matrix image can be acquired in approximately 50 ms. This limitation is due to the T2 of the myocardium being only approximately 40 ms. Multishot EPI may be used for better spatial resolution.

IMAGING TECHNIQUES

There are two general approaches to cardiac MRI. ECG-gated, spin echo (SE), and gradient echo (GRE) techniques were the first applications for cardiac imaging and continue to be the standard.

The quality of the ECG gating signal must ensure quality images. Proper placement of the ECG electrodes and the positioning of the ECG cables are necessary. No loops are allowed. Figure 26-1 illustrates proper ECG electrode placement.

Pulsing gradient fields can significantly distort the ECG signal during imaging. It is recommended that the three or four ECG lead wires be braided to reduce these effects. Also, check to ensure that the signal is gating on the R-wave and not the T-wave for optimal image quality.

 Faster imaging within a single breathhold provides improved temporal resolution.

ECG gating allows the periodic heart motion to be stopped, like a strobe light at a disco dance. In conventional multislice imaging, TR is long and echo time (TE) sufficiently short so that a single acquisition for each slice is obtained within one TR. ECG-gated imaging is similar

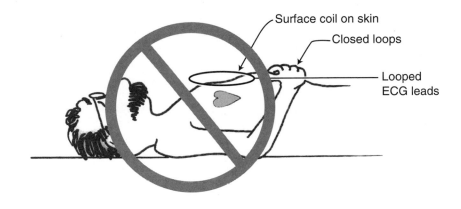

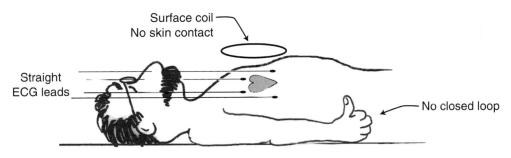

Figure 26-1   Proper electrocardiograph *(ECG)* electrode placement for cardiac-gated imaging. Closed conductive loops, even of anatomy, should be avoided.

except the TR approximates the cardiac cycle length.

Most patients have heart rates between 60 and 120 beats/min. These rates correspond to TRs of 1000 ms and 500 ms, respectively.

Question: If the cardiac frequency is 60 beats/min, what is the time of the required cycle and therefore the required TR?

Answer: 60 beats/min

$$= 60 \text{ beats}/60 \text{ s}$$
$$= 1 \text{ beat}/1000 \text{ ms}$$

hence: TR = 1000 ms

Because of the short TR, such images are heavily T1 weighted (T1W). A common approach is to make the images more T2 weighted (T2W) by skipping one or more heartbeats and increasing the TR accordingly.

Of course, the TE also needs to be lengthened; otherwise, we will have a long TR, short TE sequence that results in a proton density weighted (PDW) image.

Pulse Sequence Selection

The type of cardiac pulse sequence chosen for a given patient is determined by the objective of the study. Cardiac anatomy is best evaluated with SE MRI. Cardiac function is best evaluated with cineradiography (cine) MRI. Myocardial perfusion requires fast GRE or hybrid EPI sequences.

MRA is usually done with time-of-flight (TOF) techniques, though velocity-encoded phase contrast (PC) is sometimes used to measure blood flow in the coronary arteries or aorta.

Cine MRI.   A cine loop of one or more cardiac cycles uses spoiled GRE or fast imaging with a short TR (less than 10 ms), a short TE (2 to 4 ms), and a 20° to 30° flip angle. Images are acquired through the cardiac cycle, but only one signal for each image is acquired per cycle.

The R wave is chosen to gate the image acquisition because it has the highest voltage. Therefore if a 256 × 256 matrix is desired for each image, 256 heartbeats will be required (Figure 26-2). If the heart rate is 60 beats/min, then just over 4 minutes is required.

The cardiac cycle can be sectioned into multiple phases. The number of lines of k-space acquired during each phase of the R-R interval, equivalent to each cine frame, corresponds to the **segmentation** of k-space. Segmentation effectively reduces the number of cardiac cycles and imaging time proportionately.

 The larger the number of lines of k-space collected in each segmentation, the faster k-space can be filled.

There is a penalty for increasing k-space segmentation to reduce imaging time. Temporal resolution is reduced, resulting in image motion blur. The number of cine frames for analysis is reduced.

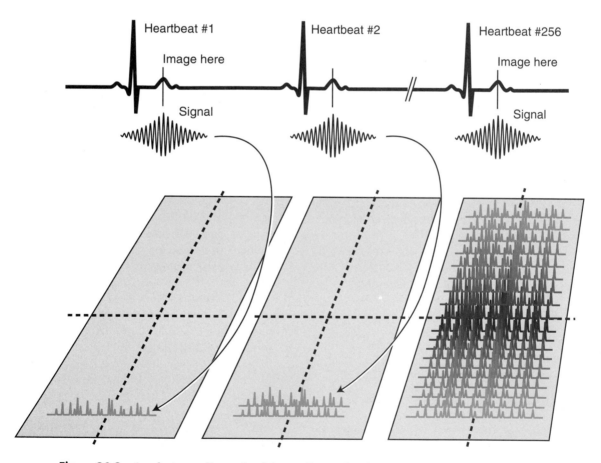

Figure 26-2   An electrocardiograph of the cardiac cycle triggers magnetic resonance imaging at each R wave. A number of heartbeats equal to the number of k-space lines are required for each image.

However, a sequence called *steady state free precession* (SSFP) has been used that has short TR (2 to 4 ms) and TE (1 to 2 ms), allowing k-space to be covered quickly. This sequence overcomes some of the previous disadvantages of cine MRI by allowing both high temporal resolution and high spatial resolution (Figure 26-3).

Echo Planar Imaging. EPI is capable of extremely fast imaging; 50 ms per image or faster is easily obtained. EPI also has a high SNR. However, EPI is compromised by chemical shift, T2*, and field inhomogeneities. Nevertheless, EPI is applied with success for cine cardiac MRI.

Multislice SE. Gated multislice SE imaging is useful for imaging cardiac anatomy. Imaging times of 2 to 4 minutes will allow 10 to 15,

256 × 256 matrix images to be acquired. Such pulse sequences are a solid addition to cine MRI. Individual slices can be obtained during a breathhold with segmented k-space techniques. When combined with dual inversion-recovery pulses, the moving blood is nulled, and crisp details of cardiac anatomy can be obtained.

Spatial presaturation pulses allow the exclusion of signal from various tissues. If many thin spatial presaturation pulses are applied to the myocardium right after the ECG trigger, they will persist for many phases of a cardiac cine sequence. This method is called **"tissue tagging."**

When the presaturation lines are applied in such a way to produce a grid of saturated tissue, the motion of the myocardium can be followed through a good portion of the cardiac

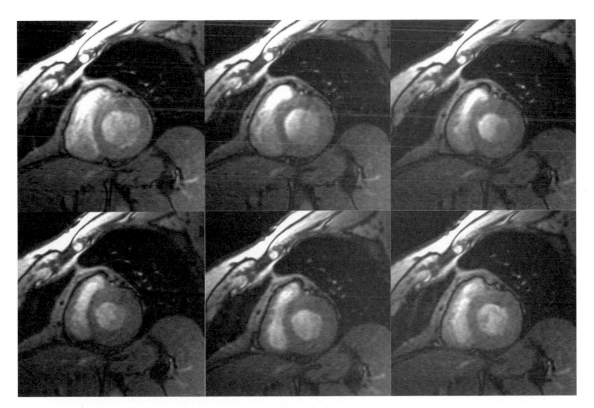

Figure 26-3   These six segmentation-gated images were obtained in six heartbeats and can be merged to form a cine loop. (Courtesy Geoff Clarke, San Antonio, TX.)

cycle, and regions of poor function can be visualized.

> When compared with the myocardium, signal from blood appears very bright with all of the faster imaging methods.

One of the nice things about conventional SE imaging is that the blood is black, allowing easy discrimination of the endocardial margins. However, conventional SE often takes a prohibitive amount of time compared with the faster cine methods.

There is a technique for "black-blood cine imaging" that uses two inversion pulses before acquisition of the cine data. The first slice-selective pulse inverts all of the spins. and the second inversion pulse realigns the spins along the positive B_Z axis.

However, the blood in the heart chambers moves into other slices between the two 180° pulses and does not receive the second inversion pulse. After an appropriate inversion time, the signal from the blood will be nulled, whereas the signal from the myocardium will be strong.

The drawback to this method is that the two inversion pulses and the inversion delay take additional time; often the number of cine phases is significantly reduced compared with white blood cell imaging.

Filling k-Space

The principal time constraint in cardiac MRI is the time required to fill k-space, which, during SE imaging, is the product of TR, the number of signal acquisitions (NSA), and the number of phase-encoding (B_Φ) steps. Reduction in any one of these parameters speeds imaging.

Spin Echo Imaging Time

$$T = TR \times NSA \times \# \, B_\Phi$$

Question: What is the time required to obtain a T2W image with the following technique: 2 signal averages, 256 phase-encoding steps, 3000 ms TR, and 100 ms TE?

Answer: $T = 3000 \text{ ms} \times 2 \times 256$
$= 1,536,000 \text{ ms}$
$= 1536 \text{ s}$
$= 25.6 \text{ min}$

The manner in which k-space is filled has been exploited to reduce imaging time. Instead of sequential filling, line by line, as with SE imaging, half Fourier imaging (HFI), segmentation of k-space, and spiral filling have been applied to fill k-space faster.

Half Fourier Imaging. k-Space exists in four distinct quadrants, each of which is related to the other (Figure 26-4). Each line in quadrant *A,* for instance, is mathematically related to the line in each other quadrant, usually as a mirror image.

If one acquires only the first half of each signal, one can compute the other half, which speeds imaging a little. This form of HFI still requires that 256 signals be acquired.

A faster form of HFI requires that only 128 signals be acquired, and the other 128 signals are computed to fill all 256 lines in k-space. Imaging time is nearly halved because usually in addition to the 128 signals acquired, an additional 8 to 12 central lines are acquired to maintain good SNR.

k-Space Segmentation. For the improvement of temporal resolution and reduction of motion artifacts, k-space can be filled in segmented rather than sequential fashion. For k-space segmentation, multiple phase-encoded signals are acquired during each heartbeat. The complete k-space is filled over 10 to 20 heartbeats, with an effective temporal resolution of approximately 50 ms, which allows cine acquisitions.

The 4 to 7 minutes required for SE cardiac MRI is reduced (3 to 5 minutes) with ECG-gated GRE imaging. This is still not fast enough for routine cardiac MRI.

With improvements in gradient coil design and performance, spoiled GRE and seg-

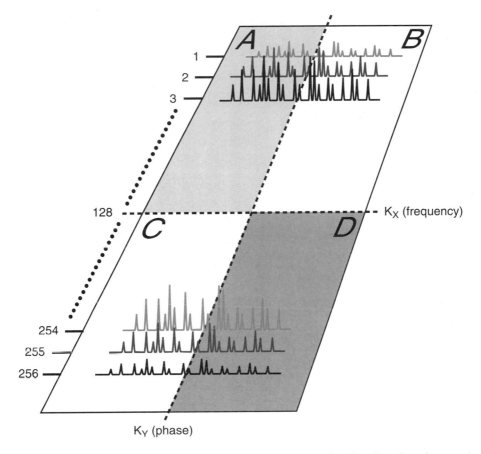

Figure 26-4 The four quadrants of k-space are mathematically related so that the remaining three can be computed from the acquisition of one quadrant.

mented k-space reduce imaging time to a single 20-second breathhold. TRs of 10 to 20 ms and TE of 2 to 7 ms with flip angles not exceeding 20° are routine. These imaging techniques result in saturation of stationary tissues and flow-related enhancement from inflowing blood.

Segmentation of k-space is shown in Figure 26-5 for a single slice. Each R-R interval is divided into several periods of the cardiac cycle. For a heart rate of 60 beats/min, 20 different segments of k-space can be measured in a 20-second breathhold. During this time, multiple cine frames can be acquired to produce the cine loop.

 Cineradiography modes are useful for evaluation of the myocardial function, ventricular volume, ejection fraction, wall thickening, and blood flow abnormalities.

Segmentation of k-space can be implemented to produce multiple image planes. In this segmentation mode each segment corresponds to a different slice, which allows an image of the entire heart in 20 seconds.

The product of the number of lines of k-space in the segmentation and the number of cardiac cycles determine the matrix size of the image. For instance, if four lines are acquired

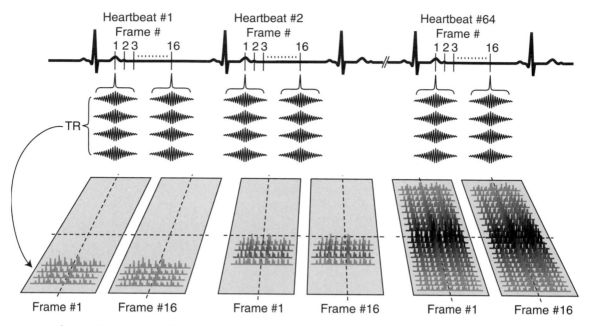

Figure 26-5 Single-slice k-space segmentation speeds image acquisition for cine imaging.

in each cycle, over a 20-second acquisition, the image matrix will be 80 × 80.

Spiral Filling. An alternative to sequential or segmental filling of k-space is spiral imaging (Figure 26-6). Spiral k-space filling uses simultaneous energization of the phase- and frequency-encoding gradients immediately after RF excitation.

The two gradients begin oscillating at low amplitudes, 90° out of phase. The amplitude of these gradients increases during signal acquisition. Filling begins at the center of k-space and spirals outward.

 With spiral imaging, the center of k-space is filled more than the periphery. This contributes to improved contrast resolution.

Spiral imaging has not yet received widespread application because of all schemes it requires special image processing. Spiral imaging was actually conceived as a method for imaging

quickly, using gradients with conventional amplitudes and ramping rates.

As such, it showed promise. However, gradient amplifier technology soon allowed imaging systems the ability to create fast ramping, powerful gradient fields that were useful for other things (like diffusion-weighting), in addition to fast imaging. Spiral imaging has not really found a foothold in any significant clinical application.

EVALUATION OF THE HEART

For most examinations, 5- to 10-mm slice thickness is adequate. With thinner slices, reduced partial volume artifact results in improved contrast resolution. However, in the heart, slice reduction may not produce the benefits found in other organs because the heart may be moving in the slice-select direction during imaging.

With a patient supine in a horizontal B_0 field, the axes of the heart and left ventricle are not parallel to the axis of the body or the B_0

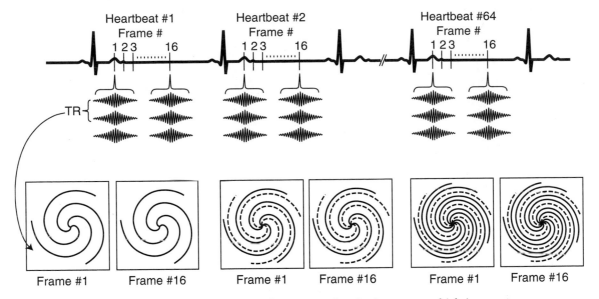

Figure 26-6 Spiral filling of k-space places more data in the center, which improves contrast resolution.

field. As a result, oblique images are necessary for proper coverage of the heart.

Cardiac Anatomy

Evaluation of cardiac anatomy is best achieved with the segmented k-space techniques previously described. Best results are obtained with a dedicated phased-array cardiac surface coil with low bandwidth (e.g., ± 32 kHz or less) for better SNR. This reduces the TR and TE and allows longer segments of k-space to be filled each cardiac cycle.

Multislice or single-slice breathhold SE MRI is best for evaluating the many types of cardiac anatomical abnormalities. Ventricular volumes, myocardial mass, and myocardial wall thickness are three of the most important measurements for staging congenital heart disease and congestive heart disease and are best evaluated with cine MRI techniques.

Regardless of the pulse sequence used to demonstrate anatomy, four anatomic planes must be imaged (Figure 26-7).

Evaluation of ejection fraction usually requires a complete set of short axis views cov-

ering the left ventricle from the base, at the mitral valve plane, to the apex. Segmental wall motion is also best evaluated with short axis views (Figure 26-8).

 There are three long axis cardiac views.

The first long axis view is of the left ventricular outflow tract (LVOT), which includes the aortic and mitral valves and the apex of the left ventricle.

The second long axis view is the two-chamber view, which provides additional images of left ventricular function and mitral valve function.

The third long axis view is the four-chamber view, which is useful for imaging the mitral and tricuspid valves and is an added measure of evaluation of segmental function. The four-chamber view should pass through the ventricular apex and the mitral and tricuspid valves.

Taken collectively, these four views (short axis plus three long axes) provide images that allow assessment of the most important

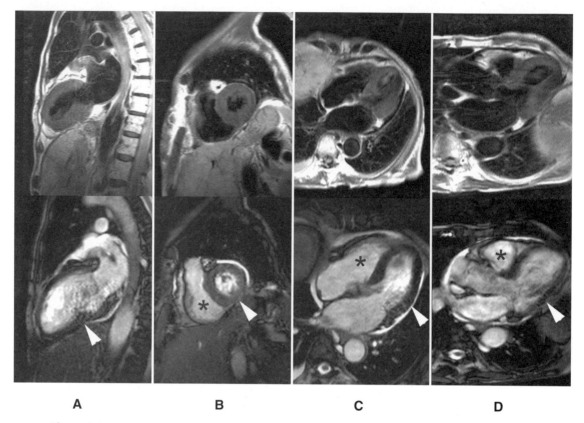

A   **B**   **C**   **D**

Figure 26-7   These images show the four basic views of the heart from left to right. **A,** Two-chamber long axis. **B,** Short axis. **C,** Four-chamber long axis. **D,** Left ventricular outflow tract. The upper row demonstrates the "black blood" spin echo technique, and the lower row demonstrates the corresponding "bright blood" gradient echo technique (in these images with the steady state free precession method). In the bottom row, the white arrowhead identifies the left ventricle, and the black asterisk shows the right ventricle. (Courtesy Eric Douglas, Houston, TX.)

cardiac structures and function. Cardiac MRI relies on specific measurements from the image data more than most other clinical applications.

The volume of the left ventricle can be determined from measurements of the cross-sectional areas of the chamber of the left ventricle, obtained from a series of short axis views. When these measurements are derived from a set of cine image data, the left ventricular ejection fraction can be calculated as the difference between the ventricular volume at end-diastole and end-systole divided by the end-diastolic ventricular volume.

The wall thickness can be measured in each short axis image, circumferentially around the ventricular chamber. The percent wall thickening is then taken as the difference between the end-diastolic and end-systolic wall thickness divided by the end-diastolic wall thickness times 100%.

 Myocardial mass can also be determined by multiplying the total myocardium volume by the density of the myocardium tissue, 1.05 g/cc.

High field strength MRI systems now include vendor-developed cardiac computer programs

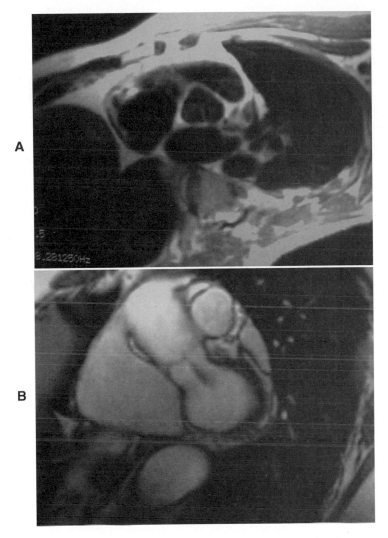

Figure 26-8 These short axis views demonstrate **(A)** black-blood technique acquired in a single breathhold with single-shot fast spin echo and **(B)** bright-blood technique with a steady state gradient echo acquisition in a single breathhold. Note the regurgitation *(black jet)* at the mitral valve. (Courtesy Bill Faulkner, Chattanooga, TN.)

to semiautomatically analyze for ejection fraction, chamber volume, and segmental myocardial function based on wall movement.

Myocardial Perfusion

EPI with a bolus administration of the paramagnetic contrast agent Gd-DTPA is fast becoming the technique of choice for evaluating the perfusion of the myocardium. This technique requires only small amounts of Gd-DTPA for each first-pass study.

The study is easily repeated to allow comparison between baseline and stress conditions. This technique is superior to radioisotope imaging because of better spatial resolution and better contrast resolution, and it is also less susceptible to artifact from soft tissue attenuation.

During perfusion imaging, the Gd-DTPA contrast is taken up much slower in infarcted tissue than in well-perfused myocardium. However, because of arterial pressure and diffusion, some contrast agent is eventually taken up by dead tissue.

The contrast material also washes out much more slowly from the infarcted region than from the healthy tissue. Thus if a T1W image is obtained during a period ranging from 10 to 30 minutes after injection of the contrast agent, the infarcted tissue will appear bright while the normal myocardium will remain dark.

Magnetic resonance contrast agent imaging is useful in evaluating abnormal wall motion. Wall motion analysis is effective for detection of ischemic and infarcted myocardium. Dobutamine-induced cardiac stress MRI has been shown to be better than ultrasound or nuclear medicine imaging for detecting myocardial wall thickening and dysfunction.

Several groups have shown that with very high-resolution MRI, the wall of arteries can be well visualized. In the case of arteriosclerosis, individual plaques can be identified, and the characteristics of the plaques, whether they are mostly fibrous or fatty, can be determined. This has led to much excitement about the possibility of using MRI to evaluate the "vulnerable plaque," that is, a plaque that will soon rupture and thereby initiate events that will lead to a blockage of the artery.

The most convincing images of vulnerable plaques thus far have been in the carotid artery, which is relatively motionless and superficial. However, investigators have demonstrated the ability to measure the wall thickness of the coronary arteries, too. Thus it is likely only a matter of time, which will bring technological improvements allowing higher SNR, before imaging of arteriosclerotic

plaques in the coronary arteries will become commonplace in a clinical setting.

Spatial Resolution. Spatial resolution in radioisotope imaging is approximately 2 lp/cm (5 mm) because of the intrinsic limitations of the gamma ray detector. On the other hand, MRI can routinely provide image resolution of 5 lp/cm (1 mm) with a 256×256 image matrix and 25 cm FOV.

Question: What is the pixel size and limiting spatial frequency of a 256×256 image matrix and 10 cm FOV?

Answer: Pixel Size $= \dfrac{100 \text{ mm}}{256}$

$= 0.4 \text{ mm}$

Spatial Frequency $= \left[\dfrac{0.8 \text{ mm}}{1\text{p}} \right]^{-1}$

$= 1.25 \text{ lp/mm}$

$= 12.5 \text{ lp/cm}$

Contrast Resolution. Cardiac MRI with radioisotopes has two deficiencies that restrict contrast resolution. The count rate is low for photon imaging because of the safety restrictions on the amount of radioactive material that can be administered. Overlying tissue, especially in obese patients, attenuates the already low signal.

On the other hand, the intrinsic values of the MRI tissue characteristics—PD, T1, and T2—have a far greater range of values than the detective quantum efficiency (DQE) of a scintillation crystal. Proper pulse sequence selection will accentuate these ranges.

Magnetic Resonance Angiography

Fluoroscopically guided cine of the coronary arteries remains the gold standard for evaluating coronary artery disease (CAD). However, approximately 30% of coronary artery angiograms are negative for CAD.

Because it is invasive, coronary artery angiography is accompanied by a finite risk of infection, infarction, and even death. MRA is a logical substitute because it is noninvasive and considerably less expensive.

 X-ray imaging of the coronary arteries has better spatial resolution than MRA.

Gradient echo TOF MRA with segmented k-space filling is successful in imaging coronary arteries down to perhaps 3 mm in diameter in a single breathhold. With such techniques laminar flow appears bright, and turbulence appears as a signal void.

Three-dimensional (3D) MRA has several advantages over two-dimensional (2D) MRA. A 3D signal acquisition has less operator error. Images acquired in 3D mode have better spatial resolution, better contrast resolution because of higher SNR, and extensive multiplanar and oblique planar image reconstruction.

CHALLENGE QUESTIONS

1. List the four leading causes of death in the United States, from highest to lowest.
2. Describe the appearance of the coronary arteries when imaged with GRE time-of-flight MRA.

3. Which has best spatial resolution when imaging contrast-enhanced coronary arteries: x-ray angiography, two-dimensional Fourier transform (2DFT) MRA, or three-dimensional Fourier transform (3DFT) MRA?
4. Which is superior for imaging the perfusion of the myocardium: radioisotope scans, x-ray imaging, or MRI?
5. List the four MRI views required for complete evaluation of the heart.
6. What minimum hardware requirements are advised for cardiac MRI?
7. Discuss the segmentation of k-space as it is used for cardiac MRI.
8. How can one enhance the T2W of SE cardiac images?
9. How is cardiac MRI speeded by the application of HFI?
10. Describe the proper positioning of ECG leads during gated cardiac MRI.

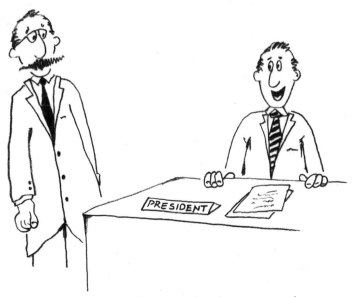

"We're very happy with your work and want to reward you.
Funds though are tight so we've decided to name our new MRI
after you. However, you'll have to change your name to Ultravision."

Part VI

Safety

Chapter 27

Contrast Agents and Magnetic Resonance Imaging

OBJECTIVES

At the completion of this chapter, the student should be able to do the following:

1. List two general approaches to magnetic resonance imaging (MRI) contrast enhancement.
2. Identify three routes for administration of MRI contrast agents and give an example of each.
3. Describe paramagnetism and how such an agent enhances image contrast.
4. Distinguish between positive and negative contrast and describe how each is produced by reduced T1 and T2.
5. Identify the blood-brain barrier and how it affects the use of MRI contrast agents.

OUTLINE

With magnetic resonance imaging (MRI), the naturally available contrast among tissues in the body is good. It was originally assumed that contrast enhancement (CE) would not be needed in MRI. Even without the use of a contrast agent, MRI is exceptionally sensitive to detecting pathological conditions. However, as the field develops, it is becoming clear that under some circumstances the addition of a contrast agent greatly increases the diagnostic value of MRI by improving disease sensitivity and specificity and by delineating pathological processes.

In some areas of the body, adjacent tissues have similar MRI appearance, and CE is needed for adequate differentiation. CE is also useful for delineating the structural integrity of the blood-brain barrier. The addition of a contrast agent allows imaging of areas of normal versus decreased tissue perfusion. In some cases, pathology can be better identified because of the different speeds with which a contrast agent enters or washes out of tumors as compared with the surrounding normal tissue.

The properties needed in an MRI contrast agent are the same as those needed for contrast agents in other imaging modalities. The agent should alter contrast at low concentrations, and its effect on contrast should be dose dependent. It must be nontoxic and nonreactive, as well as rapidly cleared from the body.

The biodistribution of a contrast agent is exceedingly important. An ideal contrast agent distributes only to the organ, tissue, or pathology of interest (Figure 27-1).

APPROCHES TO CONTRAST ENHANCEMENT

The normally occurring MRI appearance of a tissue depends on both the physical characteristics of the tissue (such as viscosity and temperature) and the chemical characteristics that influence proton density (PD), spin-lattice relaxation (T1), and spin-spin relaxation (T2).

Although changing a physical property of a sample is useful for in vitro studies, it is generally not safe to use a sufficiently large change in a living organism to make this approach useful in vivo. However, it is possible to safely alter the chemical characteristics of living tissue sufficiently to change the MRI parameters and therefore image appearance.

In MRI, the image contrast is influenced by a number of factors, including the hydrogen content (PD), spin-lattice relaxation, and T2 flow through the area being examined and the magnetic susceptibility of the tissue. If any of these parameters are changed by the addition of a contrast agent, the magnetic resonance (MR) image appearance is also changed.

When the use of an MRI contrast agent causes the tissue of interest to appear brighter, positive CE occurs. The CE is negative if the tissue of interest is darker when a contrast agent is used.

Although MRI contrast agents have traditionally been used for positive contrast, it is becoming more common to use them to reduce contrast, as in susceptibility-weighted cerebral perfusion imaging. Box 27-1 presents one classification for MRI contrast agents.

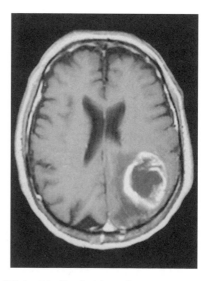

Figure 27-1   Biodistribution of a contrast agent in an astrocytoma. (Courtesy Michael Mawad, Houston, TX.)

Altering Hydrogen Content

The most obvious approach to CE is to alter the hydrogen content (PD) of tissue. Examples of this approach are water loading to increase the total signal from the kidneys and bladder and administering diuretics to decrease hydration of tissue.

An alternative approach is to remove the source of the signal entirely by administering a hydrogen-free contrast agent that fills the area of interest. Another approach is to use oxygen. Unfortunately, although oxygen is paramagnetic, the effect is too weak for clinical use.

The amount of MR signal arising from tissue can also be changed by altering the ratio of water to fat in that tissue. The relaxation characteristics of fat and water are quite different, so greatly increasing the amount of fat can increase the available signal. This approach has been used for imaging of the gut, with oral administration of fat-containing compounds such as mineral oil.

Altering the Local Magnetic Field

Motion Reduction. One approach to changing the magnetic environment perceived by spins is to administer an agent that greatly slows the normal motion of hydrogen. Normally, a hydrogen ion is tumbling quickly enough that any variations in the local magnetic environment are averaged (rather like the blurring in vision that a person experiences when spinning around rapidly).

However, if the hydrogen ion is slowed, local magnetic field variations become perceptible. This causes a shortening of the relaxation times, particularly T2. This approach is limited but has been applied with some success to CE of the gastrointestinal tract.

Paramagnetic/Superparamagnetic Agents. The most versatile approach to altering the local magnetic environment of spins is to administer an agent that is paramagnetic or superparamagnetic. The paramagnetic agents are most commonly based on gadolinium, dysprosium, or manganese. The paramagnetic property is the result of unpaired electron spins in certain electron orbital shells of transitional metals or lanthanides. For example, contrast is improved after administration of gadolinium-diethylene-triamine-pentaacetic acid dimeglumine (Gd-DTPA) (Figure 27-2).

Iron oxide particles are the superparamagnetic agents used. Such particles have high magnetic susceptibility and create a relatively large regional gradient magnetic field. Such a gradient readily influences water molecules diffusing close to the iron oxide particles. Reduced T1 and T2 result, with the degree of CE dependent on many parameters, including particle composition, size and concentration, and pulse sequence used.

All currently approved clinical contrast agents fall into this category. Paramagnetic and superparamagnetic agents are all metal ions or crystals that act like small bar magnets because they possess one or more electrons whose magnetic field is not canceled by another electron of opposite spin.

When such agents are placed in a magnetic environment, such as when they are administered as part of an MRI procedure, magnetization is induced within the contrast agent. A hydrogen atom that is close experiences the

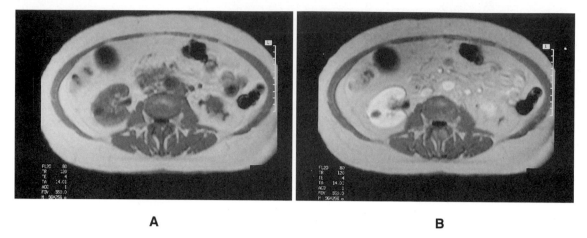

A   B

Figure 27-2 A cyst in the right kidney is apparent in the unenhanced image **(A)** but more clearly demonstrated in the 90-second postcontrast image **(B)**. (Courtesy Todd Frederick, Dallas, TX.)

magnetic field of the contrast agent in addition to the applied static magnetic field (B_0). This increase in perceived magnetic field alters both T1 and T2. Therefore such nuclear species are referred to as *relaxation centers* (Figure 27-3).

 MRI contrast agents reduce T1 and T2 relaxation times.

These contrast agents are not visualized directly by MRI, but rather, alter the MR signal indirectly by shortening relaxation times. The magnitude of the effect on each relaxation time varies with the paramagnetic or superparamagnetic species and its concentration in tissue. In general, low concentrations affect T1 more than T2 because of intensified spin-lattice interaction. At high concentration, the resulting T2 shortening is more significant because relative T2 values vary more than T1 values.

The use of CE is helpful for imaging many areas of the body. Applications of CE magnetic

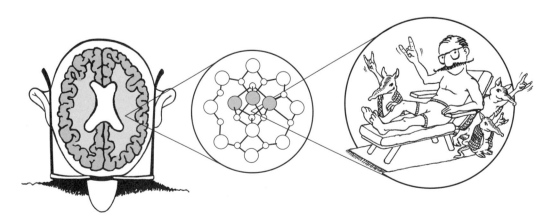

Figure 27-3 Paramagnetic agents contain relaxation centers.

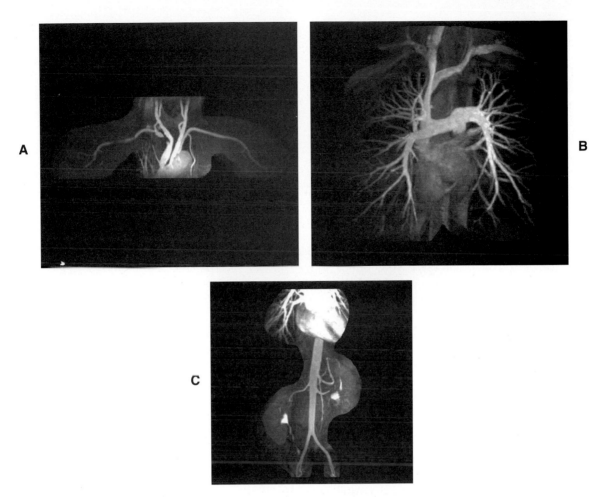

Figure 27-4   These images—**A,** subclavian contrast enhancement (CE) magnetic resonance angiography (MRA) demonstrating a right subclavian occlusion, **(B)** pulmonary CE MRA, and **(C)** renal CE MRA—demonstrate the versatility of CE MRA. (Courtesy Todd Frederick, Dallas, TX.)

resonance angiography (MRA) are used for many vessels of the body (Figure 27-4).

An additional generality deals with radiofrequency (RF) pulse sequence selection to optimize the CE. Paramagnetic contrast agents are most effective with T1 weighted (T1W) RF pulse sequences and result in an increase in signal and therefore positive CE. Conversely, superparamagnetic contrast agents affect T2 more than T1; therefore T2 weighted (T2W) RF pulse sequences are more appropriate. The

result of the use of these contrast agents is a reduced, signal intensity—negative CE.

AVAILABLE CONTRAST AGENTS

Contrast Agents Specific for Magnetic Resonance Imaging

In 1988 the first commercial contrast agent (Magnevist, Berlex Laboratories, Wayne, NJ) was clinically introduced. Magnevist is Gd-DTPA or gadopentetate dimeglumine.

Three additional contrast agents are specifically approved for use in clinical MRI. These are gadoterate meglumine (Dotarem, Guerbet Laboratories, Aulnay-sous-Bois, France), gadoteridol (ProHance, Bristol-Myers Squibb Diagnostics, Princeton, NJ), and gadodiamide (Omniscan, Sanofi-Winthrop Pharmaceuticals, New York, NY). All of these contrast agents contain the paramagnetic metal ion gadolinium, which has seven unpaired electrons in its outer shells.

Chemical Structure and Toxicity. A major difficulty in the development of any of the paramagnetic metals as contrast agents has been to diminish the toxicity of these compounds to clinically acceptable levels. The LD_{50} (lethal dose for 50% of subjects) of gadolinium chloride in rats, for example, is less than 1 mM/kg after intravenous administration. The gadolinium is still present in the body several days after administration.

If these metals are allowed to interact with the human body, they are quite toxic. A concentration of gadolinium as low as 1 mM/kg is sufficient to cause obvious neurotoxicity in brain.

It is necessary to bind agents to another substance that decreases their interactions within the body to decrease the immediate toxicity of potential paramagnetic contrast agents and to increase the speed with which they are cleared from the body. When gadolinium is bound to the chelating agent DTPA (diethylenetriamine-pantaacetic acid) (Figure 27-5), the LD_{50} in rats changes from 1 to 10 mM/kg, and the compound is eliminated from the body within hours.

The term **chelating** refers to the binding of one substance with another. The acute toxicity of the paramagnetic contrast agents approved for clinical MRI is quite low. Few adverse reactions have been reported.

 Gadolinium is chelated to DTPA to reduce toxicity.

Route of Administration and Biodistribution. The paramagnetic contrast agents currently

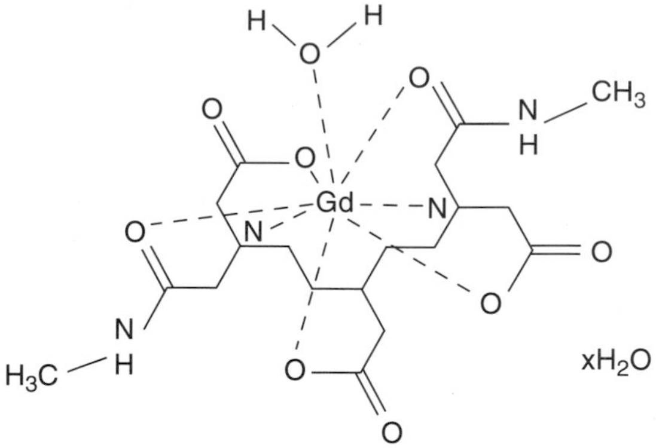

Figure 27-5 Chemical structure of gadolinium-DTPA.

available for clinical MRI are administered intravenously and distributed into the blood and extracellular space. Therefore they are considered nonspecific agents in that they are not taken up by a particular organ, tissue, or lesion type.

All paramagnetic contrast agents clear from the body rapidly after administration. The elimination half-life is generally in the range of several hours.

Effect on Magnetic Resonance Signal Intensity

These contrast agents reduce both T1 and T2 relaxation times. The relaxation time changes cause a decrease in signal intensity on T2W and T2*W images and an increase in signal intensity on T1W images.

In most clinical applications, T1W images are used for contrast-enhanced studies. Areas of increased signal intensity indicate the presence of the contrast agent.

Sometimes a T2W or T2*W image is used, in which case the presence of the contrast agent is indicated by a decrease in signal intensity. If the concentration of contrast agent in an area becomes extremely high, it is possible for the effect on the T2 to dominate even the T1W image, causing a loss of signal intensity on both types of images.

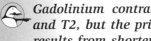 *Gadolinium contrast agents shorten T1 and T2, but the principal image contrast results from shorter T1.*

CE is often equated with bright tissue. With the use of paramagnetic contrast agents, the desired effect, bright tissue, is the result of the shortening of T1 relaxation time. Therefore imaging techniques that emphasize T1 relaxation should be used to maximize the efficacy of the contrast agent. The pulse sequences frequently used are short repetition time (TR), spin echo (SE) sequences, and inversion recovery sequences.

OTHER POSSIBLE CONTRAST AGENTS

Clay Minerals

The inert clay minerals kaolin and bentonite have been used for clinical MRI of the gastrointestinal tract. Kaolin and bentonite are administered orally in an aqueous suspension where they mix with the gastric contents and pass through the gastrointestinal system (Figure 27-6). They are nontoxic and classified as safe for general use by the Food and Drug Administration (FDA). Kaolin is used routinely

as an antidiarrheal agent (Kaopectate). These substances shorten T1 and drastically shorten T2. At doses reasonable for clinical use, T2 can be shortened sufficiently to result in a signal void on both T1W and T2W images.

Iron

Iron in the form of ferric ammonium citrate (Geritol), when administered orally, has been used with some success for contrast-enhanced imaging of the gastrointestinal tract. This is a paramagnetic substance that acts to decrease relaxation times in the same manner as other paramagnetic contrast agents. Ferric ammonium citrate has an extremely low toxicity and is categorized as quite safe.

CLINICAL APPLICATIONS

There are differences in the way contrast agents are used for different pathological conditions and organs. Intravenous agents distribute throughout the body quite rapidly, and the total relaxation time shortening is greatest when the concentration of the agent is greatest. Thus an image acquired soon after contrast administration shows the greatest change in signal intensity.

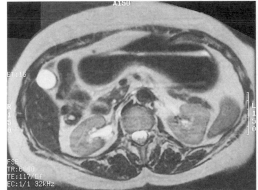
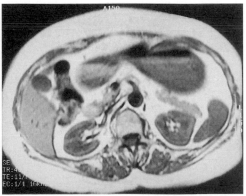

Figure 27-6 These images through the inferior aspect of the right lobe of the liver—**A,** FSE T2W and **B,** CSE T1W—show three levels in the stomach, air, water, and a barium bentonite mixture. (Courtesy Michael Davis, Boston, MA.)

However, acquiring the postcontrast MRI immediately after administration does not necessarily give the maximum contrast between the pathology and surrounding tissue. The reason is that the contrast agent washes out of normal tissue faster than out of abnormal tissue. Thus in some applications, a delayed image is preferred.

Tumor Localization and Characterization

Contrast agent administration is used extensively to improve tumor localization and characterization. The postcontrast administration appearance of the tumor depends on the tumor type, tumor location, and the timing of the postcontrast MRI. In most cases, the contrast agent is used to increase the signal intensity of the tumor on T1W images.

CE allows visualization of extremely small tumors and improves delineation of the tumor margin. Highly vascular tumors show the most CE. In breast and liver imaging especially, both early and delayed images may be useful, depending on the suspected pathological condition. In some cases, there is also evidence that CE may allow differentiation of benign from malignant lesions.

Blood-Brain Barrier Integrity

Normally, contrast agents cannot enter the central nervous system. They are unable to cross the blood-brain barrier (BBB) that protects the brain from substances in the blood. An exception is the pituitary gland, which does not have a BBB.

However, many types of pathological conditions disrupt the BBB. Contrast agents can enter brain tissue in areas in which the BBB is disturbed, resulting in increased visibility of many types of brain abnormalities. In some cases, lesions that cannot be seen otherwise become visible. Visualization of small lesions, such as early metastases, may require delayed imaging or an increased dose of contrast agent.

Tissue Perfusion

An exciting new application of contrast agents in MRI is the combining of contrast agent administration with a very fast image acquisition. This allows dynamic studies to be performed that can aid in assessing organ and tissue function.

Contrast-enhanced perfusion sensitive imaging has the potential to allow evaluation of regional blood flow, blood volume, and tissue perfusion. These techniques have already been used to delineate areas of decreased or absent blood flow in the brain and heart.

Angiography

Although most magnetic resonance angiography (MRA) is presently performed with special image acquisition pulse sequences, it is also possible to obtain angiograms by combining the information from normal and contrast-enhanced images. Bolus injection with fast imaging allows for digital subtraction angiography and multipass imaging of the vessels. This method is particularly applicable to angiography of the brain because the BBB keeps the contrast agent within the vasculature.

Normally, T1W images are used for angiography, so presence of the contrast agent increases the signal from the blood. This increases the contrast between the vasculature and surrounding tissue. A disadvantage of this technique is that arteries are not easily distinguished from veins.

FUTURE DIRECTIONS

Many new approaches to CE for MRI are being actively explored. It is expected that in the future, radiologists will have a variety of different contrast agents available, many of them much more specific in their effects than those presently approved for clinical use.

Several paramagnetic contrast agent candidates in which the biodistribution is altered are under development. For example, binding a paramagnetic contrast agent to microspheres or albumin is being used to create contrast agents that stay within the blood. Also, binding to monoclonal antibodies is being attempted in an effort to target specific diseases. Binding to liposomes of different types has potential for targeting particular organs.

In addition, paramagnetic contrast agents formulated for oral rather than intravenous administration are being tested for gastrointestinal imaging.

Several contrast agent candidates are based on iron oxide particles. Agents for both oral (gastrointestinal imaging) and intravenous (blood pool and reticuloendothelial system imaging) administration are being tested. Work is also under way to make agents that target particular receptors or pathological conditions.

A fluorocarbon contrast agent candidate (perfluorohexybromide) is being developed that evaporates at body temperature. When it is administered orally, it forms a gas in the gut, thus producing a signal void. The gas is radiopaque, has a faster transit time than barium, and appears inert and nontoxic on initial testing.

These developments indicate that with clever applications of chemistry, the role of contrast agents in MRI will only increase in the future, as new compounds are developed to improve image quality for a variety of diagnostic roles.

CHALLENGE QUESTIONS

1. What are some desired characteristics of any medical imaging contrast agent?
2. Why should iron oxide particles make a good MRI contrast agent?
3. How are contrast agents classified according to their route of ingestion?
4. What is the general appearance of tissue after MRI contrast-enhanced imaging?
5. What is the role of the BBB in contrast-enhanced brain imaging?
6. What is the principal MRI contrast agent?
7. Do superparamagnetic and paramagnetic contrast agents produce positive or negative contrast?
8. As a general rule, what is the effect of MRI contrast agents on PD, T1 relaxation, and T2 relaxation?
9. The DTPA in gadolinium-DTPA is a chelating agent. What is that?
10. Why is chelation important? Why not administer the gadolinium in atomic or ionic form?

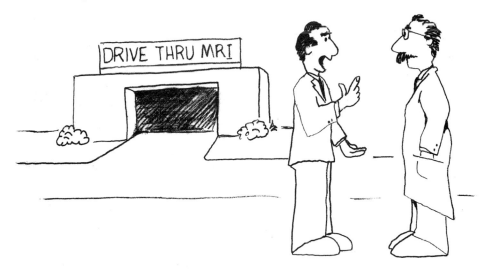

"I don't understand all the mechanics but surely
we can make this work!"

Chapter 28

Magnetic Resonance Artifacts

OBJECTIVES

At the completion of this chapter, the student should be able to do the following:

1. Identify the three principal causes of magnetic resonance imaging (MRI) artifacts.
2. Define the difference between patient-related and system-related artifacts.
3. Recognize image aliasing, chemical shift, and motion artifacts.
4. Describe the partial volume artifact and how to reduce it.

OUTLINE

An *image artifact* is a pattern or structure in the image caused by a signal distortion related to the technique of producing an image. Therefore it is an unwanted pattern or structure that does not represent the actual anatomy. Image artifacts can be misleading and interfere with diagnosis.

The complexity of magnetic resonance imaging (MRI) has unfortunately brought with it many new, confusing imaging artifacts. Luckily, many can be interpreted easily and do not interfere with diagnosis. However, the addition of each new imaging technique or pulse sequence brings the possibility of new artifacts.

The MRI artifacts illustrated here fall into several categories. The outline in Box 28-1 adopts a scheme of three principal classes of MRI artifacts, each of which can be identified as patient related or system related. None of these artifacts are characteristic of a particular manufacturer or model of MRI system.

MAGNETIC AND RADIOFREQUENCY FIELD DISTORTION ARTIFACTS

MRI requires an exceptionally uniform, homogeneous, primary magnetic field. Magnetic field homogeneity of ± 1 ppm (parts per million) is achieved by many current MRI systems.

 A homogeneity of ± 1 ppm means that a 1-T magnetic field does not vary by more than ± 1 μT throughout the imaging volume.

Distortion of the magnetic field can be caused by the patient or problems with the MRI system. A poorly shimmed magnet, gradient magnetic field miscalibration, chemical shift of the Larmor frequency, tissue magnetic susceptibility, and ferromagnetic materials can all result in distortion of the magnetic field.

Patient Related

Ferromagnetic Materials. Metals have different effects on the local magnetic field depending on the type and quantity of ferromagnetic components they contain. Metallic artifacts may range from almost none, as with titanium, to a rather severe effect, as with iron.

Ferromagnetic materials can produce not only a local signal loss but also a warping distortion of the surrounding areas. An example of such field distortion is provided by the friendly "cone-head" seen in Figure 28-1.

Box 28-1	*Classification of Magnetic Resonance Imaging Artifacts*

I. Magnetic and RF Field Distortion Artifacts
  A. Patient related
    1. Ferromagnetic materials
    2. Body shape and conductivity
    3. Extension of body outside magnetic field
    4. Chemical shift
  B. System related
    1. Primary static magnetic field inhomogeneity
    2. Gradient magnetic field inhomogeneity
    3. RF coil inhomogeneity
    4. Gradient coil switching/timing inaccuracy
II. Reconstruction Artifacts
  A. Patient related
    1. Aliasing (wraparound)
    2. Partial volume averaging
  B. System related
    1. Truncation
    2. Quadrature detection

III. Noise-Induced Artifacts
  A. Patient related
    1. Voluntary motion
    2. Involuntary motion
      a. Bowel peristalsis
      b. Respiration
      c. Cardiac and vessel pulsation
      d. Swallowing
    3. Fluid motion
      a. Blood flow
      b. Cerebrospinal fluid flow
      c. Urine movement
    4. Misregistration
  B. System related
    1. Frequency line/point
    2. Phase line/star
    3. Extraneous RF
    4. Off-resonance turning

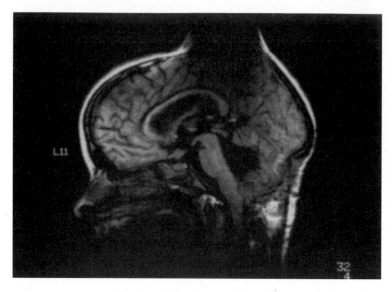

Figure 28-1 A small band of metal in this patient's ponytail produced this "cone-head" artifact. Although the region of interest was not affected by the artifact, the images were incinerated to avoid publicity about unanticipated adverse bioeffects of magnetic resonance imaging.

The typical ferromagnetic material artifact has a partial or complete loss of signal at the site of the metal. Such metal can distort the local magnetic field sufficiently so that the Larmor frequency for local spins is outside the frequency range of the imaging system. Furthermore, metal contains no hydrogen; the result is signal void at that location.

Sometimes a partial rim of high signal intensity may be seen at the periphery of the signal void, which allows differentiation of metal from other causes of focal signal loss. Usually, the degree of anatomical information loss due to such an artifact is less than that seen on computed tomography (CT) images, because the loss is local and not streaked across the image as in CT.

However, ferromagnetic material artifacts can actually cause very subtle, yet significant artifacts. The classic example is orthodontic braces, which cause severe signal dropout from the mouth and jaw. However, they can also cause artifacts in the brain by confusing the slice selection process.

 Distortion of the magnetic field results in a susceptibility artifact.

Exceptions to this are usually caused by the screws in some metallic orthopedic devices, but occasionally distortion is produced by small metallic objects such as buttons, snaps, zippers, or barrettes (Figure 28-2). The distortion of the surrounding tissue is the result of the metal-induced change in the local magnetic field. The magnetic field lines are distorted, resulting in a change in the local Larmor frequency (Figures 28-3 to 28-5).

More mundane but relatively common metallic materials that may be encountered include belt buckles, keys, mascara and other makeup, foreign bodies in the eye or elsewhere, and even certain types of nylon found in clothing, such as gym shorts and warm-up suits (Figures 28-6 to 28-9).

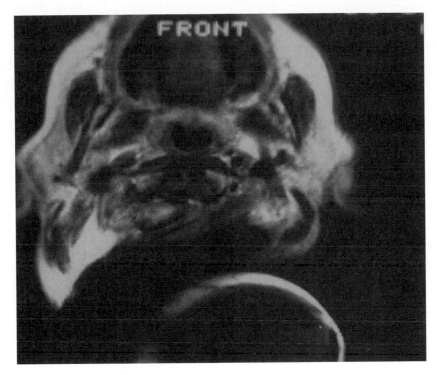

Figure 28-2 The metallic zipper in this patient's shirt produced the noticeable loss of signal, as seen on this image. The high signal rim at the edges of the void is typical.

Body Shape, Conductivity, and Extension. The patient's shape, electrical conductivity, and filling of the radiofrequency (RF) coil all become factors in creating inhomogeneity of both the primary static magnetic field and the transmitted RF pulse. Extension of a body part outside the area of maximum field homogeneity will frequently cause a metallic-like artifact at the edges of this area. This curvilinear artifact conforms to the shape of the magnetic field at the edges and may have a characteristic pattern for an individual magnet system.

Chemical Shift. Chemical shift artifacts are present wherever contiguous tissues have considerably different molecular organization. The artifact is seen as a bright rim of signal at one interface and a dark rim on the opposite side of the particular organ, oriented in the frequency-encoded direction. The most prominent examples seen are at interfaces of fat and the other body tissues.

The molecular environment within fat causes hydrogen nuclei to precess at a slightly lower frequency than those in other soft tissues. The hydrogen electron of water is bound more tightly to oxygen than that of fat is bound to carbon. This hydrogen electron provides a magnetic shield to the proton spin that is stronger for the carbon-bound hydrogen than the oxygen-bound hydrogen.

 The chemical shift between fat and water protons is 3.5 ppm.

The result is a slightly higher Larmor frequency, 3.5 ppm, for soft tissue spins compared with fat spins. For example, at 1 T the 3.5-ppm difference results in a frequency difference of 149 Hz.

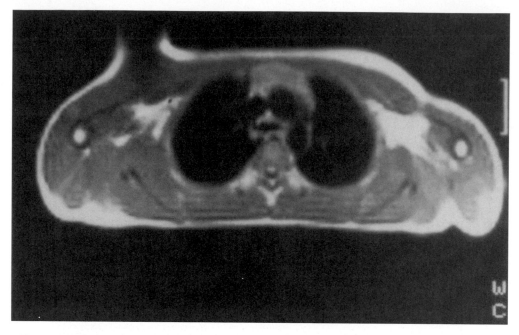

Figure 28-3   An electrocardiographic lead makes a small, localized distortion of the anterior chest wall.

At 1.5 T the frequency difference is 224 Hz, resulting in even more dephasing.

Two components within a voxel with slightly different resonance frequencies provide a hyperintense signal if they have the same phase. They will cause a hypointense signal because of signal cancellation if the magnetization of these two components is of opposed phase. Therefore fat will be slightly displaced because spatial localization is based on the hydrogen spin frequency of water. The artifact is seen only at interfaces where the signal of fat is shifted into or away from the signal of the darker, water-based soft tissues.

The prominence of the chemical shift artifact intensifies with increasing magnetic field. Therefore stronger gradient magnetic fields are required so that imaging can be done with larger bandwidth for high-field strength systems to reduce the visibility of this artifact.

 It is the bandwidth that controls the prominence of the chemical shift artifact.

The chemical shift artifact is most prominent at the border of the kidneys and perirenal fat around the bladder and at the interface of retro-orbital fat with the optic nerve and muscles (Figure 28-10). This shows up in the frequency-encoding direction on conventional images and in the phase-encoding direction in echo planar imaging (EPI).

A second type of chemical shift artifact mostly shows up on gradient echo (GRE) images. The echo time (TE) can be set so that the fat and water signals are imaged either in phase or out of phase. When they are imaged in phase, maximum signal is achieved. However, when they are imaged out of phase, the signal from fat within a voxel partially cancels the signal from water and creates a boundary artifact around many organs.

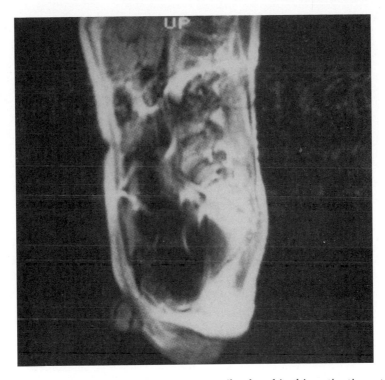

Figure 28-4   A metallic stent, which was temporarily placed in this patient's ureter, caused image degradation along the entire path from the kidney to the bladder.

System Related

There are also many system-related causes of magnetic and RF field inhomogeneity. The primary coil and each secondary coil may contribute to such artifacts.

 Zipper artifacts can occur at any position along the frequency- or phase-encoding gradients.

The primary static magnetic field can never maintain perfect stability and may vary regionally from day to day. In a similar manner, each of the hardware components used to transmit and receive RF signals and manipulate the gradient magnetic fields can do so with limited consistency. The images produced by surface coils and GRE magnetic imaging techniques are especially sensitive to magnetic field inhomogeneities.

Zipper artifacts parallel to the frequency-encoding axis can be caused by residual transverse magnetization, stimulated echoes, and therefore, incomplete spoiling. Zipper artifacts parallel to the phase-encoding gradient can be caused by multiple sources of RF leakage and feed through.

RECONSTRUCTION ARTIFACTS

Frequently observed MRI artifacts relate to RF pulse sequence techniques used and computer reconstruction algorithms. They include aliasing, partial volume averaging, truncation, and quadrature artifacts.

Patient Related

Aliasing.   The aliasing artifact is one of the most commonly encountered of this group. It

Text continued on p. 384

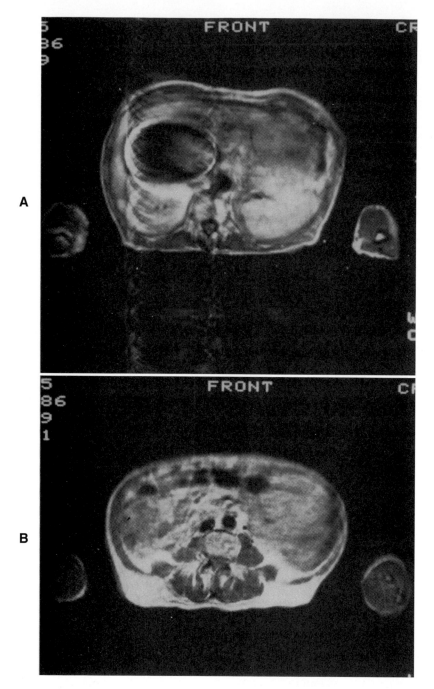

Figure 28-5   Multiple surgical clips and a Gianturco immobilization coil were in place at the time of this examination. **A,** The immobilization coil causes a relatively large signal void within the liver. **B,** Some clips show only small amounts of signal dropout, as seen in the lower abdomen of the same patient.

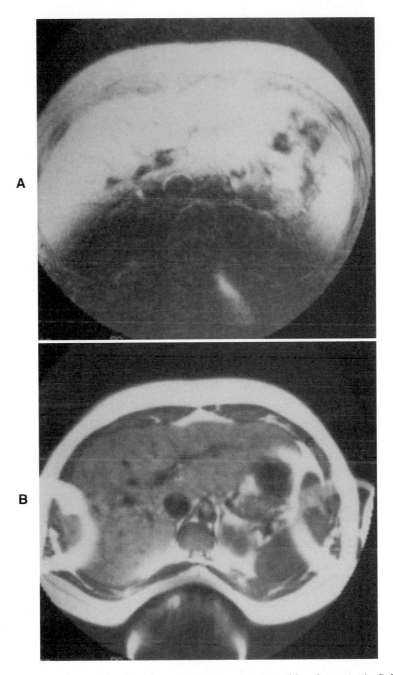

Figure 28-6 Gradient echo imaging causes accentuation of local magnetic field inhomogeneities produced by ferromagnetic materials. **A,** The large area of signal dropout results from two small metallic bra clips that were pulled up between this patient's scapulae. **B,** A spin echo image obtained through the same level shows a more typical and less prominent metallic artifact. A wraparound aliasing artifact of the arms onto the abdomen is also present.

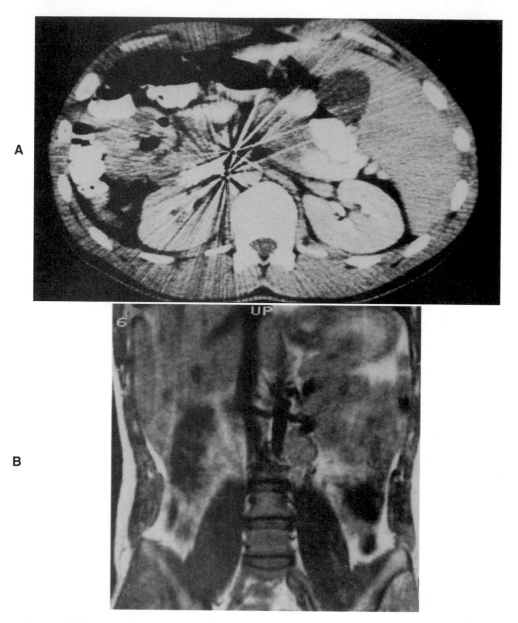

Figure 28-7 **A,** A computed tomography image of the abdomen that is nondiagnostic because of the artifacts produced by surgical clips in the postoperative bed. **B,** The magnetic resonance image of this same patient reveals the recurrent pheochromocytoma. A small signal void immediately above the mass resulted from one of the clips.

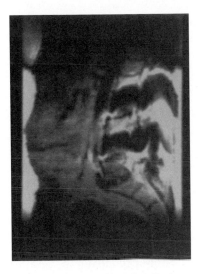

Figure 28-8 Metallic orthopedic devices can produce severe distortion and signal loss. The screws in the Harrington rods caused this image to be nondiagnostic.

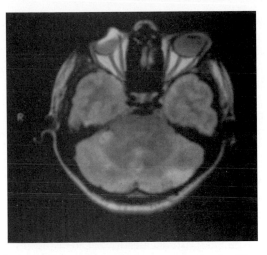

Figure 28-9 Ferrometals may cause significant artifacts, such as distortion of the orbital globes produced by eye shadow.

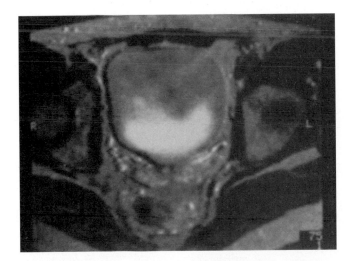

Figure 28-10 The dark rim of signal along the right bladder wall occurs because of a chemical shift artifact at the interface between pelvic fat and bladder urine and wall. The left side of the bladder is brighter, which could occasionally be mistaken for edema or tumor infiltration of the normally darker bladder wall. The bright signal within the posterior urine-filled bladder is an entry slice flow phenomenon more commonly seen in blood vessels. (Courtesy Wlad Sobol, Birmingham, AL.)

occurs when portions of the patient's body are outside the field of view (FOV) but within the area of RF excitation. Therefore RF signals that cannot be properly interpreted are produced.

When hydrogen nuclei outside the area of interest are excited, the signal they return is interpreted to have originated from within the imaging FOV. It is then projected over the real portion of the image on the opposite side of its actual location.

 Aliasing results in a wraparound artifact.

The aliasing artifact occurs because the phase angles of the external nuclei are essentially equal to the nuclei in the imaging volume but on the opposite side of the image. The reconstruction algorithm dutifully places these signals where they should be (Figure 28-6). This "wraparound" artifact is always in the phase-encoding direction; however, manufacturers

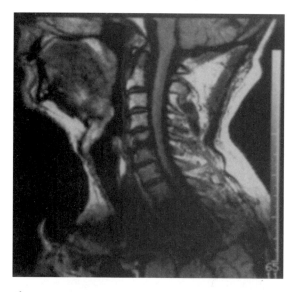

Figure 28-11 The top of the head overlaps the lower neck in this image obtained with a circumferential neck coil. When a portion of the body is outside the coil, it can wrap around the bottom of the image.

have solved this problem with the use of reconstruction filters. An example is seen in Figure 28-11, in which the top of the head (which was outside the RF coil) projects over the upper thorax and lower neck.

Partial Volume Averaging.   This artifact is similar to that engaged in CT imaging. Partial volume averaging results whenever the particular structure of interest is contained within two contiguous slices. The artifact is worse with thick slices and large voxels.

 The use of thin slices reduces the partial volume artifact.

However, thin-slice imaging requires more time for signal averaging because it must attain an adequate signal-to-noise ratio (SNR), and more slices are necessary. Furthermore the adequacy of the gradient magnetic coils or of pulse crafting may not be equal to the task of precisely defining such thin slices.

System Related

Truncation.   *Truncation* is a geometrical term that describes the cutting off or lopping of the vertex of a cone or cylinder (Figure 28-12). The remaining part is the truncated part.

The **truncation** or "ringing" artifact seen in Figure 28-13 appears as multiple, well-defined curved lines regularly conforming to the anatomical boundary. The truncation artifact is more pronounced when the number of phase-encoding acquisitions is small.

Truncation occurs in areas where there is a great difference in signal intensity, such as interfaces of fat and air or fat and cortical bone. The sharp contrast boundaries of these interfaces consist of high spatial frequencies. With a small matrix, there are not enough data to represent such high frequencies accurately. The orientation of the artifact can be along both frequency- and phase-encoding axes.

Truncation artifacts can be particularly bothersome in spinal imaging, where the cord can be distorted or a false syrinx produced.

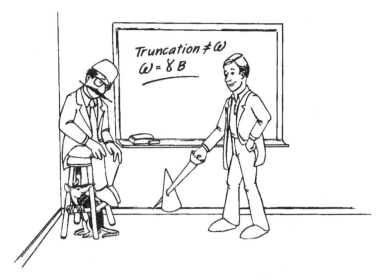

Figure 28-12   This illustrates the meaning of the term *truncation.*

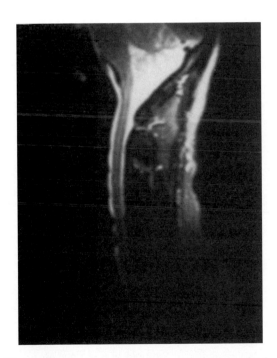

Figure 28-13   This truncation artifact has multiple, evenly spaced, curvilinear lines of bright and dark signal that follow the contour of the back of the head. When the lines project in both the phase- and frequency-encoding directions, the artifact is not the result of motion.

Truncation artifacts can be reduced by increasing the number of phase-encoded steps or reducing the FOV.

Quadrature Detection.   A zero line or **zipper artifact** is caused by RF feed through from the RF transmitter along the frequency-encoding direction at the central or reference frequency of the imaging sequence. It is typically seen on images in which only one average is acquired because no signal is obtained in the centerline of the matrix.

The result is a segmented line extending across the middle of the FOV in the frequency-encoding direction and having a zipperlike appearance (Figure 28-14, *A*). Occasionally, a single point, either bright (Figure 28-14, *B*) or dark (Figure 28-14, *C*), is the only manifestation of this artifact.

A similar-appearing line artifact can be produced by RF noise from extraneous sources and is sometimes called a *free induction decay* (FID) line (Figure 28-15). The source of such RF emissions can be any electrical appliance or broadcast authorized by

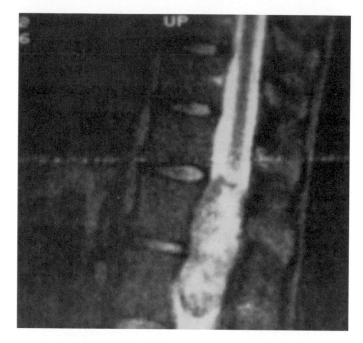

A

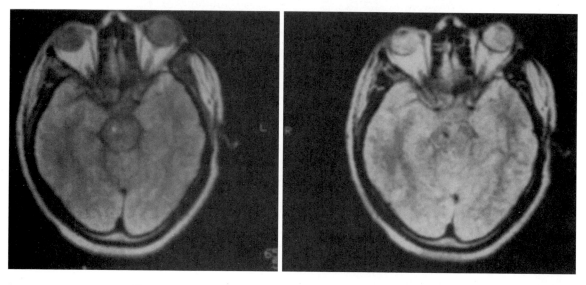

B   **C**

Figure 28-14 **A,** The "zipper" artifact is always at the center of the field of view but not necessarily through the center of the patient. **B,** A central point of brightness, as shown over the right midbrain, could potentially cause a misdiagnosis. **C,** The central point artifact can also be dark, as seen on this second echo image.

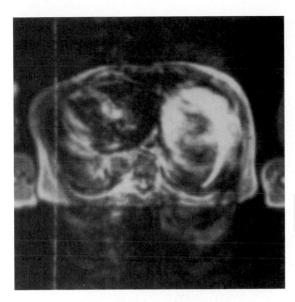

Figure 28-15 Lines produced by random radiofrequency (RF) noise can occur whenever RF shielding of the room is inadequate. Extraneous RF noise at two frequencies shows up on this image.

the Federal Communications Commission operating at the frequency of the magnet. This artifact is not normally located on the centerline.

NOISE-INDUCED ARTIFACTS

Patient Related

Motion. An additional group of artifacts is caused by voluntary, involuntary, and even microscopic physiological motion. As with photography, a picture of a moving object cannot easily be taken.

A magnetic resonance (MR) image is severely degraded if motion occurs during the imaging time. This is especially true if the motion occurs near the middle of the acquisition. Physiological motion of the blood, heart, larynx (swallowing), diaphragm, bowel, and cerebrospinal fluid (CSF) in the brain and spinal canal can cause various types of motion artifacts.

Most motion artifacts result in a poorly defined, smeared appearance of the image in the area of motion. Repetitive motion of a linear or curvilinear surface, such as the diaphragm or heart, can produce the typical "ghosting" or irregular wavelike lines of increased and decreased signal. The artifact appears parallel to the phase-encoding gradient regardless of the direction of the motion. The reason is that there is much more time in the phase-encoding direction (hundreds of milliseconds) than in the frequency-encoding read direction (tens of microseconds).

 Ghost artifacts occur when a tissue moves in a periodic fashion.

Techniques for decreasing motion artifacts without increasing imaging time have been developed for abdominal imaging. These include various corrective algorithms, physical restriction of the motion of the anterior abdomen, and rapid imaging techniques that can be performed during breathholding (Figure 28-16). Use of short repetition time (TR) and TE with multiple acquisitions produces good images by averaging the motion artifacts (Figure 28-17).

The problems with artifacts produced by swallowing and bowel peristalsis are less easily handled but are generally not as severe as those caused by vascular and respiratory motion. Fast imaging techniques that are based principally on GREs appear to provide a partial, if not complete, solution to such artifacts. Furthermore the direction of the phase-encoding gradient can be changed with most systems, rendering the artifact less bothersome.

The CSF flow in the region of the foramen of Monro and Magendie can produce bright foci in the region of the midbrain and brain stem. This signal occurs in the phase-encoding direction and may mimic various lesions such as infarcts, multiple sclerosis plaques, and gliosis.

The flow of CSF in the cervical thecal sac can also produce high signal artifacts overlying the cord, which can obscure this area or be mistaken for pathological conditions. This

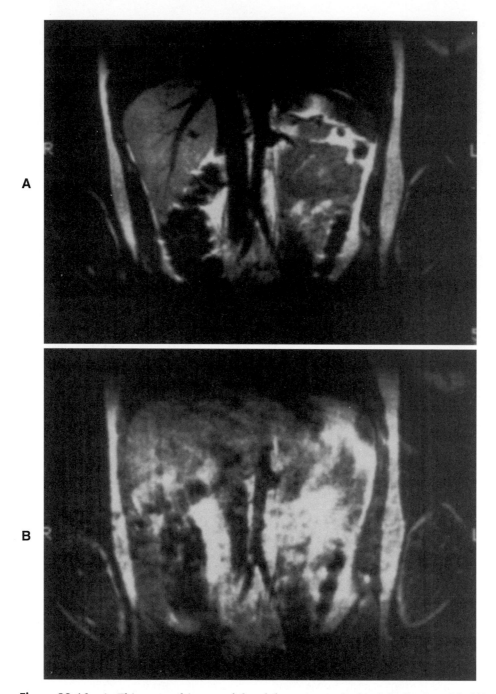

Figure 28-16   **A,** This coronal image of the abdomen was obtained during breathholding. Notice the complete absence of blurring that is usually seen near the diaphragm. **B,** A similar image obtained in an equal amount of time during quiet respiration shows poor definition of the subdiaphragmatic structures.

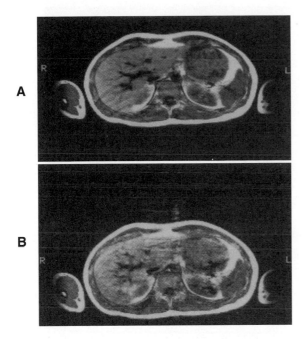

Figure 28-17 A, The motion artifact can be masked because it is, for the most part, a random signal that subtracts out in multiple, average images. **B,** A comparison of the same patient with only two averages shows a considerable amount of distortion from respiratory motion.

artifact is relatively easy to recognize because it is more linear and parallel with the spine on sagittal images, projecting in the phase-encoding direction (Figure 28-18).

Blood flow artifacts can be extremely useful because most vessels are seen as black on conventional spin echo (SE) pulse sequences. The blood returns a relatively strong signal on proton density weighted (PDW) and T2 weighted (T2W) images if it is stationary or flowing slowly (Figure 28-19), but the artifact created by its motion produces the typical signal void instead.

A problem can occur when flowing blood is oriented diagonally within the imaging plane. In this case, the nuclei remain in the imaging FOV so that the emitted RF signal is received even though there may be rapid flow. The resultant displaced blood signal parallels the dark blood vessel and appears as an adjacent bright line (Figure 28-20).

Misregistration. If patient motion occurs between a mask image and a subsequent image, the subtracted image contains **misregistration artifacts.** The same anatomy is not

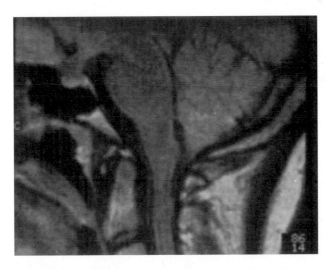

Figure 28-18 The loss of cerebrospinal fluid signal at and immediately below the aqueduct and foramen of Magendie mostly results from the rapid dephasing of spins caused by turbulent flow.

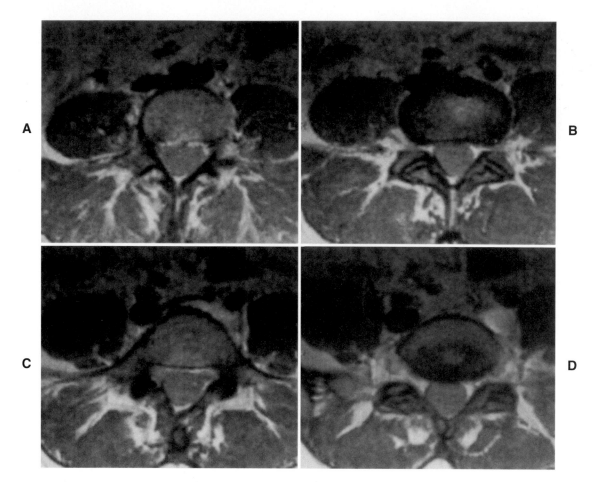

Figure 28-19   These four contiguous images, from (**A**) superior to (**D**) inferior, show the normal, black signal void in the inferior vena cava and right iliac vein resulting from rapidly flowing blood. The left iliac vein is compressed as it passes beneath the left iliac artery. It has a relatively bright, intraluminal signal in the more slowly flowing portion, which is distal to the point of compression.

registered in the same pixel of the image matrix.

This type of artifact can frequently be eliminated by reregistration of the mask, that is, by shifting the mask by one or more pixels so that superimposition of images is again obtained. However, reregistration can be a tedious process.

Often when one area of an image is reregistered, another area will become misregistered.

This can be controlled on some systems by region of interest (ROI) reregistration. Many systems can reregister not only in increments of pixel widths but also down to $^1/_{10}$ pixel width.

System Related

The **off-resonance artifact** is simply the degradation of the image as a result of inex-

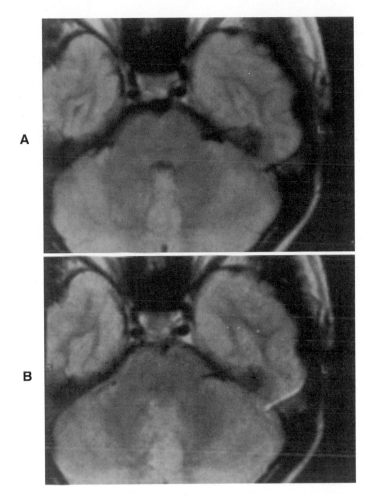

Figure 28-20 **A,** A petrosal vein is seen traveling obliquely through this transaxial image of the brain. This demonstrates a normal signal void. **B,** The second, even echo of this four-echo sequence shows a double linear track at the site of the vein. Even echo rephasing of the blood signal has occurred, accounting for the bright line, but it has been displaced laterally.

act tuning of the RF transmitter and/or receiver to the Larmor frequency, resulting in overall noisy images. This mainly occurs when imaging small structures off the magnet isocenter, such as elbows or hands.

A "bleeding" artifact results when inexact duplication of the RF pulses occurs or the gradient magnetic fields between each acquisi-

tion are incorrectly formed (Figure 28-21). This produces slight inaccuracies in the placement of signals into the appropriate pixel; the result is a smeared image of wavelike patterns similar to ghosting from motion. The off-resonance artifact can also appear similar to the truncation artifact, but not as regular and well-defined.

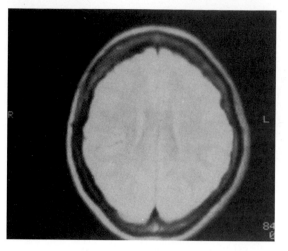

Figure 28-21 The "bleeding" artifact can be mistaken for a displacement of signal as a result of motion; however, this artifact is a more diffuse smearing of signal, both within and outside of the body.

CHALLENGE QUESTIONS

1. Define image artifact.
2. What is an off-resonance artifact, and how does it appear?
3. How can a partial volume artifact be reduced?
4. Describe a magnetic susceptibility artifact.
5. What is a misregistration artifact?
6. What causes the chemical shift artifact?
7. What is a ghost artifact?
8. Describe the cause and appearance of a zipper artifact.
9. What is a wraparound artifact?
10. Define the term *truncation*.

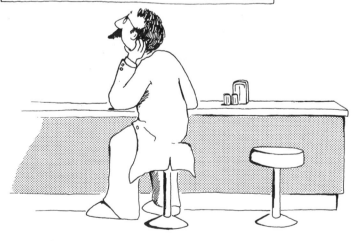

Chapter 29

Biological Effects of Magnetic Resonance Imaging

OBJECTIVES

At the completion of this chapter, the student should be able to do the following:

1. Differentiate between stochastic and deterministic effects.
2. Identify the three magnetic resonance imaging (MRI) energy fields potentially capable of producing a harmful response.
3. Describe the possible human responses to each of the three MRI energy fields.
4. Define SAR and identify recommended exposure limits.
5. Identify the cause of the banging noise in MRI.
6. Discuss hazards imposed by ferromagnetic projectiles.

OUTLINE

Many noninvasive medical imaging modalities are currently available, such as x-ray imaging, radioisotope imaging, ultrasonography, and magnetic resonance imaging (MRI). Being noninvasive, each of these modalities is inherently safe. Ionizing radiation can induce malignant disease and genetic mutations, although the risk of such responses is extremely low.

 Ultrasonography and MRI prevail in safety considerations because neither uses ionizing radiation.

Human response to ionizing radiation follows a linear, nonthreshold, dose-response relationship (Figure 29-1). *Nonthreshold* means that no dose of ionizing radiation is considered to be absolutely safe. Even the smallest dose carries a risk of response, although such risk may be lower than that from other everyday risks.

At low radiation doses, the increase in response is exceedingly low. Only after rather high radiation doses (e.g., 0.25 Gy or greater) would the anticipated response be detectable.

Such responses to ionizing radiation are stochastic. There is no threshold dose, and the response is an increase in incidence, such as cancer or leukemia, rather than severity.

Exposure to the energy fields of MRI, both individually and collectively, results in a fundamentally different type of dose-response relationship (Figure 29-2). Such a dose-response

relationship is known as a *threshold, nonlinear relationship.*

It is inappropriate to use the term *dose* when describing the energy fields associated with MRI. *Intensity* is a better term, because it implies bathing a patient in an agent, rather than administering a certain quantity of the agent to the patient.

Regardless of the type of MRI energy field considered, there is a level of intensity, the threshold intensity (I_T), below which no response is elicited. Below I_T, MRI is entirely safe. Above I_T, the response to MRI exposure first increases slowly and then more rapidly until 100% response is observed. A response that exhibits a threshold and a dose-related severity is a deterministic response.

 Responses to MRI are deterministic.

Because MRI is still developing, all of the radiobiological questions are not completely answered. It does appear that MRI, as it is currently used, is safe for all workers and patients. Experimental observations suggest that I_T for all of the MRI energy fields is considerably higher than the intensities used for clinical examinations.

MAGNETIC RESONANCE IMAGING ENERGY FIELDS

Although MRI is considered safe, radiobiologists will be busy for many years to stretch their ability to detect human responses to the

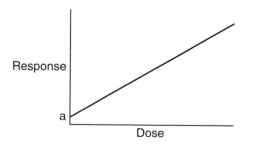

Figure 29-1 The dose-response relationship for ionizing radiation is linear. It is also nonthreshold, suggesting that even the smallest radiation dose carries a risk, albeit insignificant. The value *a* represents the natural incidence of the response.

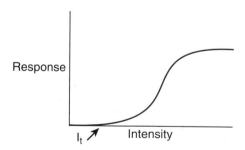

Figure 29-2 The response after exposure to the energy fields of magnetic resonance imaging is threshold and nonlinear in form.

energy fields used. It is certain that the delayed determination that x-ray exposure can cause cancer and leukemia will not be repeated with MRI, because the energy fields are nonionizing.

The potential health hazards of MRI lie in the static magnetic field, (B_0), the transient gradient magnetic fields (B_{SS}, B_Φ, B_R), the radiofrequency (RF)–pulsed electromagnetic field, or a combination of these. Radiobiological data already show that, individually, such fields are innocuous at the levels currently used for MRI.

In addition to following a threshold intensity-response relationship, these fields exhibit a time-intensity relationship (Figure 29-3). The I_T applies to continuous exposure. Above this threshold, shorter exposure times produce the same response. What is not fully understood is whether these MRI energy fields have adverse health effects when combined.

Before there is a discussion of suspected biological effects of MRI in human beings, an examination of each of the MRI fields and their potential effects on other biological systems is

necessary. The three MRI energy fields interact with matter differently (Table 29-1).

Static Magnetic Field

The static magnetic field is probably the best-recognized MRI energy field. Although people cannot sense a magnetic field, they know that it exists because of forces that attract and repel small magnets, such as kitchen latches and other everyday permanent magnets. Consequently, it is also clear that one interaction between a static magnetic field and matter results in a force that can turn certain types of matter (ferromagnetic material) into projectiles or missiles.

Additionally, tissue can be rendered weakly magnetic, or **polarized**, by exposure to a strong static magnetic, field (B_0). This induced tissue magnetism cannot be sensed. Furthermore, in the presence of a static magnetic field, tissue magnetization (M) can only be measured with great difficulty in MRI. Once removed from the influence of a static magnetic field, tissue relaxes to its normal state without a hint that it was previously magnetized.

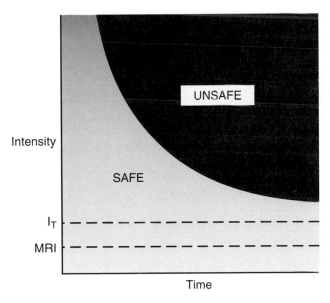

Figure 29-3 Individually, the magnetic resonance imaging energy fields follow this type of time-intensity relationship to produce a human response.

TABLE 29-1	Principal Mechanisms of Interaction of the Three Magnetic Resonance Imaging Energy Fields with Tissue
Magnetic Resonance Imaging Energy Field	**Mechanism of Interaction**
Static magnetic field (B_0)	Polarization
Transient gradient magnetic fields (B_{SS}, B_Φ, B_R)	Induced currents
RF field (RF_t)	Thermal heating

There is no scientific evidence to show that intense static magnetic fields produce harmful effects in mammals. Mechanisms have been suggested and subjected to considerable investigation but the result remains negative.

There are few studies of the effects of long-term exposure of mammals to intense static magnetic fields that use proper controls and large sample sizes. Some experiments have been designed to detect growth abnormalities, biochemical disruption, and malignant disease induction in rodents at magnetic field strengths up to 5 T. All such observations have been negative.

Other reports deal with the effects of intense static magnetic fields on cultured cells. These reports do not suggest any adverse effects on cell growth for magnetic fields up to 7 T. Such experiments involve conventional culturing of human fibroblasts. Lengthening the exposure time does not produce a positive response either.

The navigational ability of adult bees and pigeons is considered to be mediated by granules of magnetite deposits in the abdominal region and in the head, respectively (Figure 29-4). These magnetic deposits serve as a built-in compass, yet experiments have not been conducted to determine whether these characteristics can be disturbed by intense static magnetic fields. Such experiments are unimportant anyway because human beings do not rely on an internal compass.

Some speculation exists concerning bioeffects of intense magnetic fields on growth rate, mutation, fertility, and blood cell count in mammals. Growth rate and mutation effects have been reported in animals and yeast, but the results have been equivocal or not reproducible. Monkeys who were exposed to a static magnetic field of 7 T for up to 1 hour experienced a transient decrease in heart rate and sinus arrhythmia; a later study failed to demonstrate these effects with a limited exposure of 15 minutes at 10 T.

The evidence for static magnetic field effects on the developing embryos of pregnant mice who were exposed at various times during gestation did not consistently show alterations in the offspring when compared with nonexposed control mice. These studies used acceptably large sample sizes and were repeated with similar negative results.

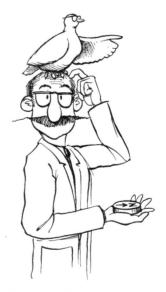

Figure 29-4 It has been shown that magnetic deposits in the head of the pigeon allow it to know which direction is north.

Transient Magnetic Field

The gradient magnetic fields used to spatially encode the magnetic resonance (MR) signals vary with time. These are often termed *moving magnetic fields* or *time-varying magnetic fields*. The preferred term is **transient magnetic field.**

A transient magnetic field is able to induce an electric current. For example, an electric current can easily be induced in a metal conductor. This is the basic principle of electromagnetic induction that generates and detects the MR signal.

Theoretically, transient magnetic fields can either stimulate or impair electric impulses along neuronal pathways in tissue. The main influence of this is the time rate of change of the magnetic field expressed as dB/dt and measured in T/s. For example, a transient magnetic field of 3 T/s results in an induced electric current density of approximately 3 μA/cm^2 in tissue.

A current density of 3 μA/cm^2 is capable of producing involuntary muscle contraction and cardiac fibrillation in experimental animals. However, the time of application was far greater than that experienced in clinical MRI.

 Transient magnetic fields can induce neurological signals.

Because some cells and tissues are electric conductors, the transient gradient magnetic fields may induce or interfere with normal conduction pathways. Depending on the intensity of the induced electric current, the normal function of nerve cells and muscle fibers may be affected. The threshold current density of transient magnetic fields depends on the tissue conductivity and the duration of time the field is energized.

The maximum transient magnetic field does not occur in the center of the magnet. There the gradient magnetic fields are near zero; they are maximum at the periphery of the imaging volume.

Radiofrequency Field

The RF field used in MRI exists in the approximate range of 10 to 200 MHz. This energy field consists of an oscillating electric field and a similar orthogonal oscillating magnetic field. These fields interact simultaneously with matter. The interaction manifests differently according to the nature of matter.

The electric field component can induce heating in matter and induce high-frequency electric currents, whereas the magnetic field component acts as a rapidly transient magnetic field. This is relevant to MRI because it has the potential for heating both superficial and deep tissues.

The electric field is generally well shielded from the patient's body by the placement of guard rings in the RF coil design. The magnetic component of the RF field is required for imaging. However, in addition to flipping proton spins, it induces eddy currents within the conductive tissues of the body. This results in heat, which increases with increasing frequency.

A rise in body temperature has been reported with exposure to RF fields; the absorbed energy causes this temperature increase. In turn, the RF frequency, exposure time, and mass of the exposed object determine the amount of absorbed energy.

The RF frequency influences energy absorption because it is wavelength dependent. Energy is most efficiently absorbed from an RF emission when the tissue size is approximately one half of the RF wavelength. The wavelengths associated with 10 MHz and 200 MHz are 30 m and 1.5 m, respectively. Shorter-wavelength RF results in more superficial heating and less penetration.

Commercial microwave ovens operate at 2.45 GHz. What is the wavelength of such radiation? . . . 12 cm. What is the size of a hot dog? . . . 12 cm.

Depending on the imaged region when an RF pulse sequence is applied to a patient, the peak power can range to 16 kW. The energy returned from the patient is very weak; it is measured in microwatts (μW). Some energy is lost to coil inefficiencies and transmits cable losses; some is reflected back to the RF power amplifier and a load attached to the back of the coil.

Some energy is transmitted through the patient without interactions, and some energy interacts with the patient and generates heat, causing a possible rise in body temperature. The amount of absorbed energy depends on the transmitted magnetic field frequency, the total power of the RF pulse, and the structure and conductivity of the exposed object.

 The physiological measure of intensity of RF energy is the specific absorption rate (SAR).

The SAR has units of W/kg and may be expressed as an average over the whole body or any specific tissue. Thus there is a whole-body and a local SAR.

The SAR may also be expressed over a long time or a single pulse. Specific absorption rate is a measure of the energy absorbed per unit time per unit mass.

Specific absorption rate is to MRI as the Gray is to ionizing radiation. The mathematical formulation of SAR is extensive and unnecessary for this discussion.

Biological effects of RF are associated with the SAR. In turn, the SAR is related to the RF power density because it varies in time (temporal) and space (spatial). Recommended exposure limits are expressed as power density. They are set approximately 100 times lower than levels known to cause a biological response.

In a guideline issued in 1998, the Food and Drug Administration (FDA) recommended that equipment manufacturers in the United States use an operating scheme put forth by the International Electrotechnical Commission (IEC). Under the standard (IEC 60601-2-33, July 1995), three modes of operation are established that relate to RF heating and dB/dt. These are the normal operating mode, the first level–controlled operating mode, and the second level–controlled operating mode; these are not directly related to any specific values but mark thresholds where concerns may arise.

The normal operation mode is what has been used for years for conventional imaging under the old FDA guideline. The first level indicates when there may be a situation of "undue physiological stress" and requires medical supervision. The second level indicates operation at a level that "may produce significant risk" and requires medical supervision and institutional review board approval.

MRI systems calculate the SAR. MRI technologists cannot continue to image if the recommended exposure limits will be exceeded. Always enter accurate patient weight to stay within the recommended limits for SAR, even if these levels are lower than levels known to cause a response.

 The SAR is highest with pulse sequences that require many 180° RF pulses, such as fast spin echo (FSE).

The basal metabolic rate for a resting adult is approximately 1 to 2 W/kg. Anatomical abnormalities in the offspring of pregnant animals have been reported when the SAR exceeded 20 W/kg during whole-body exposure. If the rate of energy absorption exceeds the rate of heat loss, the body temperature increases. When such temperature increases last for long periods, adverse biological effects result.

Exposure to microwave radiation, which involves frequencies higher than those used in MRI, causes a similar rise in body temperature. In mice, such exposure has been associated with decreased fertility and testicular degeneration. Such reports have not been confirmed by repetitive experiments.

Combined Magnetic Resonance Imaging Fields

In large-scale or long-term studies in experimental animals exposed to the combined fields of MRI negative results have consistently been reported. However, not all such experiments involved exposure to all three MRI fields, and the number of studies is limited.

Mutagenic or lethal effects in *Escherichia coli* were not observed when the bacterial cells were exposed to typical MRI fields for up to 5 hours. When human peripheral blood lympho-cytes grown in tissue culture were exposed to MRI, no significant differences to chromoso-mal lesions or sister chromatid exchanges were found between the exposed and control groups. Similar cytogenetical studies have been conducted with several mammalian cells (e.g., HeLa cells and Chinese hamster cells) with MRI exposure. Negative results were reported in all studies in terms of chromosome aberrations, sister chromatid exchanges, and DNA synthesis.

The effect of MRI on the early development of an amphibian system also resulted in the absence of harmful bioeffects. These studies were conducted with frog spermatozoa, eggs fertilized during second meiotic division, and embryos during cleavage. All were subjected separately to 30-MHz continuous wave RF in a static magnetic field of 0.7 mT for 20 min-utes. These specimens were compared at sim-ilar stages with specimens in unexposed groups. Researchers compared the damage in genetic material, interference with meiotic cell division, and impaired development of the embryos; no significant differences were observed. This suggests that MRI exposure at these intensities does not cause detectable, adverse effects in the amphibian system.

Low-Frequency Electromagnetic Fields

Though not directly applicable to the high-frequency electric and magnetic fields of MRI, considerable public attention has turned to the electric and magnetic fields associated with 60-Hz electric power distribution and use. Consequently, low-frequency electromagnetic fields (EMFs) also receive considerable scien-tific attention.

The approximate electric and magnetic field intensity associated with conventional electric power is shown in Figure 29-5. Note the relative intensity of the magnetic field of the earth. Study results of these energy fields are largely negative.

The Oak Ridge Association of Universities Expert Panel on EMF has expressed the follow-ing on the subject:

We have never stated that a causal association between EMF [electromagnetic fields] and cancer is impossible or inconceivable; we have indicated that the evidence for such an association is empirically weak and biologically implausible. We have not pro-posed that research concerning the health effects of EMF be discontinued; in fact, we have indicated areas of some scientific interest that warrant con-sideration for future research. However, given the decreasing resources available for basic health and science research, we believe that in a broader per-spective there are currently more serious health needs that should be given higher priority.

HUMAN RESPONSES TO MAGNETIC RESONANCE IMAGING

Before the advent of MRI, a considerable amount of research effort was put into studying these electric, magnetic, and electromagnetic energy fields. With the introduction and clinical use of MRI and the properly focused concern for its safe application, more studies have been undertaken at the cell, animal, and human level.

Work in this area began in the early 1960s when some farmers in upstate New York com-plained that cows grazing in pastures through which high-voltage transmission lines ran pro-duced less milk than cows in pastures without these transmission lines. These reports were followed by additional concerns about aber-rant animal behavior, allegedly resulting from the energy fields of these high-voltage trans-mission lines. These early reports led to inves-tigations regarding the possibility of such effects.

One study at Oak Ridge National Laboratory involved the construction of an enclosure to house eight cows at a time in controlled elec-tric and magnetic fields (Figure 29-6). This and other studies showed that the farm animals were unaffected by both the electric field and the magnetic field imposed by electric power transmission lines.

The energy fields produced in clinical MRI are less intense than those associated with

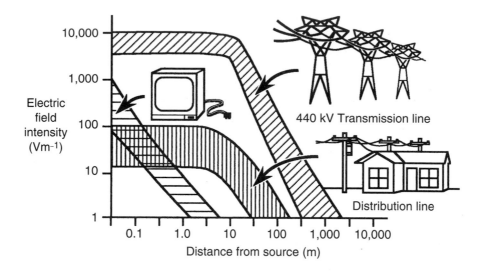

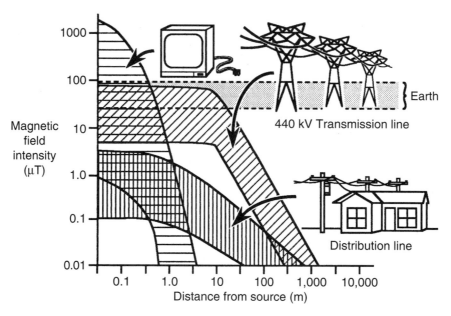

Figure 29-5 Electric and magnetic field intensities associated with electric power.

proximity to electric power devices. However, the frequency of the MRI RF is much higher than the frequency of 60-Hz electric power.

Two of the three MRI energy fields—transient magnetic fields and RF fields—have been shown to induce responses in human beings. Such responses only occurred at exceedingly high intensities. There are no known effects from the static magnetic field.

However, transient magnetic fields induce magnetic phosphenes, stimulate healing in bones, and cause cardiac fibrillation. RF expo-

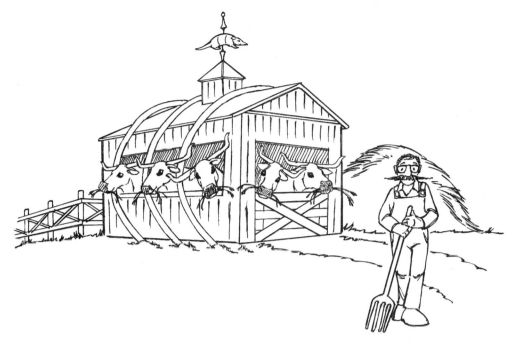

Figure 29-6 Enclosure for housing cows in a controlled electric field and magnetic field environment.

sure heats tissues, induces blood dyscrasia, and forms cataracts. Note that all of these responses are acute.

 There are no known long-term effects of MRI fields.

The extent of SAR tolerance in a subject primarily depends on oxygen supply and vascularity. The brain, kidneys, and liver are all tissues with high vascularity. The lens of the eye has poor vascularity and a lower oxygen supply. Therefore it is suspected that the lens is more susceptible to biological damage by RF energy.

Effects of Static Magnetic Field

Even at 4 T, magnetic forces and torques on tissues are small when compared with ordinary gravitational and inertial forces. The highest static magnetic field that human beings can comfortably tolerate is probably much more intense than 4 T.

When patients and volunteers have been imaged with these 4-T magnet systems, some responses have been reported. These include metallic taste, twitching, some disequilibrium, and phosphene induction. Presumably, the transient magnetic fields caused these responses.

When the examinations ended, the responses stopped. Researchers conducting these 4-T studies do caution that patient motion should be minimized in these high field imaging systems.

Effects of Transient Magnetic Field

Magnetic phosphenes are flashes of light that can sometimes be perceived with the eyes closed. D'Arsonval first reported magnetic phosphene induction in 1896. The introduction of MRI rekindled research in this area.

Electric stimulation of the sensory receptors of the retina as a result of transient magnetic fields causes this phenomenon. The threshold for the induction of magnetic phosphenes in human beings is approximately 3 T/s at low frequencies. Magnetic phosphene induction in the RF region has a threshold of approximately 20 T/s.

Bone healing accelerates if a low-frequency coil is positioned over a fracture. Although a precise mechanism of action is unknown, this method works and is an accepted adjunctive therapy. Treatments that last for several minutes are repeatedly given during a 2-week to 5-week course. Apparently, gradient magnetic fields stimulate bone healing.

Ventricular fibrillation is another potential hazard of electric currents induced by transient magnetic fields. This happens when the current density in cardiac tissue is above 0.5 mA/cm^2 and applied for longer than 3 seconds. The threshold for such an effect is thought to be 0.1 mA/cm^2.

Such disruption of the heartbeat may cause a drop in blood pressure; however, ventricular fibrillation ceases and the heartbeat returns to normal when the induced electric current is interrupted. However, this response has only been observed in patients with pacemakers.

Each of these responses, which can be induced by transient magnetic fields, has a threshold that is a complex function of frequency, waveform, pulsatile nature, and duration. Presumably, each response follows the time-intensity relationship shown in Figure 29-3.

Effects of Radiofrequency Field

The hazard of exposure to RF radiation is associated with heating. Thermal effects on tissue are related to frequency and waveform. The hazard is one of cooking, as in a microwave oven. Such effects have been observed in both experimental animals and patients.

Heating of avascular structures, such as the lens of the eye, produces cataracts. This has been demonstrated experimentally in animals and has been observed in human beings. Some evidence suggests that ship-bound sailors who worked near radio antennae and were exposed to high-intensity RF subsequently had cataracts.

Exposure to intense RF has been shown to result in nonspecific blood changes, principally lymphocytic depression. This was thought to be the case some years ago when U.S. embassy personnel in Moscow were alleged to have been exposed to RF by sources outside the embassy.

Large-scale, epidemiological studies of human beings, with respect to the RF fields of MRI, have not been done. To show any such effects, dedicated and experienced researchers would need to conduct a well-controlled, long-term study using a sufficiently large population of individuals exposed to MRI. A prospective study of patients exposed to clinical MRI is currently lacking.

RECOMMENDED GUIDELINES

The first studies conducted on MRI patients date back to early 1981. Since then, millions of patients have been imaged by MRI. The most predictable results of exposure to the MRI fields include an increase in temperature, physiochemical changes, and induction of electric currents.

None of these changes or any such adverse, acute effects have been reported in patients undergoing clinical MRI evaluation. However, as many as 5% of all patients experience claustrophobia; another 10% sleep during the examination!

In light of the rapid progress in the application of MRI in medical diagnosis, dose limits of each component field of a clinical MRI system have been recommended by the U.S. Center for Devices and Radiologic Health and by the British National Radiological Protection Board (Table 29-2).

The American National Standards Institute (ANSI) standard for whole-body exposure in comparison with the limitations that were used by the former Soviet Union is shown in Figure 29-7. These standards acknowledge that biological responses are related to the power density and the frequency.

In 1983 the International Radiation Protection Association (IRPA) recommended interim guidelines on limits of exposure to RF EMFs. These guidelines are established for occupationally

TABLE 29-2	Clinical Magnetic Resonance Imaging Exposure Limits Recommended by the United States Center for Devices and Radiologic Health and the British National Radiological Protection Board

	Recommended Limits	
MRI Energy Field	**United States**	**Great Britain**
Static magnetic field	<3.0 T	<2.5 T
Transient magnetic field	<3.0 T/s	<20.0 T/s
RF field		
Whole body	<0.4 W/kg	<0.4 W/kg
Any 1 g of tissue	<2.0 W/kg	<4.0 W/kg

exposed persons and the general public. These limits are based on the SAR values shown in Table 29-3; the resulting RF exposure limits are shown in Table 29-4.

The basal metabolic rate for human beings is approximately 1 W/kg at rest. During exertion, the metabolic rate may increase to 15 W/kg.

GENERAL SAFETY CONSIDERATIONS

Radiologists use their knowledge of the potential human bioresponses to the energy fields of MRI to ensure safety for their patients and personnel. The following safety precautions are not discussed in a particular order.

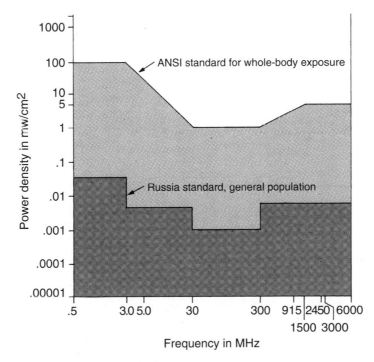

Figure 29-7 Recommended limits of radiofrequency power densities are related to frequency.

TABLE 29-3	Specific Absorption Rate Levels from Which Radiofrequency Exposure Limits Are Derived

Population	Whole-Body Exposure	Tissue Exposure (1 g)
Occupational	0.4 W/kg	4.0 W/kg
General public	0.08 W/kg	0.8 W/kg

TABLE 29-4	Recommendations of the International Radiation Protection Association (IRPA) for Exposure Limits to Radiofrequency Radiation

Frequency Range (MHz)	Power Density Limit (W/m^2)	
	Occupational	General Public
0.1 to 1	100	20
>1 to 10	100/f	20/f
>10 to 400	10	2
>400 to 2 K	f/40	f/200
>2 K to 300 K	50	10

Patient Evaluation

When patients arrive for an MRI examination, they should complete a patient information form to make sure no contraindications are present. However, completion of the form is not enough because patients do not know what is and what is not important enough to keep them from having an MRI examination. The receptionist or MRI technologist should spend sufficient time with each patient to explain the nature of the examination and to determine the patient's condition (e.g., pregnancy, pacemaker, prosthesis, metallic implant, occupational history).

 Patient screening is essential to ensure patient safety during MRI.

Claustrophobia. Patient anxiety can cause difficulty in successfully completing an MRI examination. Claustrophobia accounts for most patient anxiety during an MRI examination.

Claustrophobia is an excessive, sometimes morbid, fear of being enclosed in a tight, narrow, or otherwise confined space. The professor shown in Figure 29-8 is clearly claustrophobic.

True claustrophobes would probably not even enter the MRI suite. Patients with mild claustrophobia need special attention to help them through the examination. This special attention begins with the referring physician who should prescreen all patients and counsel those who might be claustrophobic.

The MRI facility should be forewarned of a possible claustrophobic patient so that more planning and attention to patient preparation is possible. The examination should be clearly explained to the patient, and every effort should be made to comfort the patient before and during the imaging procedure.

It is helpful to have a member of the family or friend remain in the magnet room during imaging. Usually, if a family member or friend maintains contact by holding onto the patient's foot and talking, the examination can be completed without incident.

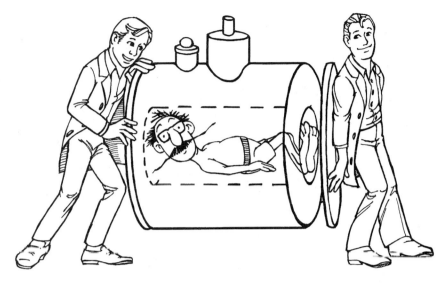

Figure 29-8 Crazed student technologists performing a routine physics experiment on a professor with claustrophobia.

The development of open MRI has eased imaging of claustrophobic patients. Previous open MR imaging systems were based on permanent magnet technology and had low field strength. Several vendors now offer open MRI models based on superconducting magnet design with B_0 up to 1 T.

Pacemaker. Cardiac pacemakers are particularly sensitive to magnetic fields. Pacemakers are designed to produce a small, electric voltage at the cardiac frequency to maintain a proper heartbeat.

Integral to the pacemaker is a device called a *reed switch,* which opens and closes in response to a small electric signal. The reed switch can be rendered inoperative, and the pacemaker fails in static magnetic fields as low as 2 mT.

 Patients with pacemakers must be excluded from the MRI suite and must not be examined by MRI.

Because of the sensitivity of pacemakers to static magnetic fields, each MRI facility should maintain a controlled environment outside of a 0.5-mT fringe magnetic field. Controlling such an environment may require additional magnetic shielding or safety exclusion fences. No public passageway or other public access should be possible in a fringe magnetic field exceeding 0.5 mT.

Biomedical Implants. There have been several tragic accidents and one death because an implanted surgical clip came under the influence of the intense static magnetic field of an MRI system. The death involved an intracranial aneurysm clip that twisted during an MRI and caused the patient's middle cerebral artery to bleed. This created a massive cerebral hemorrhage.

If a surgical clip is ferromagnetic, it will experience a torque induced by the static magnetic field and twist in the tissue. The magnitude of the torque is primarily determined by the strength of the external magnetic field; the degree of ferromagnetism; and the size, shape, and mass of the clip. The potential for harm increases with an increase in any of these characteristics.

Surgical clips that were made before 1980 should be considered ferromagnetic. Since 1980, manufacturers of surgical clips have produced only nonferrous surgical clips. If it is determined during the patient interview process that a clip is present in a critical tissue, then the examination should not proceed until determining that the clip is nonferrous.

Because many patients undergoing surgery will be MRI candidates in the future, surgical protocol should require surgeons to positively identify all metal implants and pay specific attention to their ferromagnetism. The name of the manufacturer, model number, lot number, and serial number for any implanted device should be documented in the patient's chart.

Implants identified as surgical steel, surgical stainless, or stainless steel are not necessarily nonferromagnetic. Many types of stainless steel are ferromagnetic.

The magnetic properties of all such devices should be determined directly and not assumed. Even published lists by manufacturers of nonferromagnetic clips may be inaccurate. It may be appropriate to delay an MRI examination until the precise magnetic state of any implant is determined.

Although the warning is not particularly specific, the FDA requires MRI systems to be labeled, "This device is contraindicated for patients who have electrically, magnetically, or mechanically activated implants. For example, cardiac pacemakers because the magnetic and EMFs produced by the MR device may interfere with the operation of these devices."

In addition to cardiac pacemakers, other items represent clear concerns and may contraindicate MRI (Box 29-1).

Early in the use of MRI, prosthetic heart valves were considered a contraindication for such examination. Valves implanted since 1982 are considered safe; earlier valves may also be safe, especially if imaged in a 0.5-T or less imaging system. The forces created by the magnetic field of an MRI system are small in comparison with those exerted by the heart. When prosthetic valves are present, magnetic uniformity is disturbed, and an image artifact (usually absence of signal) occurs in the region of the valve.

In addition to the possibility of mechanical displacement is the possibility of a biomedical implant dislodging. The possibility for the RF field to induce electric currents or produce focal heating at the implant also exists. Neither of these potential responses has been exhibited either experimentally or clinically.

Contrast Reactions.   At this time, four products are available to enhance the contrast of an MR image. Each of these is a chelate of gadolinium, a paramagnetic element. Magnavist, the Berlex product, was the first on the market, and the competitors include ProHance, produced by Bristol-Myers/Squibb; Omniscan, produced by Sterling-Winthrop; and Dotarem, produced by Guerbet Laboratories.

Each of these effectively enhances tissue contrast. Also, each has been scrutinized for safety. Iodinated contrast agents used in x-ray imaging result in approximately one serious

Box 29-1	*Devices That May Be a Contraindication for Magnetic Resonance Imaging*
Aneurysm clips	Hemostat clips
Biopsy needles	Implantable drug infusion pumps
Bone growth stimulators	Internal defibrillators
Bullets	Intravascular stints
Cardiac pacemakers	Neurostimulators
Cochlear implants	Occular implants
Dental implants	Orthopedic implants
Halo vests	Penile implants
Heart valve prosthesis	Vascular clamps

complication per 100,000 doses administered. The performance of these MRI contrast agents is somewhat better.

Complications that may occur include nausea, pariorthodal edema, nasal and ear lobe swelling, neurential spasm, total body erythema, breathing difficulties and anaphylactoid reactions. Essentially, those responses attributed to iodinated MRI contrast injections only occur at a lower frequency.

The use of MRI contrast agents with pregnant patients requires special attention and should probably be avoided unless the added image quality is clearly justified. Apparently, the Gd-DTPA easily crosses the placenta, is swallowed by the fetus, and passes through the fetal urinary tract. Research results in this area are still equivocal.

Auditory Concerns. When an electric current is rapidly applied to a gradient coil, the coil heats and expands. When the current is off, the coil contracts. This alternate expansion and contraction causes the banging noise heard during MRI examinations.

This banging noise created by the switching of gradient magnetic fields can approach levels up to 95 dB. This is not far below the threshold of pain, 120 dB, so ear protection may be required (Table 29-5).

Some patients undergoing an MRI have experienced a temporary hearing loss. Hearing protection is readily available with earplugs of various designs. Such protective devices should be offered to all patients.

There are a number of music headset systems designed to muffle gradient noise and soothe patients at the same time. Such anti-noise systems are highly recommended.

Ferromagnetic Projectiles

Clearly, the most recognizable potential hazard to an MRI examination is the potential for injury by projectiles. Regardless of size, ferromagnetic material can come under the influence of the static magnetic field and become a projectile or missile.

Because of the attractive force of the primary magnetic field, ferromagnetic materials accelerate to the bore of the magnet if they are not properly shielded. If an employee or a patient is in the way, injury can occur. Many such injuries and two deaths have been reported. Box 29-2 lists various items that have been reported as projectiles in MRI.

It is essential for MRI administration to conduct safety in-service sessions for other hospital personnel. Nurses, porters, and housekeeping personnel can most often become victims of the adverse effects of the static magnetic field. An incident can occur when least expected because of inattention or lack of information.

 Ferromagnetic projectiles are a significant MRI hazard.

Be on the alert for such objects as scalpels, oxygen tanks, sandbags, and jewelry. Nurses and physicians often carry surgical instruments; patients often wear jewelry. These

TABLE 29-5	Typical Decibel Levels for Familiar Sounds
Decibel Level	**Description of Sound**
130	Threshold of pain
120	Front row seats at a Metallica concert
110	Fourth-of-July fireworks
100	Texas A & M University vs University of Texas football game
90	Hard Rock Cafe
80	Loud radio
70	Motorcycle ride
60	Conversational speech
50	Crackling fire
40	Typical home
30	Bambi's babies
20	Mirror Lake campsite
10	Final exam classroom
0	Ants dancing

Box 29-2	*Objects Reported as Projectiles in a Magnetic Resonance Imaging Facility*
Ankle weights	Mop bucket
Calculator	Nail clipper
Cigarette lighter	Oxygen tank
Clipboard	Pager
Floor buffer	Pole for intravenous bag
Forklift tines	Pulse oximeter
Gurney	Scissors
Hairpin	Steel-tipped shoes
Hearing aid	Stethoscope
ID badge	Traction sandbag
Insulin pump	Vacuum cleaner
Jewelry	Various tools
Key	Watch
Knife	Wheelchair
Mop	Writing pen

small items can be particularly hazardous because of the potential for puncture wounds.

Patients are often taken to MRI for examination on a gurney and covered by a sheet. There have been several reported instances in which transporters placed oxygen tanks on the gurney. Imagine everyone's shock when the patient is rolled up to the MRI couch, and the oxygen tank is sucked into the magnet!

Regardless of what the number of in-service programs is and how much caution is taken to train personnel, floor-cleaning instruments (e.g., buffers and polishers) seem to have an affinity for MRI magnets. Several cases have been reported where such appliances have been attracted to and trapped in the magnetic field.

Sandbags used for positioning and stabilization of patients often contain not only sand but also iron pellets.

PREGNANCY AND MAGNETIC RESONANCE IMAGING

There is no evidence to suggest that MRI is harmful to a pregnant patient or a fetus. Nevertheless, the use of MRI during pregnancy is approached with great caution. Researchers continue to study potential bioeffects.

One potential problem associated with MRI during pregnancy is heat. Although it is highly unlikely that a fetus would sustain a measurable elevation in temperature, it is known that heat is teratogenic. However, this property is no different from that created by exposing the pregnant woman to a steam room, a hot tub, or a heating pad.

 MRI-induced heat is a potentially harmful agent.

If MRI is the only imaging modality to provide necessary information to the clinician for the proper managing of the pregnant patient, then the examination should be conducted because clinical techniques do not significantly elevate tissue temperature. If the attending physician needs the information from the MRI examination, the examination should proceed after the physician consults with the radiologist to select the appropriate pulse sequence.

If an ultrasound examination can provide the required information, that should be the examination of choice. On the other hand, if an examination is essential and the choice is between x-ray examination and MRI, then on the basis of safety alone, MRI should get the nod as the appropriate examination.

As with diagnostic ultrasound examination, the stage of pregnancy should not affect the decision to be examined with MRI. If an ultrasound examination of the abdomen or pelvis of a pregnant patient has been unsuccessful in identifying suspected abnormalities, MRI may be appropriate if it is likely that the information gained will materially affect the management of that patient.

MRI may also be appropriate for examinations of the brain and spine during pregnancy when other modalities involve higher risk. Even x-ray examination may be appropriate for pregnant patients when considering the known risk. Most patients who receive radiation therapy treatments to the trunk of the body and subject the fetus to considerable levels of ionizing radiation do carry the fetus to term.

Pregnant technologists operating MRI systems are perfectly safe when working in the environment of the MRI. Such technologists are exposed only to fringe fields and not to the principal imaging fields. The RF and transient magnetic fields are essentially confined to the imaging volume of the patient and actually only exist during imaging.

 Occupational exposure to the energy fields of MRI is safe.

The static magnetic field outside the imaging volume is measured in millitesla, which is well below the intensity suspected of being capable of producing an effect. MRI technologists are exposed to a static magnetic field several orders of magnitude lower than that to which a pregnant patient might be exposed. Consequently, there are no known or suspected hazards of operating an MRI system; therefore, restrictions on pregnant MRI technologists or radiologists are unnecessary.

An ongoing mail survey of MRI technologists conducted by Kanal and Shellock has provided support for the presumed safety of such operators, even during pregnancy. The miscarriage rate, frequency of complication, and condition of the newborn were the same for MRI technologists as for the general population. There is no measurable effect on any newborn that is attributable to the mother working with MRI.

CHALLENGE QUESTIONS

1. What type of dose-response relationship best applies to the energy fields used in MRI?
2. Discuss the special concerns we have regarding pregnant MRI technologists.
3. Tissue responses to the energy fields used in MRI are said to be deterministic. What does that mean?
4. What is the one potential health hazard for pregnant MRI technologists?
5. What is the possible consequence of prolonged exposure to an intense B_0 field?
6. List the general concerns and describe the nature of each for the safety of the MRI patient.
7. Are there any potential health effects from the gradient magnetic fields?
8. Define SAR and identify the recommended maximum whole-body exposure level.
9. What is the principal potential response to patient irradiation with RF energy?
10. What units are used to measure the three energy fields involved with MRI?

Chapter 30

Managing a Magnetic Resonance Imaging System

The time to begin preparing for the daily operation of a magnetic resonance imaging (MRI) facility is at least 1 year before the scheduled turnover date from the manufacturer. The reasons for this long planning time become clear as soon as all that needs to be accomplished before the first patient enters the magnet is considered. A fair amount of research and thought are required in producing a workable clinical environment (Figure 30-1).

For the establishment of a properly functioning MRI facility, the time from conception to operation may take up to 2 years. In Chapter 13, it is pointed out that the first step in this process is selection of the imaging system. Then, site selection and design of the facility are the next processes. Approximately 1 year before operation, attention should be focused on personnel, equipment, and administration.

First, all of the necessary ancillary equipment must be identified and purchase orders submitted. Then, a competent staff must be hired and sufficient time allowed for adequate training of these new employees. Staff scheduling must be arranged and imaging protocols established; service and safety arrangements are also necessary.

ANCILLARY EQUIPMENT

Routine daily magnetic resonance (MR) operations require a certain level of ancillary equipment support. As patient care becomes more and more intense, such as with sedation or anesthesia, ancillary equipment becomes more sophisticated. Considerable thought should be given to services that will be offered at a particular site, and then appropriate selection of equipment can be made. Box 30-1 lists the equipment necessary for the initial start-up and operation of most MRI systems. This list is offered as a planning guide.

Everything that goes into the magnet room must be nonmagnetic.

Nonmagnetic equipment for use with an MRI system is now readily available from several suppliers. The primary materials used in such equipment are sturdy plastics, aluminum, wood, and high-grade stainless steel. Other metals and

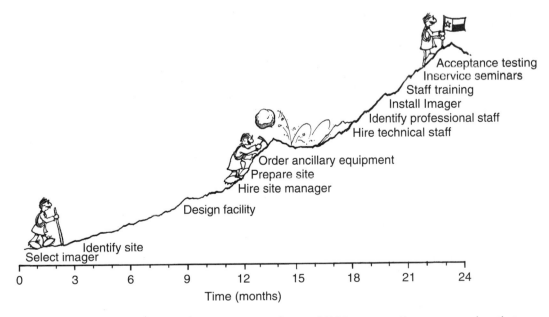

Figure 30-1 The steps and time sequence for establishing magnetic resonance imaging (MRI) have been compared with climbing a mountain, though MRI may take more time.

Box 30-1	*Ancillary Equipment Necessary for Magnetic Resonance Imaging Start-up*

Fire extinguisher(s)
Gurney(s)
Wheelchairs(s)
Intravenous pole(s)
Step stool
Oxygen tank (if there is no piped-in oxygen)
Wooden chair(s)
Tools
Respirator (that will work in the magnetic field)
Stethoscope
Plastic bucket, mop
Central vacuum (if there is carpet)
Patient monitoring (e.g., blood pressure, pulse rate)

alloys are also nonmagnetic, but it is always best to check any large metal object with a small magnet before it enters the imaging room.

Nonmagnetic gurneys are available from many x-ray supply companies. Nonmagnetic stretchers are more difficult to find and considerably more expensive but are more versatile and adaptable because they have more options, such as a raised head and adjustable height. Nonmagnetic wheelchairs are also available, as are nonmagnetic intravenous poles and step stools.

Stainless steel or aluminum oxygen cylinders, holders, and respirators are required. The cylinders can be obtained from either a local gas supply company or the cryogen supplier. Specify that the tanks be labeled "nonmagnetic" and verify that replacement tanks are the same. A respirator that works in the magnetic field is primarily plastic with no metal gauges. The fittings should be nonmagnetic brass or aluminum.

Tools can be purchased from the MRI vendor or other companies that provide nonmagnetic supplies for research laboratories. Nonmagnetic fire extinguishers should be kept in the area to prevent any unfortunate accidents during an emergency; a local supply company should be consulted for this.

Apparatus is required for monitoring sedated patients, elderly patients, and any patient with impaired communication skills. One sedated patient each day is a representative average. Minimal patient monitoring requires nonmagnetic devices for assessing blood pressure, pulse rate, and blood oxygen level.

When considering the purchase of ancillary equipment, the administrator should not overlook the role played by small equipment in the front office area of a busy MRI facility. Today's competitive world requires an electronic office for general communications and for prompt magnetic resonance (MR) report delivery and filing.

HUMAN RESOURCES

Staffing

Staffing differs among facilities and also between a hospital and an imaging center. The number of staff depends principally on the patient load. Table 30-1 identifies a representative start-up staff for both a hospital and an imaging center. After a few months of operation, it may be necessary to increase hours and days of imaging. Many MRI facilities eventually operate 18 hours a day, 6 days a week. This creates a great demand for MRI technologists and radiologists to perform complete diagnostic examinations in the most efficient and timely manner. It may be necessary to schedule staggered shifts rather quickly after start-up.

What training and experience should be required for MRI operation? Increasingly, more formal programs are available to train competent technical personnel, specifically in MRI. In addition, many continuing education seminars are offered. Training provided by MRI vendors is usually excellent but tailored to specific equipment.

 Operation of an MRI system after only on-the-job training is unacceptable.

Radiologic technologists with extensive experience in computed tomography (CT) are an obvious choice to be MRI technologists. Such individuals have already demonstrated com-

TABLE 30-1	Representative Staffing for Start-up of a Magnetic Resonance Imaging Facility

| | Number | | |
Staff Member	Hospital	Clinic	Duties
Radiologist	2	2	Image interpretation
Imaging technologist	4	2	Magnetic resonance imager operation
Receptionist	3	2	Scheduling, filing, typing
Radiology nurse	1	0	Patient support

petence as imaging technologists by completing a minimum 2-year training program and passing the examination of the American Registry of Radiologic Technologists (ARRT). Their experiences in patient care, patient positioning, anatomy, and computer operation can shorten the learning time required for operating an MRI system. Ultrasound and nuclear medicine technologists are also likely choices.

For the technical staff to develop the necessary competence to not only operate the MRI system but also exercise independent judgment about imaging techniques, they should receive appropriate continuing education. It is very important for MRI technologists to have a basic understanding of what occurs during MRI so that they can provide adequate physician assistance. Technologist certification in MRI by the ARRT is now required in keeping with appropriate standards of care.

The physical basis for MRI is totally different from that for x-ray imaging. Thought processes equating more dense tissue to white and less dense tissue to black on a radiograph cannot be applied to MRI. Thus MRI is much more complex. Technologists and physicians need to think in terms of signal intensity.

Strong signal intensity results in a bright image, and weak signal intensity results in a dark image. A complicating factor is that MR signal intensity can be completely reversed depending on the nature of the MRI pulse sequence.

Becoming comfortable with and understanding the physical principles of MRI are another matter. The technical staff must develop the necessary competence to exercise independent judgment about imaging techniques as they operate the MRI system. Each staff member must receive continuing education on a regular basis, with the support of a site administrator who remains committed to continuing education.

Scheduling

Experience has shown that approximately 30 to 45 minutes per examination should be allowed initially. Early experiments with radiofrequency (RF) pulse sequences and patient positioning require considerable time. However, with experience the average examination time can be shortened considerably. At that time, the scheduling of technologists can be somewhat altered. Fast imaging pulse sequences that shorten examination times considerably are now routine.

The extremely competitive market for MRI mandates the ability to offer same-day service and expeditious report turnaround time. It is not unusual for a patient to leave a site, having had the MRI examination completed, with a copy of the films and at least a preliminary report. The radiologist must be in a position of readiness to accommodate the referring physician by being available for consultation.

Patient scheduling should not be so tight that those who arrive on time must wait. In today's competitive atmosphere, patients who arrive on time and are properly prepared should not have to wait.

 Any hint of quality medical care can be dashed by causing patients to wait.

Technologist Scheduling. During the initial start-up phase, every aspect of the procedure is slow because of such factors as unfamiliarity with operating controls, difficulty in setting up imaging protocols, and selection of appropriate hard copies. Depending on the institution, this period lasts 1 to 6 months. The technologists should become involved and be a part of the final product. The entire department benefits from this interaction. Time and effort expended initially will bring rewards later.

Patient Scheduling. Seldom should it be necessary to repeat an examination of a patient. This not only increases the workload but also disrupts the schedule. Nevertheless, reexamination is sometimes required because of an inability to complete the examination.

Occasionally, upon review of the images by the radiologist, the appearance of a questionable area requires reexamination. The patient is contacted, and additional imaging is carried out as soon as possible. In general, 15 to 30 minutes of image time can be expected. The patient should be handled carefully and should be made to feel as comfortable about the return visit as possible.

The magnet should not remain idle because of misinformation or scheduling inefficiency. All outpatients should be called the day before their scheduled examination for confirmation of appointment. At that time, it should be verified that patients know the time of their appointment and given instructions and directions to the MRI facility. Time should be taken to answer questions or discuss fears they may have. Such attention will help tremendously in ensuring their arrival on time.

 Every effort should be made to prevent the "empty table syndrome."

It is helpful to schedule similar examinations back to back. If possible, separate segments of each day should be scheduled for head, body, and surface coil imaging. This eliminates the need for switching equipment or coils from patient to patient and saves considerable time. An efficient facility should strive to have the next patient enter the examination room as the previous patient exits.

Request Form. No patient should be examined without a proper request completed by the referring physician (Figure 30-2). As much medical information as possible should be provided with the request. In addition to giving standard identification data, the requesting physician should provide pertinent information from the clinical history of the patient and specific information about the reason for MRI.

In particular, the referring physician should be required to determine and state that the patient has no intracranial aneurysm or bypass clips, cardiac pacemaker, artificial limb, metal prosthesis, or metal fragments. If the presence of any such items is questionable, radiography or CT images should be obtained to confirm their absence. This should be done before the MRI procedure is scheduled.

Consent Form. When any hardware or software of the MRI system is not approved by the Food and Drug Administration (FDA), the FDA requires that a consent form be obtained from each patient. Regardless, it is advisable to obtain a consent form from each patient. Figure 30-3 presents such an informed consent form. In addition to providing general information and identification, the form must state that the patient understands the nature of the examination and ensure that all the patient's questions have been answered.

Of particular importance, the patient should be required to respond to the same questions posed to the clinician regarding clips, pace-

Precessional Saints Memorial Hospital   MRI Information Request Form

Date Received _____ by _____ Nursing Ext. _____   Date Scheduled _____

Patient Name _____
                                      Last   First   Middle Initial

Date of Birth _____ Sex _____   Previous MRI _____
                            Month   Day   Year

Hospital # [ ][ ][ ][ ][ ][ ][ ][ ][ ][ ]   Region of Interest _____

Patient Location _____   Referring Physician _____

Patient Age _____ Weight _____ Lb.   Height _____ Ft. _____ In. _____

Travel by: Walk   Wheelchair   Stretcher

Does patient require: O$_2$ I.V.   Infusion Pump   Other

If OP: Home phone _____   Work _____

Pertinent Clinical Hx:

_____

_____

_____

Specific reason for MRI:

_____

_____

Eye make-up must be removed before MRI examination.

Y   N   Subject in good state of health

Y   N   Subject states she is not pregnant

Y   N   Subject is able to give voluntary informed consent, or is accompanied by someone legally responsible to do so

          Review of medical history with patient indicates absence of:

Y   N   Intracranial aneurysm or bypass clips   Y   N   Metal fragments, shrapnel, bullet fragments

Y   N   Cardiac pacemaker, neuro / bio stimulator   Y   N   Permanent eyeliner (cosmetic tattooing)

Y   N   Artificial limb / joint prosthesis   Y   N   Previous heart surgery

Y   N   Cardiac valve prosthesis   Y   N   Middle ear prosthesis

Y   N   Other: _____

I have asked _____ the above questions and explained to him / her the nature of the MRI examination.

M.D. / RN / RT signature _____   Date _____

M.D. / RN / RT name (print) _____

Figure 30-2 A representative magnetic resonance imaging request form.

```
┌─────────────────────────────────────────────────────────────────────────┐
│                                                                           │
│                                          Magnetic Resonance Imaging (MRI) │
│   Resonance Regional Medical Center              Patient Informed Consent │
│   ─────────────────────────────────────────────────────────────────────  │
│                                                                           │
│   Your physician has ordered an MRI examination as part of the diagnostic tests for your medical evaluation.  This procedure │
│   can provide information which will enhance your diagnosis.  The procedure is accomplished by using a strong magnetic field, │
│   radiofrequency waves and a computer to generate the image.   No x-rays or radioactive materials are necessary. │
│                                                                           │
│   MRI systems have been in use for many years with no harmful side effects reported, except in patients with intracranial │
│   metal.  Your participation in this examination is voluntary and you may withdraw at any time.  Because of the nature of the │
│   magnetic field, it is necessary to know if you have had certain surgeries or traumas which could have resulted in any metal │
│   implants in the body.  Please inform the technologist or nurse if you have any of the following (check the appropriate lines): │
│                                                                           │
│   Yes No                                                                  │
│   ☐  ☐   1. Cardiac valve prosthesis                                      │
│   ☐  ☐   2. Cardiac pacemaker or pacer wire implants                      │
│   ☐  ☐   3. Intracranial aneurysm or bypass surgery                       │
│   ☐  ☐   4. Middle ear prosthesis                                         │
│   ☐  ☐   5. Neuro or bio-stimulator                                       │
│   ☐  ☐   6. Joint or limb prosthesis                                      │
│   ☐  ☐   7. Old shrapnel or welding wounds or accidents                   │
│   ☐  ☐   8. Other internal metal                                          │
│   ☐  ☐   9. Is there any possibility of pregnancy                         │
│                                                                           │
│   Qualified medical and technical personnel will be in attendance throughout the entire procedure. │
│                                                                           │
│   All data collected in this study is confidential as part of your patient record.  If the data is used for research studies or publica- │
│   tions, no patient identification will appear.  This information will be used only for educational, research, and scientific purposes. │
│                                                                           │
│                                                                           │
│   Signed _____       Date _____ │
│                     Patient's Name                                        │
│                                                                           │
│   Child's Assent _____       Date _____ │
│                     (If seven or older)                                   │
│                                                                           │
│   _____       Date _____ │
│                     Parent / Guardian                                     │
│                                                                           │
│   _____       Date _____ │
│                     Witness                                               │
│                                                                           │
└─────────────────────────────────────────────────────────────────────────┘
```

Figure 30-3 A typical consent form to be completed by the patient.

makers, prostheses, and other metal devices. A basic explanation of MRI should be provided to the patient. A brief and clearly stated pamphlet would be sufficient. The patient should be made aware that MRI is a benign examination and that there are no adverse effects.

Patient Preparation. Before the examination, the procedure should be explained and the patient told what the examination time will be and that it is important to remain still and relaxed.

The patient should be assured that the examination does not hurt but that loud thumping noises may be heard. Eating and drinking should be avoided for 2 hours before the examination for patient comfort for a standard MRI. Imaging the gallbladder and pancreatic ducts requires avoiding anything by mouth (n.p.o.) for 6 to 8 hours. The patient should be reminded that this is a diagnostic examination and not a treatment.

Image quality can be substantially improved and image artifacts significantly reduced if patients are properly screened and prepared for the MRI examination. Screening begins with pamphlets to educate the referring physicians, their staff, and patients.

Patient education continues throughout a series of interviews with the receptionist and technologists. Sometimes the radiologists are also involved in these interviews.

The top priority of the MRI technologist should be to educate the patient about the nature of the MRI examination to obtain the greatest cooperation from the patient. This is necessary for minimizing voluntary motion. The patient should realize that it is important to remain as still as possible during the imaging process. This means that the patient should be relaxed and should breathe normally. Earplugs that attenuate the noise but allow loudly stated instructions to be heard are often helpful.

To allay patients' fears of being forgotten once inside the magnet, a technologist should inform patients that they are kept under observation in several ways and that they may signal to the technologist at any time. Microphones and even a mere gesture of a moving foot or hand to alert the technologist are helpful. A marginally claustrophobic patient may be encouraged to complete an examination if brought out of the magnet after signaling for a short break.

IMAGING PROTOCOLS

Once the MRI system is operational and qualified imaging technologists are on staff, it will be evident that the choices presented for collection of images from a patient are almost endless. Most imaging systems are fairly versatile and allow for wide variations in pulse sequences.

The ultimate goal is to find optimal pulse sequences for each patient and for each suspected pathologic condition. The MRI technologist must work closely with the radiologist.

Each manufacturer has its own recommended protocol for a given circumstance; the radiologist has specific needs in mind, too. Nevertheless, it is the primary responsibility of the technologist to learn how to manipulate the operating console controls to optimize each examination.

 Imaging protocols should be continuously reviewed and updated.

The number of available MRI pulse sequences is enormous. In general, the technologist selects the pulse sequence that provides the most information in the least amount of time. Often, two pulse sequences are used: proton density weighted (PDW) images for anatomy and T2 weighted (T2W) images for pathology.

MRI is valuable because of the enhanced contrast resolution resulting from differences in the basic MRI parameters of proton density (PD), T1, and T2. Most pathologic processes cause changes in T1 and T2; therefore pulse sequences are generally tailored to emphasize such changes. Table 30-2 shows ranges of values for repetition time (TR), echo time (TE), and inversion time (TI) for several pulse sequences designed to emphasize a given MRI parameter.

During spin echo (SE) imaging, increases in T1 tend to reduce signal intensity, and increases in T2 tend to increase signal intensity. Therefore it is rarely sufficient to use a single SE for imaging. The technologist usually obtains an early SE image and a late SE image to avoid having an abnormality appear isointense with normal tissue.

Because T1 and T2 values for the brain are long and for cerebrospinal fluid (CSF) even longer when compared with those for other body tissues, pulse sequences for imaging of the central nervous system (CNS) are usually not appropriate for body imaging. Table 30-3 presents representative imaging protocols.

TABLE 30-2	Radiofrequency Pulse Sequences That Emphasize the Principal Magnetic Resonance Imaging Parameters				
MRI Parameter	RF Pulse Sequence	TR (ms)	TE (ms)	TI (ms)	Flip Angle
PD	Spin echo	2000	30-50		
T1	Spin echo	500	Up to 20		
T1	Inversion recovery	2000	30-50	100-500	
T2	Spin echo	2000	80-150		
T2	Gradient echo	100	10		20°

With experience, these protocols can be varied to accommodate suspected pathology.

Technologists and radiologists will want to try different pulse sequences until one is found that best works for their magnet and patient population. Technologists must be open to change and learn from experiences.

IMAGING SYSTEM MAINTENANCE

An MRI system is a highly complex instrument that requires regularly scheduled preventive maintenance and unscheduled service for repairs as needed.

The warranty period for parts and labor for an MRI system should be at least 1 year. Longer service contracts are available but at considerable expense. Warranty service is expected to occur during normal working hours, though after-hour arrangements can be made at a higher hourly labor rate. Even with this added expense, this situation is often preferable and more cost-effective than foregoing patient imaging and the revenues generated through normal operations.

TABLE 30-3	Suggested Protocols for Start-up Imaging			
Examination			TR (ms)	TE (ms)
PDW			1400-2000	30
T1W			500-600	5-20
T1W (90-500 ms TI)			1500-2000	30
T2W			2000-6000	80-150
T2*W (20°-30° flip angle)			500-1100	30
Brain		Transverse	2000	40/80
Spine		Transverse	1000	35/70
		Coronal	800	40/80
		Sagittal	800	40/80
Chest		Coronal	1000	30/60
		Transverse	1500	30/60
Abdomen		Transverse	800	30/60
		Coronal	500	25/50
Pelvis		Coronal	800	25/50
		Transverse	1000	30/60
Extremities		Sagittal	700	40/80
		Coronal	700	40/80

Preventive Maintenance. The sophisticated support systems for the main magnet require the most attention during regularly scheduled preventive maintenance. Failure of any electronic components can seriously affect the quality of the image and can disrupt imaging entirely. The magnet must be constantly fine-tuned to keep the quality of the MR signal high to produce images with maximum signal and minimum noise.

Several support systems for the magnet may include items that require regular preventive maintenance as specified by the manufacturer. These systems may include a chilled water system, a Halon system, oxygen alarms, compressed air and pumps, and air conditioning systems. A mobile MRI is equipped with generators that will also require service.

Many of these items have components that are not normal off-the-shelf items and may have a long lead-time for replacement. Therefore it may be necessary to have some components available for replacement at the site to preclude unnecessary downtime resulting from equipment failure and parts delivery.

Before operation of an MRI system, the person responsible for service and preventive maintenance must be identified. That individual should then be charged with scheduling such maintenance and deciding what backup parts and systems should be available on site.

Regular preventive maintenance on the MRI system includes diagnostics on the software and checks of the RF subsystem. Changes in RF frequency do occur. Each system normally has a 10- to 20-Hz drift each day. The gradient sensitivity and offset can drift, and readjustment of the free induction decay (FID) may be necessary to maintain image quality.

Cryogen levels should be monitored, and any differences in cryogen boil-off should be noted for possible problems. For safety procedure checks, the emergency shutdown and quench buttons should be verified as operational.

Occasionally, the patient couch should be taken out to check the cowling and the inner bore for small ferromagnetic objects.

Before the MRI system is purchased, an estimate of maintenance costs after the warranty period has ended is helpful. Negotiations for service should be done as the system is purchased so that a realistic picture of operating expenditures is available in the planning stages.

Repairs. The components that require the most attention are the electronics. Once the magnet is energized, it does not require service except for the superconducting magnet, which requires cryogen replacement. Unless a quench occurs, the magnet should not require repair. Nevertheless, the electronic components of the MRI system are the primary elements of the repair and service process. The system experiences the normal problems with disk and tape drives that exist with any other computer-assisted technology.

Because of the sensitivity of an MRI system and the complex problems associated with repair and service, several items are necessary to monitor the service provided. The following items provide some controls for the cost of repairs:

Length of Time Required for Repair. Time spent for repairs should be only due to the failure of the equipment. Service personnel should not add time to the service report for such things as filling out the service report. All times should be logged in and out by the service personnel.

Repair Completed, Problem Unsolved. Many hours may be spent trying to isolate the event that causes the problem. It is not uncommon to put the imaging system out of service several times to correct the same problem. There should be an awareness of how long this is happening and expert repair help should also be requested.

Training and Competence of Service Personnel. Most often, more than one service engineer is required to correct a problem. If additional engineers are on site for training or experience and are not productive, there should be no charge for the additional personnel.

Communication and Headquarters for Extended Service Problems. Some persistent problems require that assistance from the factory be available for resolution.

Response Time to Reported Service Problems. Time for repair of problems should not include the travel time of service personnel to the facility. It is wise to negotiate for a minimum response time for a service engineer to respond to requests for assistance. If service is required over the weekends, this item should be addressed during the purchase negotiations.

Availability of Parts Locally. Parts for the MRI system should be available locally but rarely are. Repair budgets should be increased significantly after the warranty period to include replacement components. Knowledge of the magnet and the components is mandatory for the MRI administrator or technologist to control repair costs.

Cryogen Replacement.   The superconducting magnet requires cryogenic gases for cooling. The principle of the superconducting magnet is to create an environment that does not require a continuous electrical energy source. The 15 or more miles of windings in the core of a superconducting magnet must be cooled to less than 20 K. This is accomplished through the construction of the sophisticated cryostat (see Chapter 11).

As long as the windings of the main magnet remain below approximately 20 K, the magnetic field is sustained at a constant field strength. Cryogen must be replaced on a regular schedule, and this is a technical problem that must be considered before operation.

Certain magnets are constructed so that only liquid helium (instead of helium and nitrogen) is required. The boil-off from the helium can be captured, condensed to liquid and reused. With this design, cryogen replacement costs are diminished. Also, cryogen fills occur less frequently; therefore, service costs are reduced. Monitoring of cryogen levels must be continuous. Abrupt loss of cryogens results in a quench that can be disastrous to the magnet.

Liquid nitrogen is a fairly stable cryogen with which to work because it vaporizes at 77 K and has a high surface tension. Liquid helium is not so stable; it vaporizes at 4.2 K.

It is necessary to obtain a contract with a cryogen supply company or the system manufacturer to arrange delivery of cryogens and service. Certain manufacturers arrange cryogen deliveries in addition to monitoring levels, ordering proper quantities, and scheduling fills and related service.

Cryogen replacement is a critical operation. It must be done by knowledgeable, fully trained personnel. Regardless of who does the replacement, proper safety procedures must be followed. Safety glasses must be worn for eye protection and heavy gloves for hand protection. All connective tubing and parts must be precooled to avoid the introduction of heat into either the cryogen transport dewars or the magnet itself.

Usually, nitrogen must be replaced regularly and some systems require helium replacement annually. These liquids vaporize during filling of the cryostat and during transport. Cryogens cannot be stored for more than several days in the transport dewars or else the dewars may be empty when the magnet is ready for filling.

Helium is obtained commercially from deposits of natural gas in Texas, Kansas, and New Mexico. Helium is separated by a process of freezing out the less volatile components, leaving the helium gas that must then be liquefied. All U.S. production of helium is under the control of the U.S. Bureau of Mines.

Spontaneous boil-off of cryogens consumes approximately 1% to 2% of the helium and 5% to 7% of the nitrogen per day on a stationary magnet. Cryogen consumption for a mobile magnet can be considerably higher, depending on whether the magnet is moved frequently or operated in a stationary location.

If the magnet is moved frequently and must be ramped up and down for moving, an additional 1% is used during the ramping. Critical cryogen levels are reached at approximately

50% of the total volume; below this level a quench is possible.

Magnet Quench

Helium is an important choice for a cryogen in magnets because of its chemical inactivity and its low density. However, this presents special problems if the liquid helium begins to warm or is exposed to room temperature. Charles' law states that at constant pressure, the volume of a given mass of gas is directly proportional to the absolute temperature. The importance of this law is apparent if the magnet should quench.

During a quench, the liquid gases vaporize, causing the main magnet windings to rise in temperature and become electrically resistive.

This results in more heat, which results in more liquid boil-off. The magnet windings cannot sustain the high current in the resistive phase and can be severely damaged. If this occurs, the magnetic field intensity drops rapidly to zero and the imaging system ceases to function.

 A quench occurs when the temperatures of the liquid gases—nitrogen and helium— exceed their respective boiling points.

It is possible for 100 to 150 l of helium and nitrogen to be vaporized in less than 1 minute. This produces approximately 4000 fl^3 of gas at room temperature and normal pressure, which can quickly displace all the oxygen in the room.

The recommendation is that superconducting magnets be equipped with an oxygen monitor that will sound an alarm if the oxygen level in the imaging room drops below 140 ppm. Normal levels of oxygen in air are 150 ppm (20%) by volume. This assumes even greater importance if the design of the magnet room does not allow the technologists to view the cryogen port directly. However, most superconducting magnets are vented through a cryogen vaporization duct to the outside of the facility to prevent an undue safety hazard to personnel and patients.

Should a quench occur, the magnet quickly loses its magnetic field and becomes inoperable. The magnet must then be recooled and restarted, which can take considerable time, assuming the magnet has not been damaged from the overheating.

 Quenching is an extremely expensive and hazardous event and must be avoided.

QUALITY CONTROL

The image must be evaluated daily to maintain image quality. This is best accomplished by using the first half-hour of the day for quality control (QC). A standard reference measurement on an MRI phantom should be done daily and the images and data saved for at least 1 month to evaluate subtle changes in image quality and signal-to-noise ratio (SNR). A reduction in the SNR may be the first indication of a problem.

Phantom images can be used to identify and evaluate artifacts that occur. Artifacts attributed to the inhomogeneity of a living system may be in error and should be cross-referenced to a phantom image for identification.

Medical physicists have developed several MRI QC test objects. The American Association of Physicists in Medicine (AAPM) has a large compendium of such test objects available on request. Table 30-4 lists the important image characteristics to be evaluated by such test objects.

Keeping the SNR at a level that produces excellent diagnostic images should be a closely monitored procedure. Even with magnetic and RF shielding, small subcomponents of the support systems can introduce interference that causes image degradation.

The American College of Radiology (ACR) has developed a very effective accreditation process. The ACR QC manual describes the special responsibilities for radiologists, technologists, and medical physicists. This manual also details the use of the ACR accreditation phantom (Figure 30-4). All MRI facilities should be ACR accredited.

TABLE 30-4	Image Characteristics to Be Evaluated with Magnetic Resonance Imaging Quality Assurance Test Objects
Image Characteristic	**Test Object Configuration**
Noise	Uniform liquid bath
Uniformity	Measure of signal throughout uniform liquid bath
Spatial resolution	Hole pattern or bar pattern
Contrast resolution	Hole pattern in various thicknesses of plastic
Linearity	Step wedge or various paramagnetic samples
Sensitivity profile	Ramped wedge or rod
Slice continuity	Ramp or helix

The industry-estimated number of clinical MRI systems in the United States at the end of 2001 was approximately 5000. As of March 2002, there were 2408 accredited MRI facilities accounting for a total of 2873 magnets. There were approximately another 500 facilities somewhere in the accreditation process. Each site must have a daily QC program with the ACR phantom (Table 30-5). The demand for these phantoms is increasing.

The radiologist's responsibility is chiefly oversight. The radiologist must ensure that the technologists and medical physicist are properly qualified and maintain satisfactory continuing education. Every 3 months the radiologist must conduct a review of the QC program and maintain records of that review.

The medical physicist is responsible for acceptance testing and an annual imaging system performance evaluation that includes many precise measurements. A sample of images used to make these measurements is shown in Figure 30-5.

SAFETY

Access to the magnet room must be strictly controlled because of potential adverse effects of visitors on the magnet and the magnetic field on visitors. Signs that caution entrance to the magnet room must be prominently dis-played in many areas in addition to the entrance door. An example of such a warning sign is shown in Figure 30-6. Many people read and then ignore such signs; therefore additional measures must be taken to control entrance to the MRI examination room. This is particularly important with permanent and superconducting magnets because their magnetic field cannot be interrupted or turned off.

Visitors' Effect on Magnet

When the MRI system first becomes energized, in-service training sessions for many departments in the hospital or clinic must be conducted. There will be much curiosity and many rumors about the magnet. The departments that require the most attention in this regard are building services, public relations, and personnel.

In-service training sessions with the supervisors of the building services department and the employees performing the work are vital to the safety of the imaging system. For example, one hospital had a central vacuum installed in the area because the magnet room was carpeted. Within a week of in-service session, a housekeeping employee decided the central vacuum was too troublesome and entered the magnet room with a conventional vacuum cleaner. Fortunately, only a chip was knocked off the cover of the magnet cowling, which is

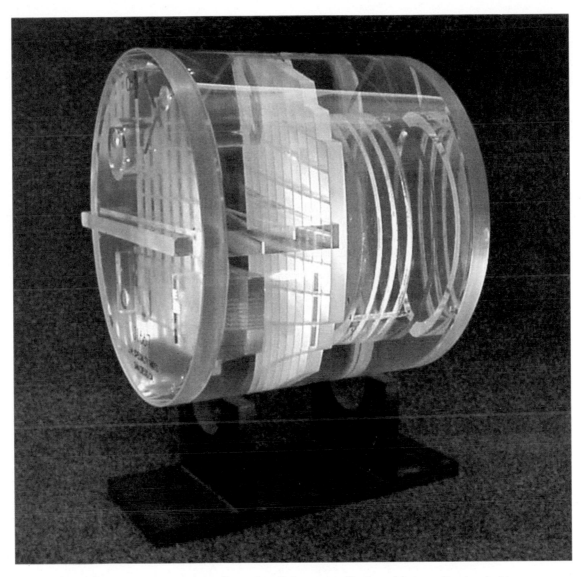

Figure 30-4 The American College of Radiology accreditation phantom. (Reprinted with permission of the American College of Radiology, Reston, Virginia. No other representation of this material is authorized without express, written permission from the American College of Radiology.)

where the vacuum cleaner struck when it was pulled out of the housekeeper's hands.

The public relations department must be made aware of the nature of the MRI system because the members will be touring the facility with visitors. Another reported incident, much more benign in nature, occurred after a magnet was first brought up to field.

There was a group of medical administrative dignitaries visiting from a nearby city who were in the preliminary stages of planning for MRI. Signs were posted prominently as to what should and should not enter the magnet room. One visitor was warned by an employee that he should not wear his analog watch into the magnetic field. The man expressed little

TABLE 30-5	Specific Tests Performed by the Magnetic Resonance Imaging Technologist and Their Recommended Frequency as Listed in the American College of Radiology Quality Control Manual

Test	Frequency
Center frequency measurement	Daily
Table positioning check	Daily
Setup and imaging interface	Daily
Geometric accuracy	Daily
High-contrast resolution	Daily
Low-contrast resolution	Daily
Artifact analysis	Daily
Film quality control	Weekly
Visual checklist	Weekly

concern because it was a gold watch. The employee responded that although gold is non-magnetic, the gears and springs of the watch are not made of gold.

 No metal can be allowed in the MRI room, unless screening shows it to be safe.

As stated earlier, MRI requires a different thought process. If care and constant monitor-

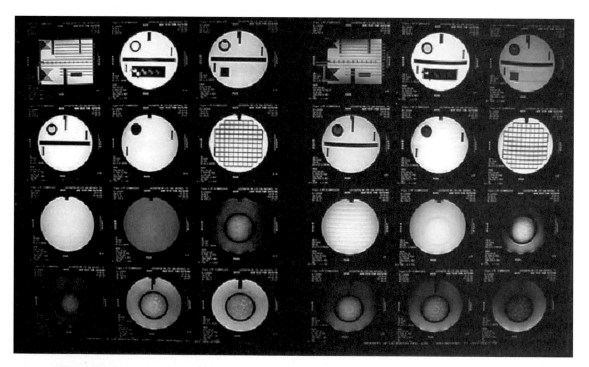

Figure 30-5 A series of images acquired with the American College of Radiology accreditation phantom to evaluate magnetic resonance imaging system performance. (Courtesy Geoff Clarke, San Antonio, TX.)

WARNING
MAGNETIC FIELD

THE FIELD OF THIS MAGNET ATTRACTS OBJECTS CONTAINING IRON, STEEL, NICKEL OR COBALT. SUCH OBJECTS MUST <u>NOT</u> BE BROUGHT INTO THIS AREA. <u>LARGE</u> OBJECTS CANNOT BE RESTRAINED.

PERSONS WITH IMPLANTS OR PROSTHETIC DEVICES SHOULD <u>NOT</u> ENTER THIS AREA. PACEMAKERS MAY BE DISABLED.

DATA ON CREDIT CARDS AND MAGNETIC STORAGE MEDIA CAN BE ERASED. WATCHES, CAMERAS, AND INSTRUMENTS CAN BE DAMAGED.

Figure 30-6 Warning sign for the entrance of the magnetic resonance imaging suite.

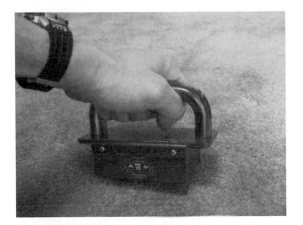

Figure 30-7 A handheld magnet of at least 100-mT strength can be used to screen objects before taking them into the magnetic resonance imaging room. (Courtesy Emanuel Kanal, Pittsburgh, PA.)

ing are not practiced, the potential for hazard is always present. Box 30-2 lists personal belongings that should be removed from visitors or patients before they enter the MRI exclusion area.

All portable metallic devices must be identified as nonferromagnetic before being brought into the imaging room of the MRI facility. A toy magnet is not adequate for such a screening task. A very strong, handheld magnet of at least 100 mT is required (Figure 30-7).

Magnet Effects on Visitors

The magnetic fringe field may have potentially harmful effects on visitors, patients, and accompanying family members. The fringe field of a superconducting MRI system should be considered hazardous. Box 30-3 identifies some people who should not be allowed access

Box 30-2	*Personal Effects That Should Be Removed from Visitors and Patients Before They Enter the 0.5-mT Exclusion Area*

Analog watches
Tape recorders
Magnetized credit cards
Calculators
Jewelry
Shoes with metal supports
Wigs
Hairpins, barrettes
Dentures (when the head or cervical spine is being imaged)

Box 30-3	*People Who Should Not Be Allowed Within the 0.5-mT Exclusion Area*

Patients with pacemakers
Patients with intracranial aneurysm clips
Persons subject to uncontrollable seizures

to the imaging room or within the 0.5-mT exclusion area. Any patient, employee, or family member entering the magnet room should be properly screened.

MAGNETIC RESONANCE SAFETY POLICIES AND PROCEDURES

After a number of serious accidents, including one widely reported childhood fatality, the ACR published recommended MR Safety Policies and

Procedures. These recommendations are based on long-established radiation safety protocols of identifying potentially hazardous areas, naming responsible personnel, limiting access, and continuously documenting and reviewing.

Zoning

The ACR recommends identifying four zones of increasing potential hazard. Figure 30-8 shows the location of these zones for a typical MR suite.

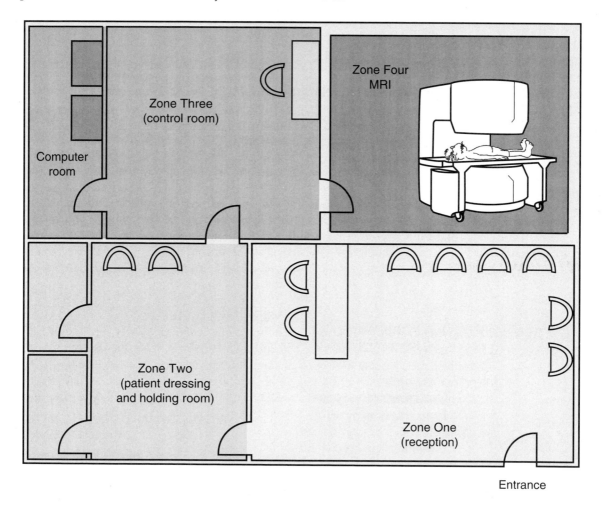

Figure 30-8 Magnetic resonance zones of increasing potential hazard for a typical magnetic resonance imaging facility.

Zone One includes all areas that are freely accessible to the general public. This would include the outside areas surrounding a free-standing MRI facility or the corridor of the hospital leading to the MRI department.

Zone Two is that area where patients and visitors are controlled and supervised by MR personnel. This would normally be the reception area and the patient preparation area.

Zone Three is the area where there is potential for injury from ferromagnetic objects and equipment. Access to this zone must be strictly controlled by MR personnel.

Such control should provide for physical restriction with a pass-key locking system to ensure that only MR personnel and properly screened and supervised non-MR personnel can enter. Zone Three is usually the control room and immediate space, such as the computer room.

 Any area within Zone Three where the fringe magnetic field equals or exceeds 0.5 mT should be clearly marked.

Zone Four is the MRI room itself. This zone should be clearly marked with warning signs and a warning light at the entrance . . . "The Magnet Is On."

The entrance to Zone Four should be visible to MR personnel at all times to absolutely ensure no unauthorized entry. Even during an emergency, such as cardiac or respiratory arrest, unauthorized and unscreened individuals must not be allowed access. It is the responsibility of the properly trained MR personnel to stabilize the patient, provide basic life support, and remove the patient to Zone Two or lower.

Magnetic Resonance Personnel

An **MR Medical Director** and **MR Safety Officer (MRSO)** should be named for each MRI facility. Often the two will be the same.

The MRSO must see that formal MR Safety Policies and Procedures are developed, implemented, and updated as necessary. Any MR safety incident or "near miss" must be reported to the MRSO, who will maintain a register of such incidents. The register can then be used to refine the MR Safety Policies and Procedures.

 The MRSO will identify two levels of MR personnel and four safety zones.

The ACR recommends that all persons entering an MR facility be identified as falling into one of three groups. There are two levels of MR personnel and a third group of non-MR personnel, including the patient.

Non-MR personnel are those who have received no MR safety training, such as the patient, visitors, and other hospital personnel. Such individuals are not allowed beyond Zone Two unless screened and supervised by Level Two MR personnel.

Level One MR personnel are those who have completed minimal MR safety training. This training will allow them to work safely within Zone Three. This group includes receptionists and patient attendees. No other hospital employees should have unrestricted access to Zone Three.

Level Two MR personnel include the MR technologists and MR radiologists. These people will have had extensive training in MR safety and MR emergency procedures. Level Two MR personnel have unrestricted access to Zones Three and Four. No work restrictions are necessary for Level Two MR personnel who are pregnant.

PATIENT PREPARATION

Although MRI is generally considered harmless, certain patients should not be imaged because of possible adverse reactions to the examination. It is not always easy to identify those patients who should be excluded because the criteria for exclusion are not obvious even to those familiar with MRI. The responsibility rests with the MR technologist to recognize the potentially unacceptable patient.

 Scheduling personnel must carefully screen patients.

Patients must remove all metallic personal belongings and devices before entering Zone

Three. This is ensured if the patient is provided with a gown having no metal fasteners for the MRI procedure.

The use of metal detectors for patient screening is not recommended. Patients who have or may have internal ferromagnetic objects, such as metal shavings or surgical clips, must be screened further.

If positive written identification and documentation of internal metal are not possible, plain film radiography should be conducted. The MRSO should make the final decision for examination of any patient with a questionable screen.

Occupational Groups

Members of several occupational groups should be viewed with suspicion before MRI examination because they may have foreign metallic objects in the body. Often the presence of such objects is unknown.

Auto mechanics, machinists, and welders come into contact with metal shavings and filings. Most people who work in such a capacity take protective measures, such as wearing safety glasses and other protective apparel. Therefore they should have no history of injury.

Exclusion of patients with intraorbital metal is common. This practice prevents injury caused by magnetic metal torquing in the magnetic field, which has been reported.

Patients who have metal fragments in their bodies may come to the MRI facility with no history of foreign body injury. Usually, these fragments are fixed in subcutaneous tissue, but the possibility of a hazard always exists.

Surgical Clips and Prostheses

Numerous neurosurgical clips and implants have been tested, and some are magnetic. It is impossible to recognize the type on any radiograph. Even if all neurosurgical clips were changed to nonmagnetic materials today, it would be impossible to know in the future whether a patient had one of the old magnetic aneurysm clips or a new nonmagnetic one.

 The patient with neurosurgical clips is not imaged unless the technologist is absolutely certain that the clips are nonmagnetic.

Middle ear prostheses are not considered hazardous to patients but may somewhat compromise the image quality. Many but not all middle ear prostheses that have been tested are nonmagnetic. Some minor image degradation in the area of the implant or prosthesis may occur.

Surgical clips and sutures in the abdomen are more of a problem. There is no contraindication to the use of MRI in the patient with surgical clips in the abdomen. On occasion, significant artifacts indicating magnetic metal clips appear. Trial and error is the only way to determine whether abdominal surgical clips will produce artifacts that are objectionable.

Joint prostheses are primarily constructed of stainless steel and do not cause a problem unless the area of interest is directly next to the prosthesis. For example, it is possible to image the lumbar spine of a patient with bilateral hip prostheses. However, it is usually not possible to obtain a complete diagnostic examination of the pelvis.

Pregnant Patients

There are no data currently available to suggest that any harmful effects occur to a pregnant patient or fetus. However, it is generally believed that until more research data are available, pregnant patients should be imaged only when alternate procedures are considered ineffective.

 Pregnancy is not a contraindication to MRI at any stage of pregnancy.

MR contrast agents should not be used with pregnant patients without the consent of the MR Medical Director or MRSO. Some adverse effects are possible; therefore each pregnant patient should be individually evaluated.

CHALLENGE QUESTIONS

1. What characteristic must be kept in mind when equipping an MRI facility?
2. A patient has a history of neurosurgery. What should be done?
3. What are the minimum qualifications for operation of an MRI system?
4. What is the basis for an exclusion area surrounding an MRI suite, and what is the intensity level of exclusion?
5. Discuss some management features designed to provide the patient with efficient service.
6. Why is regularly scheduled in-service training necessary for hospital personnel?
7. Discuss some helpful ways to ease the claustrophobic patient through an examination.
8. Discuss the recommendation for quality control for an MRI facility.
9. What steps should be planned in the event of an unintended quench?
10. Why is an informed consent required from a patient undergoing MRI?

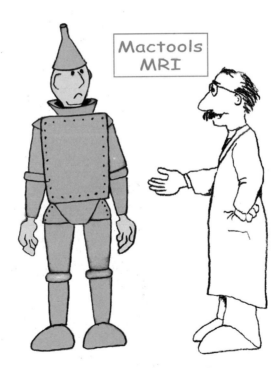

"I really would like to accommodate you but you're going to have to find another way to see if you have a heart"

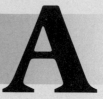

The Bloch Equations

Within a few weeks after Felix Bloch's announcement in 1946 regarding the discovery of *nuclear induction*, now known as *nuclear magnetic resonance (NMR)**, he published a set of equations describing NMR. The most remarkable feature of this set of three coupled differential equations is Bloch's clear explanation. In addition to providing a description of the NMR experiments, the Bloch equations are applicable to other areas of physics. Scientists compare the power of these equations with that of the Maxwell equations, which relate electric and magnetic fields to electric charges and currents, as well as forming the basis for the theory of electromagnetic waves.

Even though NMR scientists in physics, chemistry, and engineering substantially alter the mathematical notation of the equations, Bloch's set of equations, which predicts the behavior of nuclear spin systems in a magnetic field, is nearly infallible. Despite the complicated appearance of the Bloch equations, an intense study session can provide insight into the behavior of spins in magnetic resonance imaging (MRI). Familiarity with spin behavior is critical to understanding thc significance of magnetic resonance measurement parameters.

*The Bloch announcement from Stanford University was one of two. A simultaneous discovery was made by Edward Purcell at Harvard University. The two men subsequently shared the 1952 Nobel Prize in physics.

Nuclear magnetization is often described as a vector in three-dimensional (3-D) Cartesian space with components M_X, M_Y, and M_Z. By convention, the Cartesian coordinate system is oriented with the Z-axis parallel to the direction of the applied field (B_0); the X and Y axes are mutually perpendicular to each other and to the Z-axis. The laws of thermodynamics set the maximum nuclear magnetization at a value M_0, and its magnitude $(M_X^2 + M_Y^2 + M_Z^2)^{1/2}$ can never exceed M_0.

Bloch postulated two relaxation times, longitudinal and transverse. He associated longitudinal with M_Z and transverse with M_X and M_Y, and then he assigned them the symbols T1 and T2, respectively. T1 and T2 are time constants for a first-order kinetics process, which can be incorporated into a set of coupled differential equations as follows:

$$\frac{dM_X}{dt} = \frac{M_X}{T2} \tag{1a}$$

$$\frac{dM_Y}{dt} = \frac{M_Y}{T2} \tag{1b}$$

$$\frac{dM_Z}{dt} = \frac{(M_Z - M_0)}{T1} \tag{1c}$$

The first two equations state that the transverse components of the nuclear magnetization decay with the time constant T2. The third equation states that the longitudinal component builds up to the value M_0 with a time constant T1.

The following are some interpretations and applications of equations 1a, 1b, and 1c. Consider a nuclear spin system at equilibrium created by placing a sample in a field B_0 for a time t, which is long in comparison with T1 and T2. The following definition applies:

$$\frac{dM_X}{dt} = \frac{dM_Y}{dt} = \frac{dM_Z}{dt} = 0 \qquad (2)$$

That is, the components of the nuclear magnetization do not change with time when the nuclear spin system is at equilibrium.

Suppose by the intervention of an external force, or perturbation, M_0 is transformed from the Z-axis to the Y-axis (Figure A-1). The time history predicted by equations 1a, 1b, and 1c can be used to interpret the Bloch equations (Figure A-2).

The graphs in Figure A-2 have been generated by stepwise solution of equations 1a, 1b, and 1c with $M_Y = M_0$, T2 $= 100$ ms, and T1 $= 500$ ms. M_Y decreases with time constant T2 and approaches zero after several T2 periods. M_X was initially zero and remains at that value. M_Z, also initially zero, increases with time until it essentially becomes M_0 after several T1 periods. Equations 1a, 1b, and 1c are the mathematical statement of the T1 and T2 relationships for the rotating frame of reference at resonance.

Note that numerical integration is a commonly used digital computing technique. The name is formidable, but the technique does not need to be. For the illustrations in this appendix, assume a time change; calculate the difference in the value of M_X, M_Y, and M_Z that occurs in the time interval; correct the M_X, M_Y,

or M_Z values; and repeat the operation. The NMR enthusiast can accomplish several such steps on a handheld calculator and then estimate the curves.

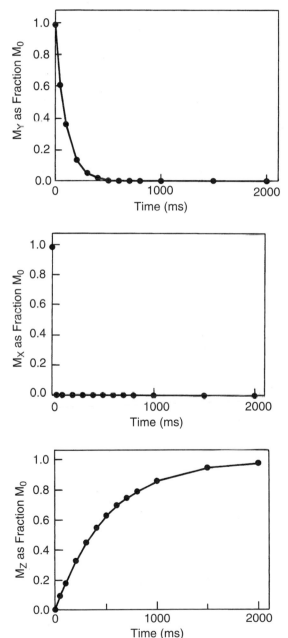

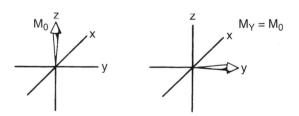

Figure A-1

Figure A-2

Remember that T1 must always be equal to or greater than T2. If this restriction is violated, the magnitude of the M_0 vector can easily exceed the thermodynamic M_0 limit. There is no known substance with T2 *greater than* T1.

Two factors allow for elaboration on equations la, 1b, and 1c. First, no method for direct observation of M_Z exists. Quantum mechanics guarantees this fundamental truth. Second, a physical means of perturbing nuclear spin systems at equilibrium has not been discussed yet. Introducing a radiofrequency (RF) field in the XY plane solves both of these limitations.

An RF field can be an applied secondary magnetic field (B_1) along the X-axis of our coordinate system. B_1 rotates the vector M_0 around the X-axis at a rate γB_1, where γ equals the gyromagnetic ratio of the nucleus under observation. Incorporation of this effect changes equations la, 1b, and 1c into the following equations:

$$\frac{dM_X}{dt} = \frac{M_X}{T2} \tag{3a}$$

$$\frac{dM_Y}{dt} = \frac{M_Y}{T2} + \gamma B_1 M_Z \tag{3b}$$

$$\frac{dM_Z}{dt} = \frac{(M_Z - M_0)}{T1} - \gamma B_1 M_Y \tag{3c}$$

Equations 3a, 3b, and 3c are simply a mathematical statement that any vector in the YZ plane is rotated by B_1 to a new location. Figure A-3 shows the effect of ωB_1 on a nuclear spin system that is initially at equilibrium.

The RF field B_1 creates a motion of M_0 around the X-axis. The trajectory of M_0 can be interrupted at will by turning off the RF oscil-lator. In this case, equations 3a, 3b, and 3c simplify to become equations 1a, 1b, and 1c, with the components M_X, M_Y, and M_Z determined by the time the RF field was turned off. After the RF field is turned off, the behavior shown in Figure A-2 results.

Until now, discussion has centered around the rotating frame at resonance. When the rotating frame is not at resonance, it requires another modification of the equations. The terms to be included are the frequency of the rotating frame (ω) and the resonance frequency (ω_0), or γB_0. A difference $(\omega - \omega_0)$ corresponding to 1000 Hz means the magnetization rotates 1000 times per second. Mathematically, rotating magnetization in the XY plane is incorporated by decreasing M_X and increasing M_Y with respect to time, as shown in equations 4a, 4b, and 4c. A comparable form exists for rotation in the YZ plane. The Bloch equations in the form of equations 4a, 4b, and 4c, which incorporate both of these features, are reliable descriptors of the magnetization vectors in a sample during an NMR observation.

$$\frac{dM_X}{dt} = -\frac{M_X}{T2} + (\omega - \omega_0)M_Y \tag{4a}$$

$$\frac{dM_Y}{dt} = -\frac{M_Y}{T2} - (\omega - \omega_0)M_Y + \gamma B_1 M_Z \tag{4b}$$

$$\frac{dM_Z}{dt} = -\frac{(M_Z - M_0)}{T1} - \gamma B_1 M_Y \tag{4c}$$

The offset terms only appear in M_X and M_Y. Numerical integration leads to the time history shown in Figure A-4.

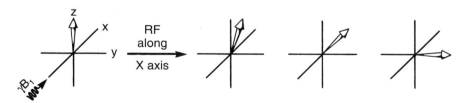

Figure A-3

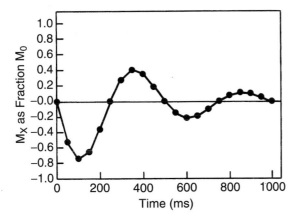

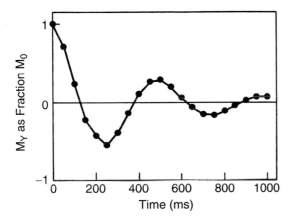

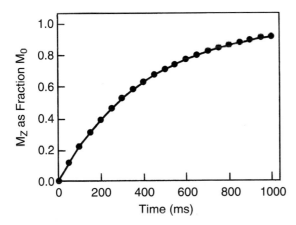

Figure A-4

In this case, the detected signal is a damped sine wave for M_X and a damped cosine wave for M_Y. This is indeed the observed quadrature NMR signal.

The parameters M_X, M_Y, and M_Z are all affected by an RF pulse. These lead to three plots analogous to those in Figure A-4. B_0 magnetization varies with time and is affected by repeated excitation. The solution to these three equations by computer and a plot of the results versus time permit the NMR user to visualize the events during an NMR observation either spectroscopically or by imaging.

What faults exist in this analysis of NMR? One drawback is the assumption of a perfectly homogeneous magnetic field. In an inhomogeneous magnetic field, each nucleus has a unique offset frequency $(\omega - \omega_0)$. The NMR signal behavior observed for this sample is the summed behavior of the various nuclei. This process, called forming the **ensemble average**, provides the intellectual bridge between the behavior of an isolated spin system and multiple spin systems found in imaging applications. The ensemble averaging procedure is not shown here, but it can and does provide a cogent explanation for the spin echo (SE) and image formation by magnetic field gradient modulation. A second omission is that the Bloch equations do not make a provision for the spin-spin coupling interaction that is always present in NMR spectroscopy.

In conclusion, the versatile Bloch equations of nuclear induction, which describe how spin systems behave in a magnetic field, lend themselves to modification and approximations suitable for interpreting magnetic resonance observations. A basic understanding of these equations is essential before the novice can become an expert in MRI interpretation.

Additional Resources

Advance Newsmagazines
www.advanceweb.com

Agfa HealthCare
www.agfamedical.com

AILab Co (Advanced Imaging Laboratory)
www.ail.co.kr

Air Products and Chemicals, Inc.
www.airproducts.com/gases/keepcold.ht

American Association of Physicists in
  Medicine (AAPM)
www.aapm.org

American College of Medical Physicists
www.acmp.org

American College of Radiology (ACR)
www.acr.org

American Healthcare Radiology
  Administrators (AHRA)
www.ahraonline.org

American Registry of Radiologic Technologists
  (ARRT)
www.arrt.org

American Roentgen Ray Society (ARRS)
www.arrs.org

American Society of Neuroradiology (ASNR)
www.asnr.org

American Society of Radiologic Technologists
  (ASRT)
www.asrt.org

Applied Radiology
www.appliedradiology.com

Armed Forces Institute of Pathology
  (AFIP)
www.afip.org

Association of Educators in Radiological
  Sciences, Inc. (AERS)
www.aers.org

Aurora Imaging Technology, Inc.
www.auroramri.com

Avotec, Inc.
www.avotec.org

Berlex Laboratories
www.berleximaging.com

Bracco Diagnostics, Inc.
www.bdi.bracco.com

Braden Shielding Systems
www.bradenshielding.com

Cybermed, Inc.
www.cybermed.co.kr

Diagnostic Imaging Magazine
www.diagnosticimaging.com

Eastman Kodak Co.
www.kodak.com/go/health

Elsevier Science
www.elsevier.com

ETS-Lindgren
www.lindgrenrf.com

FONAR Corp.
www.fonar.com

Fujifilm Medical Systems USA, Inc.
www.fujimed.com

Gammex RMI
www.gammex.com

GE Medical Systems
www.gemedicalsystems.com

Health Physics Society
www.hps.org

Herley Medical Products
www.amtinc.com

Hitachi Medical Corp.
www.hitachimed.com

IGC-Medical Advances, Inc.
www.medadv.com

Image Systems Corp.
www.imagesystemscorp.com

Indiana University Radiology Education and
Research Institute
www.indyrad.iupui.edu

John Wiley and Sons, Inc.
www.wiley.com

Konica Medical Imaging, Inc.
www.konicamedical.com

Lippincott, Williams and Wilkins
www.lww.com

Magnacoustics, Inc.
www.magnacoustics.com

Medical Technology Management Institute
www.mtmi.net

Medrad, Inc.
www.medrad.com

MRI Devices Corp.
www.mridevices.com

MRI Safety, Bioeffects and Patient Management
www.mrisafety.com

National Council on Radiation Protection and
Measurements
www.ncrp.com

Nuclear Associates/Inovision Radiation
Measurements/Syncor
www.victoreen.com

Nycomed Amersham
www.us.nai.com

The Phantom Laboratory
www.phantomlab.com

Philips Medical Systems
www.medical.philips.com

ProScan MRI Education Foundation, Inc.
www.proscan.com

Radiological Society of North America
www.rsna.org

Resonance Technology, Inc.
www.mrivideo.com

RT Image c/o Valley Forge Press
www.rt-image.com

Saunders/Mosby/Churchill
    Livingstone/Butterworth-Heinemann
www.us.elsevierhealth.com

Schiller Medical SA
www.schiller.fr

Section for Magnetic Resonance Technologists
    (SMRT)
www.ismm.org/smrt

Society for Cardiovascular Magnetic
    Resonance (SCMR)
www.scmr.org

Society of Interventional Radiology (SIR)
www.sir.org

Springer-Verlag New York, Inc.
www.springer-ny.com

Thieme Medical Publishers, Inc.
www.thieme.com

Toshiba America Medical
    Systems
www.medical.toshiba.com

Tyco Healthcare
www.mallinckrodt.com

University of California, San
    Francisco
www.radiology.ucsf.edu

Practice Examinations

The following are two practice examinations of Type A test items (i.e., a stem followed by four distracters and one answer). Most national examinations and credentialing organizations use Type A test items exclusively.

The mix of test items follows that adopted by the American Registry of Radiologic Technologists (ARRT) so that each practice examination contains test items in each category equal to those prescribed by the ARRT.

The ARRT Content Specifications for the Examination in Magnetic Resonance Imaging break down as follows:

A. Patient Care and MRI Safety	17 questions
C. Data Acquisition and Processing	62 questions
D. Physical Principles of Image Formation	43 questions
Total Test Items	122 questions

Specification B, Imaging Procedures, is not covered in this textbook and therefore is not covered in these practice examinations.

You should take these examinations one at a time, separated by additional study of the textbook material. The goal should be to score 100% on the second practice examination.

MRI EXAM I

1. When use of an MRI contrast agent causes tissue to appear brighter, which of the following has occurred?
   a. negative contrast
   b. neutral contrast
   c. positive contrast
   d. relaxation contrast
   e. proton density contrast

2. Relaxation centers are regions of
   a. increased magnetization.
   b. increased proton density.
   c. increased susceptibility.
   d. reduced T1 relaxation.
   e. reduced T2 relaxation.

3. When exposed to intense static magnetic fields, cultured human cells
   a. die prematurely.
   b. grow more rapidly.
   c. grow more slowly.
   d. show no effect.
   e. stall in G_0.

4. The main potential for biological response from RF is
   a. carcinogenesis.
   b. induction of currents.
   c. polarization.
   d. suppression of relaxation time.
   e. tissue heating.

5. Electric current density induced by transient magnetic fields is measured in
   a. ampere per square centimeter.
   b. ampere per second.
   c. tesla per centimeter.
   d. tesla per second per centimeter.
   e. tesla per second.

6. The threshold for induction of magnetic phosphenes at low frequencies is approximately
   a. 1 T/s.
   b. 3 T/s.
   c. 10 T/s.
   d. 30 T/s.
   e. 100 T/s.

7. The human responses reported during imaging with a 4-T system are presumed to be due to
   a. ferromagnetic projectiles.
   b. increased time of exposure.
   c. the radiofrequency field.
   d. the static magnetic field.
   e. transient magnetic fields.

8. Bone fracture healing is helped by
   a. high-frequency RF.
   b. low-frequency RF.
   c. polarization.
   d. static magnetic fields.
   e. transient magnetic fields.

9. At the start of an MRI examination, patient anxiety is generally due to
   a. claustrophobia.
   b. drowsiness.
   c. improper preparation.
   d. irritability.
   e. sleeplessness.

10. Approximately what percent of all patients exhibit some claustrophobia?
    a. 1
    b. 5
    c. 10
    d. 20
    e. 50

11. Operation of a successful MRI facility must include
    a. calling each outpatient the day before the scheduled examination.
    b. explaining the operating console to the patient.
    c. having the patient show up 1 hour before examination time.
    d. requiring the radiologist to interview the patient before examination.
    e. sending a postcard to remind each patient of the scheduled examination time.

12. Continuing education of MRI technologists is
    a. desirable.
    b. essential.
    c. required by law.
    d. unimportant.
    e. unnecessary.

13. Pulse sequences optimized for imaging the CNS are usually not appropriate for body imaging because for CNS compared with body tissues,
    a. PD is too low.
    b. T1 and T2 are long.
    c. T1 and T2 are short.
    d. T1 is long and T2 is short.
    e. T1 is short and T2 is long.

14. If a quench occurs and helium escapes, the principal effect on the MRI technologist will be
   a. Donald Duck's voice.
   b. lowered body temperature.
   c. skin rash.
   d. sticky hair.
   e. superficial burn.

15. Proper quality control for an MRI system requires that test object imaging be performed at least
   a. daily.
   b. weekly.
   c. biweekly.
   d. monthly.
   e. anually.

16. The principal hazard to patients and personnel in an MRI facility is the biological effect of
   a. ferromagnetic projectiles.
   b. the main magnetic field.
   c. the RF field.
   d. the sound level.
   e. the transient magnetic field.

17. A clearly marked exclusion area should be identified at the
   a. 0.1-mT fringe field.
   b. 0.3-mT fringe field.
   c. 0.5-mT fringe field.
   d. 1-mT fringe field.
   e. 5-mT fringe field.

18. After a 90° RF pulse, the signal received from the patient is
   a. a free induction decay.
   b. a gradient echo.
   c. a spin echo.
   d. magnetically transferred.
   e. zero.

19. The term *pulse sequence* refers to
   a. gradient magnetic field pulses and RF pulses.
   b. only gradient magnetic field pulses.
   c. only RF pulses.
   d. RF pulses and static magnetic field pulses.
   e. static magnetic field pulses and gradient magnetic field pulses.

20. The time to echo (TE) is the time between the
   a. 180° RF pulse and the next 180° RF pulse.
   b. 180° RF pulse and the next 90° RF pulse.
   c. 180° RF pulse and the spin echo.
   d. 90° RF pulse and the 180° RF pulse.
   e. 90° RF pulse and the spin echo.

21. The inversion recovery pulse sequence consists of a train of
   a. $\alpha° \ldots \alpha° \ldots \alpha° \ldots$
   b. $180° \ldots 90° \ldots 180° \ldots 90° \ldots$
   c. $90° \ldots 180° \ldots 180° \ldots$
   d. $90° \ldots 180° \ldots 90° \ldots 180° \ldots$
   e. $90° \ldots 90° \ldots 90° \ldots$

22. Which of the following pulse sequences involves all three: TR, TE, and TI?
   a. echo planar
   b. gradient echo
   c. inversion recovery
   d. saturation recovery
   e. spin echo

23. As M_{XY} relaxes to zero,
   a. gradient magnetic field decreases.
   b. nothing happens.
   c. signal intensity decreases.
   d. signal intensity increases.
   e. spin echo is produced.

24. After the relaxation of net magnetization to equilibrium, the MR signal
   a. is constant at an intermediate level.
   b. is decreasing.
   c. is saturated.
   d. is zero.
   e. oscillates at the Larmor frequency.

25. At equilibrium, if a 90° RF pulse is used, which of the following MR signals will be produced?
    a. free induction decay
    b. gradient echo
    c. relaxation signal
    d. spin echo
    e. stimulated echo

26. Control of TE is exercised by control of
    a. proton density.
    b. T1 relaxation time.
    c. T2 relaxation time.
    d. the 180° RF pulse.
    e. the 90° RF pulse.

27. With the inversion recovery pulse sequence, MR images are constructed from
    a. free induction decay.
    b. gradient echoes.
    c. inversion echoes.
    d. spin echoes.
    e. stimulated echoes.

28. In MRI, the role of the Fourier transform is to
    a. change the MR signal into a frequency spectrum.
    b. measure the amplitude of the MR signal.
    c. measure the frequency bandwidth of the MR signal.
    d. precisely shape the magnetic field.
    e. separate T1 from T2.

29. The Fourier transformation of a spin echo results in data in the
    a. amplitude domain.
    b. frequency domain.
    c. length domain.
    d. time domain.
    e. volume domain.

30. The result of a Fourier transform in MRI is called a/an
    a. amplitude function.
    b. image function.
    c. object function.
    d. source function.
    e. transform function.

31. In MRI, smooth objects are represented by
    a. a narrow range of frequencies.
    b. a wide range of frequencies.
    c. high frequencies.
    d. low frequencies.
    e. zero frequency.

32. The mathematical tool used to analyze the frequency content of an object is the
    a. backprojection method.
    b. Cartesian number rule.
    c. Fourier transform.
    d. imaginary number rule.
    e. induction transform.

33. Noise in an image is generally more apparent when which of the following are present?
    a. high amplitude signals
    b. high spatial frequencies
    c. long relaxation times
    d. low spatial frequencies
    e. short relaxation times

34. The raw data of an MR signal contains what components of the spatial frequency?
    a. angle and frequency
    b. intensity and frequency
    c. magnitude and phase
    d. phase and angle
    e. X and Y coordinates

35. In general, when one samples the data of the spatial frequency domain with emphasis on the higher spatial frequencies, the
    a. contrast resolution will be less.
    b. examination will take longer.
    c. field of view will be larger.
    d. signal-to-noise ratio will be less.
    e. spatial resolution will be less.

36. The physiological motion of a nervous action potential takes approximately how much time?
    a. 1 ms
    b. 200 ms
    c. 500 ms
    d. 1 s
    e. 5 s

37. When an image is constructed, the matrix size is equal to the number of different
    a. B_0 values used.
    b. frequency-encoding gradients applied.
    c. phase encoding gradients applied.
    d. RF pulses transmitted into the patient.
    e. slice selection gradients applied.

38. The STIR sequences can be designed to suppress the signal from fat because fat has a
    a. high PD.
    b. long TE.
    c. long TR.
    d. short T1.
    e. short T2.

39. *Temporal resolution* is a term applied to
    a. tables of temperature.
    b. temporary resolution.
    c. the accurate determination of temperature.
    d. the change in contrast resolution with body temperature.
    e. time-related events.

40. For a 128 × 128 image matrix to be constructed, which of the following must be applied with 128 different values?
    a. frequency-encoding gradients
    b. phase-encoding gradients
    c. proton density amplitudes
    d. RF pulses
    e. slice selection gradients

41. The FLAIR pulse sequence is a
    a. Find Late Activity in Recovery.
    b. Fluid Attenuated Inversion Recovery.
    c. STIR sequence with a longer T1.
    d. STIR sequence with a shorter T1.
    e. STIR sequence with high PD.

42. When a sequence of pulses reduces longitudinal relaxation by the same amount that is recovered between pulses, the result is
    a. a saturated state.
    b. a steady state.
    c. an equilibrium state.
    d. T1 amplification.
    e. T2 amplification.

43. The gradient echo pulse sequence can be identified as:
    a. $\alpha° \ldots \alpha° \ldots \alpha° \ldots \alpha° \ldots$
    b. $180° \ldots 180° \ldots 180° \ldots 180° \ldots$
    c. $180° \ldots 90° \ldots 180° \ldots 90° \ldots$
    d. $90° \ldots 180° \ldots 90° \ldots 180° \ldots$
    e. $90° \ldots 90° \ldots 90° \ldots 90° \ldots$

44. T2* is shorter than T2, principally because of
    a. differences in T1.
    b. differences in T2.
    c. proton density variations.
    d. the influence of irreversible magnetic field inhomogeneities.
    e. the influence of reversible magnetic field inhomogeneities.

45. Long repetition times (TRs) result in
    a. accelerated T1 relaxation.
    b. accelerated T2 relaxation.
    c. increased PD.
    d. longitudinal magnetization that is close to equilibrium.
    e. transverse magnetization that is close to equilibrium.

46. An alpha pulse is a/an
    a. pulsed gradient magnetic field.
    b. pulsed signal reception.
    c. RF pulse between 90° and 180°.
    d. RF pulse less than 45°.
    e. RF pulse less than 90°.

47. A pulse sequence diagram should contain all of the following lines of data except
    a. MR signal acquired.
    b. phase-encoding gradient magnetic field.
    c. proton density profile.
    d. slice selection gradient.
    e. transmitted RF pulse.

48. For completeness, an MRI pulse sequence diagram should contain how many lines of information?
    a. one
    b. two
    c. three
    d. four
    e. five

49. The two properties of any picture element are
    a. character and position.
    b. contrast and spatial.
    c. depth and character.
    d. position and size.
    e. size and depth.

50. A pulse sequence is
    a. a mathematical algorithm.
    b. a spatial rendering of the MR signal.
    c. a time line diagram of MR operation.
    d. the name of a controlling subassembly of an MR imaging system.
    e. the result of a Fourier transformation.

51. Spatial localization of signals in an MR imaging system is identified by
    a. B_0 intensity.
    b. collimation.
    c. filtration.
    d. signal encoding.
    e. signal enhancement.

52. Regardless of the type of magnet, the Z-axis is always
    a. across the patient.
    b. horizontal.
    c. parallel with the B_0 field.
    d. parallel with the long axis of the patient.
    e. vertical.

53. For spins to be excited in a given slice of tissue, the RF pulse must
    a. be omitted.
    b. be repeatedly energized.
    c. be turned on for a longer time.
    d. match the Larmor frequency at B_0 plus B_{XYZ}.
    e. match the Larmor frequency at B_0.

54. The Q value of an RF pulse is expressed as the
    a. bandwidth divided by the resonant frequency.
    b. resonant frequency divided by the bandwidth.
    c. resonant frequency times the bandwidth.
    d. square of the bandwidth.
    e. square of the resonant frequency.

55. The effect of the pulsed phase-encoding gradient on the phase of spins along a column is
    a. nothing.
    b. to decrease the phase perpendicular to the gradient.
    c. to impress a phase shift along the gradient.
    d. to increase the phase perpendicular to the gradient.
    e. to reduce proton density effects along the column.

56. The gyromagnetic ratio for hydrogen is equal to
    a. 21 megahertz per tesla.
    b. 21 tesla per megahertz.
    c. 42 megahertz per tesla.
    d. 42 tesla per megahertz.
    e. 63 tesla per megahertz.

57. Which one of the following RF pulses should produce the thinnest slice in a 1-T imaging system?
    a. 21 ± 0.5 MHz
    b. 42 ± 0.1 MHz
    c. 42 ± 0.5 MHz
    d. 63 ± 0.1 MHz
    e. 63 ± 0.5 MHz

58. The number of multiple signals that are averaged is represented by
    a. ACQ.
    b. Bug.
    c. FID.
    d. SAR.
    e. SAT.

59. Referring to the figure below, which letter in the pulse sequence represents free induction decay?
    a. A
    b. B
    c. C
    d. D
    e. E

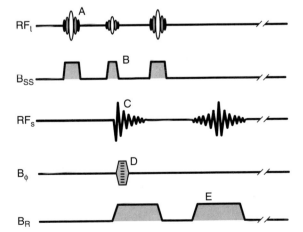

60. During a single TR of a partial saturation pulse sequence,
    a. a stimulated echo is formed.
    b. an image can be constructed.
    c. one gradient echo will be generated.
    d. one line of the spatial frequency domain is produced.
    e. one spin echo will be generated.

61. The purpose of the 90° RF pulse in an inversion recovery pulse sequence is to
    a. enhance the proton density.
    b. lengthen T1 relaxation.
    c. lengthen T2 relaxation.
    d. lengthen T2* relaxation.
    e. rotate the net magnetization onto the XY plane.

62. What is the time required for double echo imaging compared with that for single echo imaging?
    a. half
    b. the same
    c. twice
    d. four times
    e. eight times

63. Which of the following influences the character of an MRI pixel?
    a. electron density
    b. mass density
    c. optical density
    d. proton density
    e. slice thickness

64. Which of the following best describes an MR image?
    a. characteristic
    b. dynamic
    c. representational
    d. static
    e. superimposed

65. Approximately, how many colors can the human eye detect?
  a. 2
  b. 20
  c. 100
  d. 200
  e. 2000

66. Which of the following types of image receptor is used for MRI?
  a. coil
  b. film
  c. piezoelectric crystal
  d. scintillation detector
  e. TLD

67. The ability to detect differences in brightness level is termed
  a. color perception.
  b. conspiquity.
  c. contrast perception.
  d. definition.
  e. visual acuity.

68. Pixel location is determined by
  a. B_0 intensity.
  b. extrinsic pressure.
  c. gradient magnetic fields.
  d. intrinsic modification.
  e. RF pulse sequences.

69. Abnormal tissue character is best exhibited by
  a. distortion.
  b. extrinsic compression.
  c. extrinsic displacement.
  d. intrinsic deformity.
  e. unexpected pixel brightness.

70. The principal parameters influencing the character of an MRI pixel are all of the following except
  a. electromagnetic induction.
  b. motion.
  c. proton density.
  d. T1 relaxation.
  e. T2 relaxation.

71. Pixel character is principally determined by
  a. B_0 intensity.
  b. extrinsic pressure.
  c. gradient magnetic fields.
  d. intrinsic modification.
  e. RF pulse sequences.

72. The principal mechanism for producing an MRI signal is
  a. electromagnetic induction.
  b. motion.
  c. proton density.
  d. spin-lattice relaxation time.
  e. spin-spin relaxation time.

73. Referring to the figure below, which tissue has the highest equilibrium magnetization?
  a. A
  b. B
  c. C
  d. D
  e. E

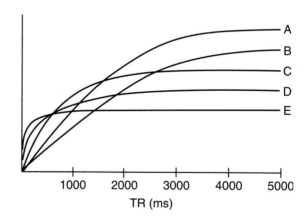

74. Referring to the figure above, at what approximate TR is the longitudinal magnetization for tissues B and C equal?
  a. 500 ms
  b. 1500 ms
  c. 2500 ms
  d. 3500 ms
  e. 4000 ms

75. Referring to the figure on p. 444, at a TR of 2000 ms, which tissue should appear darkest?
    a. A
    b. B
    c. C
    d. D
    e. E

76. In a conventional spin echo pulse sequence, after the 90° RF pulse,
    a. $M_{XY} = \alpha M_0$.
    b. $M_{XY} = 0$.
    c. $M_{XY} = M_0$.
    d. $M_Z = \alpha M_0$.
    e. $M_Z = M_0$.

77. Referring to the figure below, which of the five tissues has the lowest magnetization at equilibrium?
    a. A
    b. B
    c. C
    d. D
    e. E

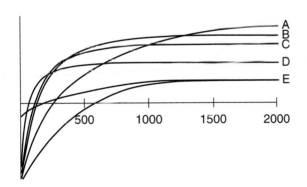

78. Referring to the figure above, at approximately 1000 ms, which tissue should appear brightest?
    a. A
    b. B
    c. C
    d. D
    e. E

79. A gyroscope wobbles because of an interaction between
    a. charge and charge.
    b. charge and spin.
    c. mass and charge.
    d. mass and mass.
    e. mass and spin.

80. In the Larmor equation, B is the
    a. frequency of precession in megahertz.
    b. gradient magnetic field.
    c. gyromagnetic ratio in megahertz.
    d. magnetic field intensity in megahertz per tesla.
    e. magnetic field intensity in tesla.

81. In the absence of an external magnetic field, the direction of a nuclear magnetic moment will
    a. be random.
    b. be straight down.
    c. be straight up.
    d. precess.
    e. spin.

82. The gyromagnetic ratio for a given nucleus
    a. has a specific value.
    b. has units of tesla per megahertz.
    c. is determined by the magnetic field.
    d. varies with B_0.
    e. varies with the frequency of precession.

83. When M equals zero, this indicates that nuclear magnetic moments
    a. are arranged opposite.
    b. are arranged parallel.
    c. are arranged randomly.
    d. are in motion.
    e. have disappeared.

84. M_0 is proportional to
    a. B_0.
    b. gyromagnetic ratio.
    c. T.
    d. T^2.
    e. the square of the proton density.

85. In both the stationary and rotating frame of reference, the Z-axis is always in the direction of the
    a. external magnetic field.
    b. gradient magnetic field.
    c. gyromagnetic ratio.
    d. relaxation time.
    e. proton density.

86. To rotate net magnetization from the Z-axis, one must use
    a. a gradient magnetic field of proper frequency.
    b. a rotating magnetic field of proper frequency.
    c. a static magnetic field of proper frequency.
    d. the proper T1 relaxation time.
    e. the proper T2 relaxation time.

87. Vector diagrams used to illustrate MRI principles are in which frame?
    a. laboratory
    b. musical score
    c. oblique
    d. rotating
    e. stationary

88. In the rotating frame, the net magnetization vector
    a. decays with T1 relaxation.
    b. decays with T2 relaxation.
    c. does not precess.
    d. is the proton density.
    e. precesses at the Larmor frequency.

89. When tissue is placed in a static magnetic field, the hydrogen nuclei tend to
    a. align perpendicular to the field.
    b. align with the field.
    c. diffuse.
    d. spin against the field.
    e. spin with the field.

90. Net magnetization is the result of which property of individual spins?
    a. the difference
    b. the motion
    c. the precession
    d. the relaxation
    e. the sum

91. Which of the following increases as M_0 increases?
    a. proton charge
    b. proton density
    c. RF pulse
    d. T1 relaxation time
    e. T2 relaxation time

92. Which of the following is not a principal MRI parameter?
    a. Larmor frequency
    b. proton density
    c. spin density
    d. T1 relaxation time
    e. T2 relaxation time

93. In addition to proton density, signal intensity is also affected by
    a. how the proton is charged.
    b. how the proton is chemically bound.
    c. proton valence state.
    d. the distribution of the proton.
    e. the mass of the proton.

94. Proton density can best be defined as hydrogen
    a. charge.
    b. concentration.
    c. configuration.
    d. relaxation.
    e. translation.

95. The T1 relaxation time is related to the time required for
    a. longitudinal saturation.
    b. M_{XY} to relax to equilibrium.
    c. M_Z to relax to equilibrium.
    d. translation saturation.
    e. transverse saturation.

96. Referring to the figure below, which tissue has the highest proton density?
    a. A
    b. B
    c. C
    d. D
    e. not enough information

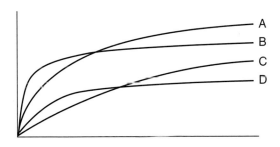

97. A given tissue has a T1 relaxation time of 750 ms. When a patient has been out of the magnet for 1.5 seconds, what will be the value of M_Z?
    a. 0.14 M_{XY}
    b. 0.14 M_Z
    c. 0.14 M_0
    d. 0.37 M_Z
    e. 0.37 M_0

98. Transverse magnetization is symbolized by
    a. B_0.
    b. B_Z.
    c. M_0.
    d. M_{XY}.
    e. M_Z.

99. Referring to the figure at the top of the next column, which point represents complete relaxation?
    a. A
    b. B
    c. C
    d. D
    e. not enough information

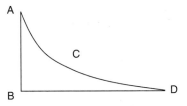

100. An FID is a result of relaxation of
    a. B_0.
    b. B_{XY}.
    c. M_0.
    d. M_{XY}.
    e. M_Z.

101. Referring to the figure below, how many FIDs are shown?
    a. one
    b. two
    c. three
    d. four
    e. five

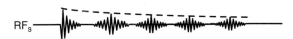

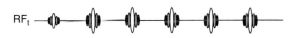

102. The maximum amplitude of a spin echo occurs
    a. at the beginning of the signal.
    b. at the end of the signal.
    c. at the midpoint of the signal.
    d. variously according to pulse sequence.
    e. variously because of motion.

103. In order to measure M_Z, one must use the following pulse sequence:
    a. $\alpha° \ldots \alpha°$
    b. $180° \ldots 180°$
    c. $180° \ldots 90°$
    d. $90° \ldots 180°$
    e. $90° \ldots 90°$

104. Magnetization of tissue along the Z-axis cannot be measured directly because
    a. M_{XY} is too small.
    b. M_Z is too small.
    c. T1 is too short.
    d. T2 is too short.
    e. the B_0 field is not homogeneous.

105. The inversion delay time (TI) is the time between the
    a. $\alpha°$ RF pulse and $\alpha°$ RF pulse.
    b. 180° RF pulse and 180° RF pulse.
    c. 180° RF pulse and 90° RF pulse.
    d. 90° RF pulse and 180° RF pulse.
    e. 90° RF pulse and 90° RF pulse.

106. The term *spectrum* is also referred to as
    a. frequency distribution.
    b. nuclear species.
    c. precession.
    d. proton density.
    e. relaxation time.

107. An NMR spectrum is obtained from a
    a. free induction decay.
    b. gradient magnetic field.
    c. precessional state.
    d. proton density.
    e. relaxation time.

108. The Fourier transform of an MR signal results in a distribution of intensity as a function of
    a. inverse time.
    b. iteration.
    c. mass.
    d. proton density.
    e. time.

109. The term *chemical shift* relates principally to a change in
    a. Larmor frequency.
    b. molecular configuration.
    c. nuclear mass.
    d. proton density.
    e. relaxation time.

110. A hydrogen NMR spectrum may have peaks because each nucleus has slightly different
    a. Larmor frequency.
    b. molecular configuration.
    c. nuclear mass.
    d. proton density.
    e. relaxation time.

111. A change in resonant frequency for similar nuclei in a given molecule is caused by
    a. electron cloud.
    b. molecular configuration.
    c. nuclear structure.
    d. proton density.
    e. relaxation times.

112. Magnetic resonance (MR) signals are converted by Fourier transformation from
    a. Cartesian coordinates to polar coordinates.
    b. frequency data to phase data.
    c. phase data to amplitude data.
    d. spatial frequency domain to spatial location domain.
    e. spatial location domain to space.

113. A digital image with a 9-bit matrix size would have how many pixels?
    a. 64×64
    b. 128×128
    c. 256×256
    d. 512×512
    e. 1024×1024

114. One gigabyte is equal to
    a. 2^5 bytes.
    b. 2^{10} bytes.
    c. 2^{15} bytes.
    d. 2^{20} bytes.
    e. 2^{30} bytes.

115. Magnetic resonance imaging (MRI) spatial resolution is normally measured in
    a. cycles per centimeter.
    b. cycles per millimeter.
    c. line pairs per centimeter.
    d. line pairs per millimeter.
    e. shades of gray.

116. In general, the contrast resolution of an object will improve as the
    a. high spatial frequencies are adequately sampled.
    b. image matrix size gets larger.
    c. low spatial frequencies are rejected.
    d. noise increases.
    e. pixel size gets larger.

117. One line pair per millimeter is equal to how many line pairs per centimeter?
    a. 0.01
    b. 0.1
    c. 1.0
    d. 5.0
    e. 10

118. A 0.5-T MR imaging system is said to have B_0 field homogeneity of $\pm$ 10 ppm. This is equal to
    a. ± 0.5 μT.
    b. ± 5 μT.
    c. ± 50 μT.
    d. ± 500 μT.
    e. ± 5000 μT.

119. The chemical shift artifact is usually
    a. along the B_0.
    b. along the RF axis.
    c. in the frequency-encoding direction.
    d. in the phase-encoding direction.
    e. throughout the slice selected.

120. An image artifact can best be described as
    a. an absent anatomy.
    b. an unwanted pattern that does not represent actual anatomy.
    c. positive or negative enhancement of actual anatomy.
    d. something absent in the patient.
    e. something left behind in the patient.

121. The partial volume artifact can be reduced by
    a. increasing FOV.
    b. increasing TR.
    c. obtaining more signals.
    d. reducing flip angle.
    e. reducing slice thickness.

122. The quadrature detection artifact occurs along the
    a. B_0 field.
    b. frequency-encoding axis.
    c. longitudinal axis.
    d. phase-encoding axis.
    e. transverse axis.

MRI EXAM II

1. The use of mineral oil to image the GI tract is an example of enhancing
   a. electron density.
   b. proton density.
   c. T1 relaxation.
   d. T2 relaxation.
   e. T2* relaxation.

2. The use of a paramagnetic agent works by changing
   a. electron density.
   b. mass density.
   c. proton density.
   d. T1 relaxation time.
   e. T2 relaxation time.

3. Transient magnetic fields are measured in
   a. tesla per square centimeter.
   b. tesla per hertz.
   c. tesla per second per meter.
   d. tesla per second.
   e. tesla.

4. Exposing pregnant mice to an intense static magnetic field causes
   a. congenital abnormalities.
   b. growth retardation.
   c. malignant disease induction.
   d. no effect.
   e. reduced maze learning.

5. Low-frequency electromagnetic fields (EMFs) relate to
   a. diagnostic ultrasound.
   b. microwave radiation.
   c. MRI.
   d. typical household electricity.
   e. ultrasonic diathermy.

6. The potential hazard to patients from RF irradiation is principally due to
   a. current induction.
   b. excitation.
   c. ionization.
   d. polarization.
   e. tissue heating.

7. It is recommended that the fringe magnetic field be access controlled to
   a. 0.1 mT.
   b. 0.5 mT.
   c. 1 mT.
   d. 5 mT.
   e. 10 mT.

8. Ferromagnetic surgical clips are hazardous because they
   a. can be pulled from the patient.
   b. cause signal drop.
   c. may heat up excessively.
   d. may rotate out of the field of view.
   e. may twist to align with the static magnetic field.

9. If the presence of foreign ferromagnetic material in the patient is questionable,
   a. CT images should be obtained.
   b. the examination should be done anyway.
   c. fluoroscopy should be done.
   d. radiographs may be taken.
   e. sonograms may be taken.

10. A consent form for an MRI examination is necessary
    a. when any imaging system components are not USFDA approved.
    b. for every examination.
    c. when it is the patient's first MRI examination.
    d. when the imaging system has been repaired recently.
    e. when the imaging system is brand new.

11. Liquid helium has a vaporization temperature of
    a. 0 K.
    b. 4 K.
    c. 19 K.
    d. 77 K.
    e. 100 K.

12. A partial saturation image made with a short repetition time is most likely a
    a. motion image.
    b. proton density weighted image.
    c. pure image.
    d. T1 weighted image.
    e. T2 weighted image.

13. Routinely, double echo imaging is used to provide
    a. magnetic resonance angiograms.
    b. proton density weighted images for anatomy and T1 weighted images for pathology.
    c. proton density weighted images for anatomy and T2 weighted images for pathology.
    d. T1 weighted images for anatomy and T2 weighted images for pathology.
    e. T2 weighted images for anatomy and T1 weighted images for pathology.

14. Joint prosthesis in an MRI patient may
    a. be a contraindication for MRI.
    b. be pulled from the patient.
    c. become ineffective.
    d. degrade the image.
    e. heat unacceptably, because of RF exposure.

15. The pregnant patient
    a. can be imaged at any time, after completion of satisfactory consent forms.
    b. can be imaged at any time, provided the results will materially affect patient management.
    c. can be imaged after a radiographic screen.
    d. should not be imaged in the first trimester with MRI.
    e. should not be imaged with MRI.

16. After a 180° RF pulse, the signal received from the patient is
    a. a free induction decay.
    b. a gradient echo.
    c. a spin echo.
    d. saturated.
    e. zero.

17. The initial amplitude of an FID is dependent on all of the following except
    a. B_0.
    b. gyromagnetic ratio.
    c. proton density.
    d. relaxation time.
    e. temperature.

18. A spin echo pulse sequence consists of the following train of RF pulses:
    a. $\alpha° \ldots \alpha° \ldots \alpha° \ldots$
    b. $180° \ldots 180° \ldots 180° \ldots$
    c. $180° \ldots 90° \ldots 180° \ldots 90° \ldots$
    d. $90° \ldots 180° \ldots 90° \ldots 180° \ldots$
    e. $90° \ldots 90° \ldots 90° \ldots$

19. In a double echo, spin echo pulse sequence, TE for the second echo is the time from the 90° RF pulse to the
    a. first spin echo.
    b. next 180° RF pulse.
    c. next 90° RF pulse.
    d. second 180° RF pulse.
    e. second spin echo.

20. The inversion delay time (TI) is the time between the
    a. 180° and the 90° RF pulse.
    b. 180° and the spin echo.
    c. 180° RF pulse and the next 180° RF pulse.
    d. 90° and the 180° RF pulse.
    e. 90° and the spin echo.

21. Of the available net magnetization, the only one that can be observed during an MR imaging process is
    a. B_Φ.
    b. B_{SS}.
    c. M_0.
    d. M_{XY}.
    e. M_Z

22. At any point in time, the intensity of the MR signal is proportional to the size of
    a. B_Φ.
    b. B_{SS}.
    c. M_0.
    d. M_{XY}.
    e. M_Z.

23. As M_Z relaxes to equilibrium,
    a. an FID is produced.
    b. nothing happens.
    c. signal intensity decreases.
    d. signal intensity increases.
    e. spins become saturated.

24. A free induction decay will be produced by which combination of RF pulses?
    a. $\alpha°$ . . . 180°
    b. 180° . . . 180° . . .
    c. 180° . . . 90°
    d. 90° . . . 180°
    e. 90° . . . 90° . . .

25. A spin echo appears
    a. immediately after a 180° RF pulse.
    b. immediately after a 90° RF pulse.
    c. immediately after an $\alpha°$ RF pulse.
    d. sometime after a 180° RF pulse.
    e. sometime after a 90° RF pulse.

26. The time to echo (TE) is
    a. one half the time from the 180° RF pulse to the next 180° RF pulse.
    b. one half the time of the 90° RF pulse to the spin echo.
    c. the time between 90° and 180° RF pulses.
    d. the time from the 180° RF pulse to the spin echo.
    e. the time from the 90° RF pulse to the spin echo.

27. The source function in MRI is a plot of
    a. 1/time vs 1/length.
    b. intensity vs 1/time.
    c. intensity vs 1/length.
    d. intensity vs length.
    e. intensity vs time.

28. In the spatial frequency domain, sharp-edged objects
    a. approach a single frequency.
    b. are independent of frequency.
    c. contain a narrow range of frequencies.
    d. contain high frequencies.
    e. have maximum signal amplitude.

29. Optimum sampling of an MR signal requires that a value be determined
    a. at least once a cycle.
    b. at least twice a cycle.
    c. at least three times a cycle.
    d. at least four times a cycle.
    e. more than five times a cycle.

30. When a representation in the time domain is transformed into the frequency domain, units are transformed from
    a. cm to cm^{-1}.
    b. cm^{-1} to cm.
    c. hertz to centimeter.
    d. hertz to seconds.
    e. seconds to hertz.

31. Slice selection during MR imaging requires a gradient magnetic field and a/an
    a. broadband RF pulse.
    b. flat RF pulse.
    c. inverse RF pulse.
    d. shaped RF pulse.
    e. single frequency RF pulse.

32. The unit cycle per millimeter is best matched to
    a. amplitude frequency.
    b. Cartesian coordinates.
    c. polar coordinates.
    d. spatial frequency.
    e. temporal frequency.

33. Which of the following must be sampled for a high-resolution image?
    a. high spatial frequencies
    b. high proton densities
    c. low spatial frequencies
    d. low proton densities
    e. short relaxation times

34. The middle region of the spatial frequency domain map is that which best determines
    a. contrast resolution.
    b. proton density information.
    c. relaxation time data.
    d. signal amplitude.
    e. spatial resolution.

35. The different orientation of the net magnetization vectors along a row of voxels represents
    a. phase incoherence.
    b. proton density.
    c. relaxation time.
    d. spatial frequency.
    e. temporal frequency.

36. Field of view (FOV) relates to the
    a. diameter of a pixel.
    b. diameter of the area that is reconstructed.
    c. diameter of the patient aperture of the imaging system.
    d. maximum diameter of the patient.
    e. size of the imaging coil.

37. The term *trajectory in k-space* refers to
    a. each angle and distance.
    b. each X and Y point.
    c. the method of sampling the amplitude spectrum.
    d. the method of sampling the spatial frequency domain.
    e. the method of sampling the temporal frequency domain.

38. When the Y gradient of a horizontal B_0 superconducting magnet is identified as the slice selection gradient, the image plane is
    a. coronal.
    b. irregular.
    c. oblique.
    d. sagittal.
    e. transverse.

39. Lines of the spatial frequency domain acquired with weak phase-encoding gradients principally contribute information about
    a. contrast resolution.
    b. irregular objects.
    c. large smooth objects.
    d. small sharp objects.
    e. temporal resolution.

40. In FSE, the zero order spin echo is that which follows the
    a. first 180° RF pulse.
    b. last 180° RF pulse.
    c. lowest amplitude pulse.
    d. strongest phase-encoding gradient pulse.
    e. weakest phase-encoding gradient pulse.

41. When the X gradient magnetic field of a vertical B_0 superconducting magnet is applied as the slice selection gradient, the image plane is
    a. coronal.
    b. irregular.
    c. oblique.
    d. sagittal.
    e. transverse.

42. Lines of the spatial frequency domain obtained with strong phase-encoding gradients are located
    a. in the center of the spatial frequency domain.
    b. interleaved throughout the spatial frequency domain.
    c. just outside the spatial frequency domain.
    d. on either side of the spatial frequency domain.
    e. on the periphery of the spatial frequency domain.

43. Gradient echo imaging is characterized by
    a. a refocusing gradient magnetic field.
    b. a single 180° RF pulse.
    c. a single 90° RF pulse.
    d. shorter T1 relaxation times.
    e. shorter T2 relaxation times.

44. After a 30° flip angle, transverse magnetization has a value of
    a. 0.01 M_0.
    b. 0.37 M_0.
    c. 0.5 M_0.
    d. 0.63 M_0.
    e. 0.90 M_0.

45. When compared with T2, T2*
    a. is always longer.
    b. is always shorter.
    c. will depend on PD.
    d. will depend on T1*.
    e. will depend on T1.

46. Stimulated echoes occur as a consequence of
    a. equilibrium magnetization.
    b. magnetization steady state.
    c. magnetization transfer.
    d. T2 relaxation.
    e. T2* relaxation.

47. At what flip angle does the transverse magnetization equal 0.5 M_0?
    a. 15°
    b. 30°
    c. 45°
    d. 60°
    e. 75°

48. A gradient magnetic field designed to inhibit the formation of a stimulated echo is called a
    a. spoiler.
    b. steady state.
    c. stimulator.
    d. transfer gradient.
    e. truncation.

49. The character of a pixel element refers to its
    a. brightness.
    b. depth.
    c. location.
    d. size.
    e. spectrum.

50. The two principal timing patterns in a pulse sequence diagram are
    a. proton density profile and exposure time.
    b. RF pulses and exposure time.
    c. RF pulses and gradient magnetic fields.
    d. temporal resolution and contrast resolution.
    e. temporal resolution and spatial resolution.

51. In an MR image, a pixel emitting an intense MR signal would be rendered
    a. black.
    b. bright.
    c. dark gray.
    d. light gray.
    e. void.

52. The contrast rendition of an MR image is principally determined by
    a. gradient magnetic field amplitude and timing.
    b. receiving coil bandwidth.
    c. RF pulse amplitude and timing.
    d. the gray scale resolution of the computer.
    e. the number of signal acquisitions.

53. The principal control of spatial resolution in an MR imaging system is determined by
    a. gradient magnetic field frequency and timing.
    b. proton density range.
    c. RF pulse amplitude and timing.
    d. the gray scale resolution of the computer.
    e. the number of phase-encoding pulses.

54. Gradient magnetic fields serve two principle purposes:
    a. pixel character and slice selection.
    b. pixel intensity and pixel character.
    c. pixel intensity and slice selection.
    d. pixel location within a slice and pixel intensity.
    e. slice selection and pixel location within a slice.

55. Spins in a coronal slice in a vertical B_0 superconducting imaging system are selectively excited when which magnetic field is applied?
    a. B_α
    b. B_β
    c. B_X
    d. B_Y
    e. B_Z

56. When two pixels exist in the same magnetic field and one is brighter than the other, it is probably brighter because of
    a. a more intense RF pulse.
    b. a stronger gradient magnetic field.
    c. higher proton density.
    d. longer imaging time.
    e. the postprocessing algorithm.

57. The frequency-encoding gradient is
    a. energized during RF excitation.
    b. energized during signal acquisition.
    c. energized after signal acquisition.
    d. pulsed at the same time as the phase-encoding gradient.
    e. that which determines spatial resolution.

58. The selection of a slice of tissue for imaging requires
    a. a gradient magnetic field plus RF excitation.
    b. absence of a gradient magnetic field.
    c. an oscillation B_0.
    d. gradient magnetic field and MR signal acquisition.
    e. RF excitation and MR signal acquisition.

59. The "spin warp" method refers to
    a. a twisted change in frequency after the gradient pulse.
    b. a twisted change in frequency during the gradient pulse.
    c. the phase shift impressed along the B_0.
    d. the phase shift impressed along the gradient.
    e. the twisted change in frequency due to the RF pulse.

60. An MR imaging pulse sequence could not work with a single 180° RF pulse because
    a. T1 relaxation would be too short.
    b. T2 relaxation would be too short.
    c. T2* relaxation would be too short.
    d. the resulting magnetization is overpowered by the B_0 field.
    e. there is no transverse magnetization.

61. Multiecho imaging in a conventional spin echo pulse sequence results in multiple sets of images having different
    a. contrast resolution.
    b. field of view.
    c. matrix size.
    d. spatial resolution.
    e. temporal resolution.

62. What time is required to produce an image having a 256 × 256 matrix from two signal acquisitions with a repetition time of 2000 ms?
    a. 17 minutes
    b. 25 minutes
    c. 34 minutes
    d. 50 minutes
    e. 8.5 minutes

63. Referring to the figure below, which letter in the following pulse sequence represents the frequency-encoding gradient?
    a. A
    b. B
    c. C
    d. D
    e. E

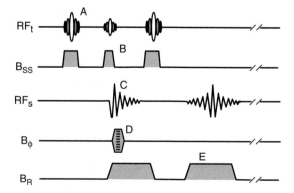

64. The MR signal observed in the partial saturation pulse sequence is a/an
    a. conventional spin echo.
    b. fast spin echo.
    c. FID.
    d. gradient echo.
    e. GRASE echo.

65. Rods of the human retina
    a. are more sensitive than cones.
    b. are used primarily for daytime vision.
    c. are used principally for photopic vision.
    d. respond to color better.
    e. respond to intense light levels.

66. The ability to perceive fine detail is called
    a. color perception.
    b. conspiquity.
    c. contrast perception.
    d. definition.
    e. visual acuity.

67. An MR image represents what tissue characteristic?
    a. electron density
    b. gyromagnetic ratio
    c. hydrogen concentration
    d. mass density
    e. optical density

68. Pixels in an MR image have two descriptors:
    a. character and color.
    b. contrast resolution and location.
    c. location and character.
    d. spatial resolution and contrast resolution.
    e. spatial resolution and location.

69. The number of principal MRI parameters matches the number of primary colors. That number is
    a. one.
    b. three.
    c. five.
    d. seven.
    e. nine.

70. When an MR image is undergoing post-processing, ROI stands for
    a. a method of observing qualitative change.
    b. a method of obtaining quantitative data.
    c. rapid organ imaging.
    d. region of interest.
    e. relaxation on inversion.

71. When the size of an anatomical structure in an MR image is being evaluated, the appropriate classifications are all of the following except
    a. distorted.
    b. intense.
    c. large.
    d. normal.
    e. small.

72. Referring to the figure below, which diagram best represents T2 relaxation?
    a. A
    b. B
    c. C
    d. D
    e. E

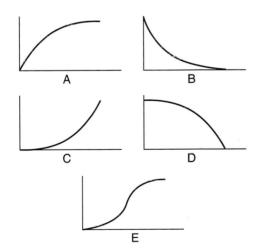

73. Referring to the figure below, which tissue has the shortest relaxation time?
    a. A
    b. B
    c. C
    d. D
    e. E

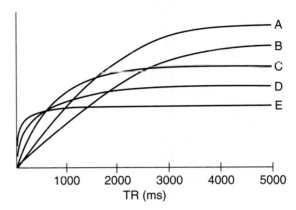

74. Referring to the figure below, at a TR of 300 ms, which tissue should appear brightest?
    a. A
    b. B
    c. C
    d. D
    e. E

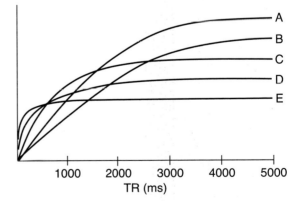

75. One reason that pure proton density images (T1 or T2) are not obtained is that it
   a. cannot be done.
   b. costs too much.
   c. requires NMR spectrometry.
   d. requires system modifications.
   e. takes too long.

76. When considering brain tissue, rank gray matter (GM), white matter (WM), and cerebrospinal fluid (CSF) in increasing order of net magnetization at equilibrium.
   a. CSF, WM, GM
   b. GM, WM, CSF
   c. GM, CSF, WM
   d. WM, CSF, GM
   e. WM, GM, CSF

77. Liquid nitrogen has a vaporization temperature of
   a. 0 K.
   b. 4 K.
   c. 20 K.
   d. 77 K.
   e. 100 K.

78. Referring to the figure below, the relaxation shown is
   a. longitudinal relaxation.
   b. motion relaxation.
   c. proton density relaxation.
   d. pure image relaxation.
   e. spin-spin relaxation.

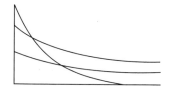

79. Referring to the figure below, which of the five tissues has the longest relaxation time?
   a. A
   b. B
   c. C
   d. D
   e. E

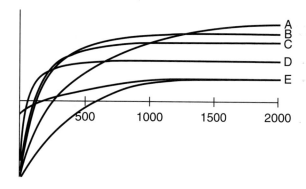

80. In a partial saturation pulse sequence,
   a. all FIDs are of equal amplitude.
   b. all spin echoes are of equal amplitude.
   c. early FIDs have a higher amplitude.
   d. early spin echoes have higher amplitude.
   e. magnetization is transferred.

81. The Larmor equation is best stated as
   a. $\omega = PD \times B$
   b. $\omega = B$.
   c. $B = PD$.
   d. $\omega = B$.
   e. $B = \omega$.

82. A nuclear magnetic moment in the presence of an external magnetic field interacts by
   a. charge and charge.
   b. charge and magnetic field.
   c. magnetic field and electric field.
   d. magnetic field and magnetic field.
   e. mass and mass.

83. Net magnetization is defined as the
    a. number of nuclei in a patient.
    b. number of nuclei in a voxel.
    c. sum of nuclear magnetic moments.
    d. sum of proton density.
    e. total number of spins.

84. Referring to the vector diagrams below, which figure properly represents net magnetization at equilibrium?
    a. A
    b. B
    c. C
    d. D
    e. E

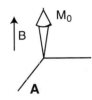 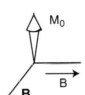

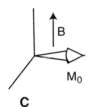 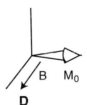

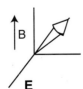

85. Net magnetization at equilibrium, M_0, is important to MRI because its value determines
    a. precessional frequency.
    b. signal intensity.
    c. proton density.
    d. T1 relaxation time.
    e. T2 relaxation time.

86. The laboratory frame of reference is also called the
    a. motion frame.
    b. precessing frame.
    c. rotating frame.
    d. stationary frame.
    e. translating frame.

87. Energy is most efficiently transferred from one system to another at
    a. mass density.
    b. precession.
    c. relaxation.
    d. resonance.
    e. proton density.

88. Two basic properties of a hydrogen nucleus important to MRI are
    a. charge and spin.
    b. mass and charge.
    c. mass and concentration.
    d. precession and mass.
    e. spin and magnetic moment.

89. Because the proton spins, it also
    a. diffuses.
    b. has a magnetic moment.
    c. induces.
    d. precesses.
    e. relaxes.

90. Which of the following contributes to the magnitude of M_0?
    a. proton charge
    b. proton density
    c. RF pulse
    d. T1 relaxation time
    e. T2 relaxation time

91. At equilibrium, no signal can be received from a patient because
    a. B_0 is constant.
    b. M_0 is constant.
    c. proton density is constant.
    d. there is no M_{XY} component.
    e. there is no M_Z component.

92. Strictly on the basis of proton density, which of the following tissues should appear the darkest?
    a. cortical bone
    b. fat
    c. lung
    d. medullary bone
    e. muscle

93. Proton density is most closely related to
    a. bound hydrogen.
    b. induced hydrogen.
    c. mobile hydrogen.
    d. relaxed hydrogen.
    e. transient hydrogen.

94. The T1 relaxation time is also known as
    a. longitudinal relaxation.
    b. precession relaxation.
    c. proton relaxation.
    d. translation.
    e. transverse relaxation.

95. The T1 relaxation time is 300 ms. What will be the value of M_Z after a patient has been in a B_0 field for 300 ms?
    a. $0.37 M_0$
    b. $0.37 M_Z$
    c. $0.5 M_Z$
    d. $0.63 M_0$
    e. $0.63 M_Z$

96. The T1 relaxation time for a given tissue is 600 ms. On removal from a magnet, what will be the value of M_Z after 600 ms?
    a. $0.37 M_0$
    b. $0.37 M_Z$
    c. $0.5 M_Z$
    d. $0.63 M_0$
    e. $0.63 M_Z$

97. After removal from the magnet for approximately five T1 relaxation times, M_Z will equal approximately
    a. Zero.
    b. $0.37 M_0$.
    c. 0.5.
    d. $0.63 M_0$.
    e. M_0.

98. Relaxation of transverse magnetization is controlled by
    a. motion.
    b. precession.
    c. proton density.
    d. T1 relaxation.
    e. T2 relaxation.

99. Relative to T1 relaxation times, T2 relaxation times
    a. are a little bit longer.
    b. are about the same.
    c. are just a little shorter.
    d. are very much shorter.
    e. vary among tissues.

100. The term *envelope of an FID* refers to the
    a. initial proton density.
    b. length the signal is straightened.
    c. line joining signal peaks.
    d. motion of the signal.
    e. total relaxation time.

101. The FID does not represent true T2 relaxation principally because of
    a. different tissues within the same voxel.
    b. magnetic field inhomogeneity.
    c. magnetic susceptibility effects.
    d. motion.
    e. proton density inhomogeneity.

102. Dephasing of spins within a region containing the same tissue occurs because of
    a. magnetic field inhomogeneity.
    b. proton density inhomogeneity.
    c. T1 relaxation.
    d. T2 relaxation.
    e. temperature.

103. The envelope of an FID is related to
    a. proton density.
    b. $T1^*$.
    c. $T1$.
    d. $T2^*$.
    e. $T2$.

104. Referring to the figure below, which diagram can best be used to estimate T1 relaxation time?
    a. A
    b. B
    c. C
    d. D
    e. E

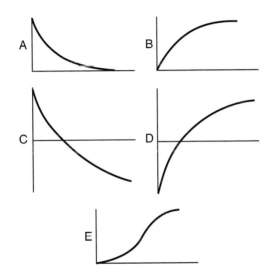

105. The M_Z can only be measured by flipping magnetization
    a. back to equilibrium.
    b. onto the XY plane.
    c. to the $+Z$ direction axis.
    d. to the Z direction.
    e. with an alpha pulse.

106. After a 180° RF pulse,
    a. $M_Z = -M_0$.
    b. $M_Z = 0$.
    c. $M_Z = M_0$.
    d. $M_Z = M_{XY}$.
    e. M_Z precesses.

107. An NMR spectrum is a graph of intensity as a function of
    a. electric potential.
    b. frequency.
    c. mass.
    d. relaxation time
    e. spin state.

108. The NMR spectrum is obtained from an MR signal through the process of
    a. backprojection reconstruction.
    b. complex restoration.
    c. Fourier transformation.
    d. iteration.
    e. signal relaxation.

109. Which nuclear species would show the highest signal intensity from an NMR spectrum of the human body?
    a. carbon
    b. hydrogen
    c. nitrogen
    d. oxygen
    e. phosphorus

110. A nuclear species may exhibit more than one peak in an NMR spectrum because of its
    a. electron configuration.
    b. mass distribution.
    c. molecular configuration.
    d. nuclear structure.
    e. proton density.

111. The change in resonant frequency among similar nuclei in the same molecule is due to slight changes in
    a. proton density.
    b. relaxation times.
    c. temperature.
    d. the local magnetic field.
    e. the transient magnetic field.

112. The separation of peaks in an NMR spectrum increases with increasing
    a. B_0.
    b. B_{XYZ}.
    c. gyromagnetic ratio.
    d. relaxation time.
    e. proton density.

113. The number 234 can be expressed in binary fashion as
    a. 01001111.
    b. 01010111.
    c. 01010111.
    d. 01101001.
    e. 01101111.

114. One kilobyte is equal to
    a. 2^3 bytes.
    b. 2^6 bytes.
    c. 2^{10} bytes.
    d. 2^{15} bytes.
    e. 2^{20} bytes.

115. The human visual system can resolve approximately how many shades of gray?
    a. 8
    b. 32
    c. 64
    d. 128
    e. 512

116. The ability to image objects with low spatial frequency is the ability to image
    a. high-contrast objects.
    b. low-contrast objects.
    c. stationary objects.
    d. very large objects.
    e. very small objects.

117. A high spatial frequency represents
    a. a short signal time.
    b. a very large object.
    c. good contrast resolution.
    d. poor spatial resolution.
    e. rapid changes of the MR signal.

118. With a 1.0-T imaging system, the soft tissue/fat chemical shift artifact occurs because of a Larmor frequency difference of
    a. 3.5 Hz.
    b. 35 Hz.
    c. 75 Hz.
    d. 149 Hz.
    e. 300 Hz.

119. A 1.0-T MR imaging system is said to have B_0 field homogeneity of $\pm$ 10 ppm. This is equal to
    a. ± 0.1 μT.
    b. ± 1 μT.
    c. ± 10 μT.
    d. ± 100 μT.
    e. ± 1000 μT.

120. The truncation artifact is more pronounced when the
    a. FOV is large.
    b. number of phase-encoding acquisitions is large.
    c. number of phase-encoding acquisitions is small.
    d. repetition time is long.
    e. repetition time is short.

121. The partial volume averaging artifact exists when
    a. a structure is contained within three or more slices.
    b. a structure is not fully contained within a slice.
    c. FOV is large.
    d. the repetition time is too long.
    e. the repetition time is too short.

122. To truncate is to
    a. deform an object.
    b. lop off part of the object.
    c. reshape an object.
    d. slice an object.
    e. stretch an object.

Answers to Challenge Questions

CHAPTER 1

1. Visible light, x-ray, radiofrequency.
2. Radiofrequencies in the range of approximately 10 to 200 MHz.
3. Felix Bloch, Stanford University (1905-1983). Bloch theorized nuclear magnetism and proposed equations to explain such a property.
4. Contrast resolution is the ability of an imaging system to distinguish one soft tissue from another. Magnetic resonance imaging excels in contrast resolution.
5. Spatial resolution deals with high-contrast objects, such as a bone-lung interface, calcified lung nodules, and breast microcalcifications. Spatial resolution is the ability to image very small high-contrast objects. The best spatial resolution in medical imaging is x-ray mammography.
6. The intrinsic tissue characteristics of proton density, T1 relaxation, and T2 relaxation are very different for different soft tissues. These differences can be detected and rendered as an MR image.
7. Sensitivity is an indication of how well an imaging modality can detect subtle changes in anatomy. Specificity is an additional descriptor relating how well the imaging system can identify the meaning of those differences in diagnosing disease or abnormal anatomy.
8. $f = \gamma B_0$, where f is the frequency of precession, γ is the gyromagnetic ratio (42 MHz/T for hydrogen), and B_0 is the intensity of the static magnetic field.
9. A vector diagram is a graphical relationship illustrating physical quantities that have not only magnitude but also direction.
10. Precession. A spinning top or gyroscope has mass; when the mass rotates, it generates angular momentum. The interaction between angular momentum and the gravitational field results in precession.

CHAPTER 2

1. Except for permanent magnet imaging systems, both the static and gradient magnetic fields are produced by an electric current in a conductor. This is the foundation for electromagnetism.
2. Magnetic resonance imaging rooms are shielded with specially designed conductors to reduce the intensity of environmental electromagnetic radiation in the radiofrequency band.
3. Benjamin Franklin first experimented with static electricity in the middle of the eigh-

teenth century. Electrostatics is the science of describing how stationary electric charges behave.

4. Both x-rays and radiofrequencies have the same velocity ($c = 3 \times 10^8$ m/s). X-rays and radiofrequencies are composed of two energy fields: electric and magnetic, oscillating perpendicular to one another. Radiofrequencies have lower frequency, longer wavelength, and less energy than x-rays do.

5. Induction is the transfer of energy from one state or frame of reference to another without touching. In contrast, conduction involves a physical medium in the transfer of such energy.

6. $E = hf$, where E is energy, h is a physical constant, termed *Planck's constant*, and f is frequency. This basically indicates that the higher the frequency of electromagnetic radiation, the higher is the energy of that radiation.

7. $E = \dfrac{F}{Q}$, where F is expressed in newtons and Q in coulombs. The newton is the unit of force $\dfrac{kg\text{-}m}{s^2}$ and the coulomb is a quantity of electrostatic charge ($1\ C = 6.24 \times 10^{18}$ electrons).

8. $v = \lambda f$, where v is the velocity in meters per second, λ is the wavelength in meters, and f is the frequency of oscillation in hertz.

9. 1. Unlike charges attract; like charges repel.
   2. The force of attraction or repulsion is proportional to the product of the charges divided by the square of the distance between them. This is known as *Coulomb's law*.
   3. Electrostatic charge is distributed uniformly on the surface of a smooth conductor.
   4. Electrostatic charge is concentrated at regions of irregularity on a nonsmooth conductor.

10. A magnetic field is a force that interacts with magnetic poles. The magnetic field is measured in tesla and a magnetic pole in ampere-meter $\left(1T = \dfrac{1N}{A\text{-}m}\right)$.

CHAPTER 3

1. Classical mechanics, often called *Newtonian physics,* deals with the interactions of large objects, such as bowling balls, automobiles, and space ships. Quantum mechanics deals with the interactions of very small objects, such as subatomic particles and electromagnetic radiation. The physical laws are different for both.

2. The rotating frame of reference. The coordinate system is rotating about the Z-axis at the Larmor frequency, and the observer is presumed in that frame.

3. The north and south magnetic poles and associated field intensity produced by spinning charged particles.

4. The oscillating magnetic field associated with a 42-MHz radiofrequency.

5. More spins are aligned with the external magnetic field, and they are in a lower energy state.

6. M_Z and M_{XY}, respectively.

7. When a patient is placed in a magnetic field, approximately 1 in 1,000,000 proton spins align, either with or against this external magnetic field. Once so aligned, the magnitude of alignment is constant and results in a net value with the external magnetic field. This net value is the equilibrium value.

8. M_0 is directly proportional to the proton density, the square of the gyromagnetic ratio, and the intensity of the external magnetic field. M_0 is inversely proportional to tissue temperature $\left(M_0 \cong \dfrac{PD\gamma^2 B}{T}\right)$.

9. Nuclear magnetic resonance spectroscopy is conducted at high magnetic fields, up to approximately 24 tesla, but the most important parameter is the frequency at which the NMR signal is received; multiples of 50 and 100 MHz are most often used.

10. M = Σμ, where M is the net magnetization, Σ is the mathematical symbol meaning to add, and μ represents each nuclear magnetic moment.

CHAPTER 4

1. The gyromagnetic ratio is different for each nuclear species. This is a GMIS* parameter and cannot be changed. *GMIS = God made it so.
2. A radiofrequency pulse that is transmitted into the patient is symbolized as RF_t. See Figure 4-11 for a visual representation.
3. The proton spins precess randomly around the axis of the external magnetic field. They are out of phase, and therefore the sum is projected along the Z-axis.
4. The free induction decay (FID) is produced by the precessing spins that are initially in phase but rapidly dephase. The resulting RF signal is at first of high intensity and rapidly falls to zero.
5. It is much too weak, and it is not time varying oscillating and therefore will not electromagnetically induce.
6. Longitudinal magnetization.
7. $M_Z = M_0$, $M_{XY} = 0$.
8. The equilibrium magnetization value, M_0, which is principally determined by the magnitude of the proton density (PD).
9. $M_Z = 0$, $M_{XY} = M_0$.
10. The angle through which the net magnetization vector has been rotated by application of an RF pulse.

CHAPTER 5

1. Because it is emitted immediately after the termination of the transmitted RF pulse and the electronics of the receiver must respond more quickly.
2. 90°-180° . . . / . . . 90°-180° . . . , etc.
3. The timing of the energizing of the radiofrequency transmitter and the gradient magnetic field coils.
4. Echo planar imaging (EPI).

5. When the repetition time (TR) is not sufficiently long to allow complete longitudinal relaxation of the spin ensemble to equilibrium.
6. See Figure 5-2 for an illustration of how the RF pulse is indicated for a gradient echo pulse sequence.
7. The time between the initial 90° RF pulse and the middle of the spin echo. This time is twice the time between the 90° RF pulse and the 180° RF pulse.
8. See Figure 5-2 for a diagram of the transmitted and received signals for a double echo, spin echo pulse sequence.
9. The time between the inverting 180° RF pulse and the 90° RF pulse.
10. A spin echo. Although the inversion recovery pulse sequence is generally identified as 180°-90° . . . 180° 90° . . . , in fact, there is an additional 180° RF pulse that follows each 90° RF pulse, and that produces the spin echo.

CHAPTER 6

1. Proton density (PD), longitudinal relaxation time, (T1) and transverse relaxation time (T2).
2. T2*, T2, T1.
3. The concentration of mobile hydrogen, proton density (PD).
4. Magnetic field inhomogeneity.
5. 63%; approximately 5 T1s.
6. Frequency is the rate at which something revolves or spins. Phase is the direction that multiple spins exhibit at any given instant.
7. The molecular species in which the hydrogen atom is embedded.
8. That envelope represents the rate at which the signal relaxes because of T2*. One needs transverse relaxation in a perfectly homogeneous magnetic field for the envelope of the signal to represent T2 relaxation.
9. Tissues with short T1 appear bright, tissues with long T1 appear dark, but high

proton density enhances the appearance of both.

10. Tissues with long T2 appear brighter than tissues with short T2; however, all tissues with higher proton density will appear brighter.

CHAPTER 7

1. The B_0 field is too intense and inhomogeneous.
2. The saturation recovery pulse sequence with varying repetition time (TR). The inversion recovery pulse sequence with varying inversion time (TI).
3. In the middle of the spin echo that was produced.
4. A spin echo.
5. An FID of long duration whose envelope would describe the true T2 of the tissue.
6. Because all of the net magnetization is along the Z-axis, which is coplanar to the external magnetic field, B_0. Some net magnetization must project onto the XY plane for a signal to be detectable.
7. See Figure 7-1.
8. An FID followed by three spin echoes, each of decreasing intensity and alternating polarity.
9. There is no signal.
10. See Figure 7-7 for an illustration of the vector diagram that represents tissue magnetization after a 90° RF pulse.

CHAPTER 8

1. A new signal of intensity versus inverse time, hertz, the NMR spectrum.
2. Aliasing or wraparound artifact.
3. k-Space.
4. At least two data points, samplings, within each cycle of the MR signal.
5. Nyquist.
6. Any bone-soft tissue interfaces, breast microcalcifications, and calcified lung nodules.
7. Yes, the more data acquired, the higher the capacity of the computer necessary, and

the longer it will take to reconstruct an image.

8. The gradient coils, which generate the gradient magnetic fields.
9. A special form of the Fourier transform particularly adapted for the computed generation of solutions where the sampled signal is truncated, allowing the computation to be completed more quickly.
10. See Figure 8-1 for a graphic representation of the Fourier transform of a square wave and a spin echo.

CHAPTER 9

1. An NMR spectrum.
2. Carbon (^{13}C), nitrogen (^{15}N), fluorine (^{19}Fl), sodium (^{23}Na), and phosphorus (^{31}P).
3. The lines in the spectrum become sharper and more distinct and more separated.
4. Lines that appear in the NMR spectrum representing the fine detail of spatial relationship among spins within the same molecule.
5. The slight change along the frequency axis of the same nuclear species because of the manner in which it is bound within its molecule. It reflects the magnetic shielding of the nucleus by the electron configuration. Chemical shift is more obvious at high magnetic field strength.
6. ± 10 ppm.
7. 3.5 ppm, when referred to TMS.
8. 42 MHz/T.
9. 225 Hz.
10. The frequency-encoded axis.

CHAPTER 10

1. The gantry, the operating console, and the computer.
2. The operating system.
3. Permanent magnet, electromagnet, and superconducting electromagnet.
4. Floating point operation.
5. The gradient coils.

6. $512 \times 512 \times 1 = 262{,}000$ bytes or approximately one-quarter megabyte.
7. A gas that has been compressed and reduced in volume so that it is now a liquid. Such a state exists only at a very cold temperature.
8. Window width, window level.
9. To provide a return path for the magnetic field and intensify the B_0 field.
10. To make the B_0 magnetic field more uniform in intensity by the use of shim coils or external ferromagnetic material.

CHAPTER 11

1. Electromagnets produce a magnetic field by an electric current conducted through wires fashioned as a solenoid. Permanent magnets produce a magnetic field by the intrinsic magnetic property of their material.
2. The temperature in the cryostat rises, exceeding that of the critical temperature of the cryogen, and the cryogen vaporizes. The cryogenic gas escapes from the imaging system, and the superconducting coils rise in temperature so that they can no longer superconduct.
3. Both permanent magnets and resistive electromagnets peak at about 0.3 T. Superconducting electromagnets had been produced with field strengths to approximately 24 T but those for imaging are limited by the FDA to 3 T.
4. 19 K, 5 K, 77 K, 273 K.
5. 21°C, 294 K.
6. A precisely machined and positioned pole face.
7. All electrical, mechanical, molecular, and quantum motion ceases.
8. It is cooled by water, there is a low intensity fringe magnetic field, and you can turn it off at night.
9. Insulator—inhibits the flow of electrons. Semiconductor—either inhibits or promotes the flow of electrons depending on electrical polarity. Conductor—promotes the flow of electrons. Superconductor—

allows the flow of electrons without the loss of energy.
10. The ability of an electrical conductor to promote the flow of electrons without resistance; there is no loss of energy, and therefore no voltage is required.

CHAPTER 12

1. Shim coils are used to adjust the B_0 magnetic field to its maximum uniformity. For MRI, uniformity is termed *homogeneity*.
2. Reduced field of view and image nonuniformities.
3. $\pm 3 \ \mu T$.
4. The spatial resolution is limited by the pixel size, and pixel size is equal to 80 mm $\div$ 512 = 0.15 mm.
5. 0.025 T/m per 0.1 s = 250 T/m/s.
6. Reduce the field of view; increase the matrix size.
7. G_X.
8. Because they are closer to the tissue-emitting signal and have a smaller signal receiving distance, the signal-to-noise ratio is higher.
9. The read gradient is always frequency encoded. It can be G_X or G_Y, depending on the need to suppress chemical shift artifacts.
10. One that is used to both transmit RF into the patient and receive the MR signal from the patient. Normally, head and body coils are homogenous; surface coils are inhomogeneous.

CHAPTER 13

1. Its weight and structural loading may dictate that it not be positioned on an upper floor.
2. 1.0 mT.
3. The absence of a fringe magnetic field.
4. Use nonmagnetic and nonconducting conduit and enclosures. When such conducting conduits are necessary, follow waveguide design to eliminate extraneous RF. Use DC instead of AC.

5. The principal advantages are high B_0 field intensity, uniformity, and signal-to-noise ratio. The principal disadvantages are the extensive fringe magnetic field, more patient confinement, and higher cost.

6. To ensure that no patients who undergo imaging have metallic plants, prostheses, or surface metal that would interfere with the quality of the MR image.

7. What would be the effect of the fringe magnetic field of the MRI system on nearby electronic equipment? What would be the effect of nearby iron, stationary or moving, on the quality of the MR image?

8. A Faraday cage is an electromagnetic shield constructed of metal sheets or mesh designed to attenuate ambient external RF from the imaging room.

9. Passive shielding uses iron to reduce the intensity of the fringe magnetic field. Active shielding uses reverse polarity windings of the electromagnet in the cryostat to reduce the intensity of the fringe magnetic field.

10. 3 kHz to 300 GHz.

CHAPTER 14

1. The size of the pixel. Pixel size is determined by the field of view divided by the matrix size.

2. Both are single numerals, the digit in the decimal number system and the bit in the binary number system.

3. The amplitude of the phase-encoding gradient.

4. Install gradient coils (G_{XYZ}) to produce gradient magnetic fields (B_{XYZ}).

5. 2^{12} = 4096 – 4096 individual gray levels are possible with such a system.

6. 2 lp/cm = 0.2 lp/mm = 5 mm/lp $\therefore$ 2.5 mm.

7. 111011 cm.

8. 256×256 = 65,536 pixels per image. Each pixel has 12-bit gray scale, that is, 1.5 bytes ($2^{12} \div 2^8$ = 1.5 bytes). That product is 98,304 bytes or approximately 100,000 bytes = 0.1 megabytes $\times$ 32 = 3.2 megabytes.

9. Postprocessing with varying window level and width allows the observer to visualize the entire 12-bit range.

10. With increasing spatial frequency, object size decreases, which makes it more difficult to resolve both spatially and contrastwise. Therefore both spatial resolution and contrast resolution are reduced at higher spatial frequencies.

CHAPTER 15

1. The measure of spatial frequency in MRI is lp/cm.

2. k-Space is the spatial frequency domain with X and Y coordinates. The X coordinates are assigned to frequency, and the Y coordinates are assigned to phase. See Figure 15-7.

3. Approximately 10 lp/cm for head and whole body and up to 20 lp/cm for the surface coil.

4. Trajectory through k-space refers to the manner in which the lines in k-space are filled. The variations of filling k-space are line by line sequentially, line by line segmentally, line by line continuously, and spiral filling.

5. Normally, this will result in a 256 × 256 image matrix. Each line represents one MR signal detected, each signal having been sampled and Fourier transformed. It would have been 256 different amplitudes of the phase-encoding gradient magnetic field.

6. Spatial resolution improves with smaller pixels, and therefore a 512-image matrix has better spatial resolution. Contrast resolution improves with larger pixels because of better signal-to-noise ratio, and therefore the 256 matrix will have better contrast resolution.

7. Magnetic resonance imaging is performed because of its superior contrast resolution. Contrast resolution is principally dependent on the low-amplitude phase-encoding signal acquisitions, which fill the central region of k-space. Therefore the central region is more important.

8. There is no one-to-one relationship. Each area in k-space contains numerical information relating to every pixel in the image.
9. Noise is rather uniform and independent of spatial frequency in MRI. Signal increases with lower spatial frequencies. Consequently, larger objects (low spatial frequencies) exhibit better signal-to-noise ratio and therefore better contrast.
10. Narrower receiver bandwidth produces higher signal-to-noise ratio and therefore better contrast resolution.

CHAPTER 16

1. Five lines, one each for (a) the transmitted radiofrequency pulse and (b) the received signal, and one line for each gradient magnetic field.
2. $20 \times 2 \times 512 = 20.5$ seconds.
3. The timing of the RF pulses and the type of pulse sequence used. Field of view and pixel size principally influence spatial resolution but not the contrast or contrast rendition.
4. See Figure 18-11 for a diagram of the RF pulse sequence for an inversion recovery image and the timing for the appearance of the MR signal.
5. There is no sharp edge to the RF pulse, and therefore some bleeding into adjacent slices can occur, resulting in image degradation; this is controlled by obtaining slices in a noncontiguous fashion.
6. $3 = \dfrac{1.73}{\sqrt{3}}$ or almost a doubling of signal-to-noise ratio.
7. At any time that the transmitted RF is energized.
8. See Figure 17-20 for an illustration of how the vector diagram appears when an ensemble of spins is partially saturated.
9. The Z-axis is always drawn parallel to the B_0 magnetic field. Therefore for a horizontal B_0, the Y-axis is vertical, anteroposterior through the patient, and the X-axis is lateral across the patient.

10. Gradient coils are hardware; they conduct electric current and are fabricated to produce a gradient magnetic field with a particular orientation. It is the gradient magnetic field that influences MR signal production and detection.

CHAPTER 17

1. Visual acuity is the ability to recognize and identify fine detail. Visual acuity is improved when ambient light levels are reduced. Image masking and low light level illumination in the reading room are essential.
2. That will result in a proton density weighted image.
3. The numerical value of each pixel in MRI represents the value of proton density, T1 and T2 for the tissue in that voxel.
4. The early echo image will be T1 weighted and the late echo image, proton density weighted.
5. Fluids have long T1 and T2 relaxation times; therefore, cerebrospinal fluid will appear bright on images with long TR (PDW) and long TE (T2W).
6. Magnetic resonance imaging uses the emission of electromagnetic radiation.
7. Inversion recovery imaging, in general, produces higher contrast images at the expense of longer imaging time.
8. The application of the three gradient magnetic fields, B_{SS}, B_Φ, and B_R and the frequency of the RF excitation pulse.
9. Alter the RF pulse sequence timing so that the net magnetization of the two tissues are not the same at the time of sampling.
10. Soft tissues have T1 relaxation times measured in hundreds of milliseconds. T2 relaxation times are tens of milliseconds.

CHAPTER 18

1. B_{SS}, the gradient magnetic field, identifies the slice. In a superconducting MRI system having a horizontal B_0 field energizing, G_Z

will produce a transverse image, G_Y, a sagittal image, and G_X, a coronal image.

2. Imaging time is greatly reduced and that reduces patient motion artifacts.

3. To restore phase coherence of the spin ensemble and produce the spin echo for signal detection.

4. Spin echo fills one line of k-space for each TR. Fast spin echo fills multiple lines of k-space with each TR by cycling multiple 180° RF pulses with varying intensity phase-encoded gradient magnetic fields (B_Φ).

5. The first Fourier transform is of the MR signal and produces a line in k-space along the frequency-encoded direction. The second Fourier transform is of the orthogonal data along the phase-encoded direction of k-space.

6. The frequency-encoded gradient magnetic field (B_R) is shaped in time to accommodate moving spins.

7. Short-term inversion recovery and absolute inversion recovery. These are two modifications of an inversion recovery pulse sequence.

8. After multiple RF pulses closely spaced, spins do not fully relax and contribute to a secondary echo. This is the stimulated echo.

9. When data or an object is reproduced as a mirror image that is symmetrical about an axis, the condition is Hermitian. In k-space, Hermitian symmetry is exhibited on either side of both axes.

10. Each echo in a train of echoes in FSE is generated under a different amplitude phase-encoding gradient (G_Φ). The effective echo time refers to that echo generated with the lowest amplitude phase-encoded gradient magnetic field (B_Φ). This is usually the middle echo.

CHAPTER 19

1. Nothing happens. The Larmor frequency at 1.5 T is 63 MHz. At any other frequency no interaction occurs.

2. 126 MHz.

3. Because it is the most abundant atom in the body, 60%, and because it has the highest gyromagnetic ratio of tissue atoms, 42 MHz/T.

4. Magnetization transfer is the transfer of tissue magnetization from macromolecules to water, resulting in improved signal-to-noise ratio.

5. Hydrogen in water precesses with the frequency 3.5 ppm or 100 Hz lower than fat in a 1-T MRI system.

6. These protons resonate at frequencies extending over a wide range depending on the molecular configuration. When these spins are ignored the result is reduced image contrast.

7. Increasing receiver bandwidth reduces the appearance of the chemical shift artifact at all B_0 field intensities but also reduces the SNR.

8. 16 kHz ÷ 512 = 31 Hz/pixel; 147 pixels ÷ 31 Hz/pixel = approximately 5 pixels.

9. The chemical shift artifact appears along the frequency-encoding gradient magnetic field (B_R) for conventional MRI and along the phase-encoding gradient magnetic field (B_Φ) for EPI MRI.

10. Use of chemical shift selection with RF pulses and dephasing with spoiler gradients to null the signal from fat. This can also be done with an inversion recovery imaging technique that uses an inversion time equal to the time when the fat spins are saturated so that they have no longitudinal magnetization to be flipped on the XY plane for signal detection (STIR).

CHAPTER 20

1. Faster imaging.

2. Gradient echo imaging with a flip angle between approximately 30° and 70° to produce the maximum signal in a given tissue.

3. A bipolar read gradient magnetic field, B_R.

4. For very short repetition times after a few gradient echoes are formed, longitudinal

magnetization reaches a constant level because the degrees of saturation and recovery are equal.

5. The initial negative pole of B_R causes rapid dephasing of spins early in the FID. The positive pole of B_R allows these spins to rephase to the level they would have experienced and then to dephase again.

6. See Figure 20-10 for a graphic representation of the difference between T2 and T2*.

7. B_0 magnetic field inhomogeneity. T2* is also influenced by chemical shift, tissue magnetic susceptibility, and in the case of GRE, the read gradient magnetic field.

8. Residual transverse magnetization, M_{XY}, is spoiled or destroyed after each signal acquisition in FLASH. Such transverse magnetization is rephased in an FISP pulse sequence. Both are steady state approaches.

9. That flip angle in GRE, which produces maximum signal intensity as a function of TR and T1 relaxation.

10. Large flip angles result in large relaxation and greater signal intensity. However, the process takes longer. Small flip angles produce less but still sufficient signal intensity for good images with a shorter repetition time and therefore faster imaging.

CHAPTER 21

1. TURBO imaging is gradient echo imaging preceded by 180° RF inversion pulse designed to enhance the T1 weighting of the image.

2. Gradient and spin echo imaging. This is a superfast imaging technique, which acquires multiple gradient echoes within a single spin echo.

3. k-Space is filled ten times more rapidly with TURBO technique, but each line of k-space has different T1 weighting because of the initializing 180° RF pulse.

4. Of inversion recovery imaging results in the most RF energy deposition because each line of k-space requires 180°, 90°, 180° RF pulse.

5. For TURBO imaging, each line of k-space is acquired with different T1 weighting. Because the low-amplitude phase-encoded signals contribute most of the contrast, they are usually acquired first to fill the central region of k-space.

6. This refers to a high-frequency filter or a high bandpass filter, which is an electronic term. The receiver electronics allow only high frequencies to be sampled, reducing the low-frequency component of the MR signal.

7. Conventional cardiac MRI is gated to the cardiac cycle, instead of acquiring one line of k-space in each cycle. Multiple lines, a segment of k-space, are filled within each cardiac cycle.

8. See Figure 21-1.

9. That the phase-encoding gradient is incremented for each TR. See Figure 21-3.

10. Three-dimensional image acquisition where the voxel size has equal dimension for each of the three sides (e.g., 0.5 mm on a side).

CHAPTER 22

1. Echo planar imaging. Images can be obtained in as little as approximately 50 ms.

2. Cardiac MRI and functional brain imaging.

3. Echo planar imaging. An entire image can be produced with a 90° RF pulse followed by a 180° RF pulse. In gradient echo EPI, you do not even need the 180° preparation pulse.

4. Because EPI is performed so quickly, chemical shift artifacts are large and appear in the phase-encoding direction. The inversion pulse for fat saturation can remove such an artifact.

5. During the formation of the spin echo, a read gradient magnetic field (B_R) is cycled, causing the spin echo to be transformed into multiple gradient echoes. An additional small phase-encoding gradient pulse, called a *blip*, is applied between

echoes so that each of the gradient echoes is acquired under a different phase-encoding gradient (B_ϕ).

6. Because the phase-encoding gradient, B_ϕ, and the read gradient, B_R, are cycled so rapidly, the transient magnetic field expressed in T/s is exceptionally large. This can produce an unwanted neural stimulation in the patient.

7. Spin-spin relaxation (T2). During the time of sampling, multiple gradient echoes are formed under the envelope of the spin echo.

8. Pulse sequence selection can be used to great advantage to accentuate either proton density or T1 relaxation or T2 relaxation.

9. An additional coil of similar geometry is placed outside of the gradient coil and energized with opposite polarity. The result is a reduction in eddy currents, which can be very bothersome in the extremely fast imaging of EPI.

10. High B_0 field intensity, 1 T or better, intense gradient magnetic fields, 25 mT/m or better, and high slew rate, 100 T/m/s or better.

CHAPTER 23

1. Most vascular blood flow is laminar; the blood in the center in the lumen is traveling faster than the blood near the walls. Plug flow exists when the blood moves across the entire vessel with the same velocity.

2. Digital subtraction angiography is better because of the contrast agent filling the vessel. Magnetic resonance angiography suffers from flow void artifact due to turbulence, but this is rapidly improving with contrast-enhanced MRA.

3. Time of flight (TOF) and phase contrast (PC) are sensitive to blood flow, and both can be well imaged with maximum intensity projection (MIP) techniques.

4. Three-dimensional MRA requires that two gradients act as phase-encoding gradients

but in different directions. The sequence is repeated for the number of times required by the matrix size.

5. Turbulence produces intravoxel dephasing, which results in loss of signal and produces a signal void within the vessel.

6. The 3DFT is better for spatial resolution at the expense of increased imaging time. However, contrast resolution may be reduced with thin-slice imaging.

7. 10 mm.

8. Flip angle and repetition time must be carefully chosen to maximize the contrast between blood and stationary tissue.

9. T1 weighted imaging, with a short TR.

10. See Figure 23-1 for a diagram of how the flow rate of blood in the aorta is a function of time during the cardiac cycle.

CHAPTER 24

1. Perfusion deals with blood flow in microcapillaries; diffusion deals with blood and water flow in tissue through the intercapillary spaces.

2. BOLD stands for *b*lood *o*xygen *l*evel *d*ependent imaging.

3. Those sequences that result in perfusion/diffusion imaging but particularly diffusion imaging.

4. Gadolinium compounds injected intravascularly are exogenous contrast agents; altered tissue states, such as hemoglobin versus oxyhemoglobin, are endogenous contrast agents.

5. Deoxyhemoglobin has shorter T2 relaxation time.

6. fMRI requires no ionizing radiation.

7. Rapid sequence images are obtained, first with oxyhemoglobin and then after a physically agitative task, which consumes oxygen causing oxyhemoglobin to change to deoxyhemoglobin. Subtracting the first image from the second results in highlighted areas of brain activity.

8. The change following stimulus from the oxyhemoglobin to the deoxyhemoglobin

state occurs with the time lapse of a few seconds. Sequential images must be obtained within that time period.

9. Exogenous fMRI requires a bolus injection, usually of a gadolinium-DTPA. Imaging must commence at the time when the bolus first enters the tissue being imaged.

10. No effect on any of the three parameters but it does shorten T2*.

CHAPTER 25

1. The time constant relating to how fast molecules will move from one medium to another because of their thermal agitation.

2. The diffusion coefficient has units of mm^2/s, whereas the b factor is measured in s/mm^2.

3. The diffusion coefficient is a property of tissue compartments. The b factor is influenced by the manner in which gradient magnetic fields are applied and therefore is dependent on the MRI system.

4. Usually, tissue that is rapidly perfused appears dark. Tissue that is not perfused appears bright.

5. One of the three gradient magnetic fields is energized very briefly on either side of the refocusing 180° pulse that produces the spin echo.

6. $\frac{S}{S_0}$ is signal attenuation. High signal attenuation represents increased diffusion.

7. $A = \frac{S}{S_0} = e^{-bD}$, where A is the signal attenuation, S_0 is the initial signal strength, and S is the signal strength after application of diffusion gradients.

8. The signal attenuation is increased exponentially. This is a straight-line relationship on a semilog graph.

9. The random movement of particles or molecules in a substance due to the temperature of that substance. Brownian motion increases with increasing temperature. At absolute zero, there is no such motion.

10. Gradient echo imaging and spin echo–echo planar imaging.

CHAPTER 26

1. Heart disease, cancer, cerebral vascular disease, and accidents.

2. Laminar flow appears bright, and turbulence appears as a signal void.

3. X-ray angiography remains the gold standard because it has superior spatial resolution; however, 3DFT MRA is closing in. The 2DFT MRA has the poorest spatial resolution of the three.

4. There is not a simple answer, but MRI is fast replacing radioisotope imaging because (1) there is little attenuation of signal by overlying tissue, (2) signal detection in MRI is much more efficient than that in radioisotope imaging, and (3) with contrast-enhanced MRI, both spatial and contrast resolution are superior.

5. Long axis view, short axis view, four-chamber view, and two-chamber view.

6. 1.5 T B_0 field intensity; cardiac phased-array coil; gradient magnetic field intensity of at least 25 mT/m with slew rates of at least 100 T/m/s.

7. With cardiac gating instead of a one-line fill in k-space during each RR interval, a segment of multiple lines is filled. This allows the entire imaging sequence to be completed in a few heart beats but reduces temporal resolution of the cine-cardiac study.

8. Skip a few heartbeats between signal acquisition and increase the TR accordingly.

9. The HFI stands for *half Fourier imaging*. In such a process, only half of the 128 or 256 lines in k-space are filled. The other half are computed as the mirror image of those filled.

10. Leads should be colinear, with the external magnetic field, B_0. They should not be in contact with the patient's skin and should have no kinks or loops.

CHAPTER 27

1. The contrast agent should improve contrast after a small volume injection, and

the level of contrast should be dose dependent. It should be nontoxic and concentrate in the tissue of interest and clear from the body rapidly.

2. When body cavities are imaged, such as the GI tract, such agents greatly disturb the magnetic field uniformity and therefore reduce T2* and improve contrast.

3. By ingestion, by inhalation, or by intravenous injection.

4. MRI contrast agents generally increase signal intensity from the affected tissue. This is termed *positive contrast enhancement.*

5. Generally, molecules of the contrast agent cannot cross the blood-brain barrier.

6. Gadolinium tagged to DTPA. The gadolinium is paramagnetic by virtue of seven unpaired electrons in various outer shells. It accelerates dephasing, shortens T2*, and reduces signal intensity.

7. Because the action of both is to accelerate dephasing, resulting in shorter T2* in large doses, signal intensity is reduced. The contrast is negative in nature.

8. There is no effect on proton density. Both relaxation times are reduced, causing a loss of signal on T2 weighted images and an increase in signal on T1 weighted images.

9. Chelation is the action of binding one atom or molecule to another. The DTPA serves as a receptor molecule to which the gadolinium can be bound.

10. The element, gadolinium, is quite toxic by itself. Chelating gadolinium to DTPA reduces its toxicity significantly.

CHAPTER 28

1. Any pattern or structure on the image that does not truly represent the anatomy being imaged.

2. If the RF transmitter/receiver is not properly tuned for that particular B_0 field, the result is a noisy image. The noise can be uniform or wavelike.

3. Increase the slice thickness and/or pixel size. Both of these options will allow more of the object to be within one voxel.

4. Ferromagnetic materials have high magnetic susceptibility and result in either signal dropout or severe image distortion.

5. Misregistration occurs when multiple images are added or subtracted as in MRA. Anatomy in one image is in an adjacent pixel in a subsequent image. Patient motion is usually the cause.

6. Water protons and fat protons do not precess at exactly the same Larmor frequency. Therefore the signal received by these two tissues is displaced on the frequency-encoding axis. Signal enhancement or signal loss can occur.

7. Ghosting occurs when there is a lack of phase stability in the MR signal. A common source of ghosting occurs when tissue moves in a periodic fashion, such as the diaphragm or the CSF; a summation artifact may be generated and appear as a ghost of the stationary tissue.

8. The appearance is just that, a zipper or regular streaklike artifact usually along the frequency-encoding axis. This is due to external sources of RF being detected by the receiving coil or undesired MR signals, such as those due to stimulated echoes.

9. This is caused by aliasing, which results from undersampling of the MR signal in the phase-encoding direction. Aliasing produces an image of anatomy of the opposite side of the body from where it should appear. Aliasing can be reduced by increasing the field of view.

10. Truncation artifacts are associated with sharp tissue interfaces. This occurs when the MR signal is so strong that it is outside of the sampling window. The appearance is of a ringing effect next to that interface.

CHAPTER 29

1. Threshold, nonlinear.

2. There is no reason for a pregnant MRI technologist to alter her normal work habits out of concern about the energy fields used with MRI. Magnetic resonance imaging is a safe occupation.

3. Deterministic responses exhibit a threshold exposure. Below that exposure, no response will occur; above that threshold, the severity of the response increases with increasing exposure time and intensity.

4. Projectiles, under the influence of the B_0 field.

5. Tissue becomes magnetized, and atoms and molecules become polarized. However, this effect is exceptionally small; it disappears rapidly on removal from the magnetic field, and there are no immediate or lasting physiological effects.

6. Possible auditory concerns from the loud thumping of the gradient coils, potential reactions to MRI contrast agents, possible mechanical twisting of magnetic surgical clips, interference with pacemaker performance, and claustrophobia.

7. Gradient magnetic fields change intensity with time. This property can result in electromagnetic induction of an electric current. The current of neurological pathways can be influenced by such gradient magnetic fields, causing a variety of physiological responses. However, none are life threatening, and all cease when imaging stops.

8. Specific absorption rate (SAR) refers to the time-related fashion in which RF energy is deposited in tissue. The recommended maximum limit is 0.4 W/kg.

9. Heating. Tissue temperature may be elevated, and under some circumstances, superficial burns are possible.

10. The B_0 field is measured in tesla, the gradient magnetic field is measured in mT/m, and the RF field is measured in hertz. The most important measure for evaluating biological response is the specific absorption rate due to RF irradiation, which is measured in W/kg.

CHAPTER 30

1. All of the mechanical and electronic apparatus to be used in and around the MRI suite must be nonmagnetic.

2. Review the patient's neurosurgical chart to ensure that no ferromagnetic surgical clips are present. If you are uncertain, a radiograph may be required to determine if clips are present. The date of the operation may help determine if such clips may be ferromagnetic.

3. At least 2 years of formal training in medical imaging and certification by the American Registry of Radiologic Technologists. Additional formal training and regular continuing education in MRI are also necessary. Certification as an MRI technologist by the ARRT should be the goal of every MRI technologist.

4. Patients with a cardiac pacemaker represent the most sensitive people because the fringe magnetic field may disrupt the operation of the pacemaker. The exclusion level is 0.5 mT.

5. A reminder phone call the day before the examination; help with completing a patient questionnaire; personal consultation about the nature of the examination; and report generation in a timely fashion.

6. To avoid the possible disruption of MRI system operation because of interference by ferromagnetic objects. Such objects can be brought into the imaging room by visitors, patients, physicians, and other hospital staff.

7. Have a friend or family member visit with the patient during the examination. Provide the patient with eyeshades and headphones. Carefully explain the nature of the examination to such a patient. In some situations, patient sedation may be necessary.

8. Accreditation of the MRI facility by the American College of Radiology is strongly advised. The cornerstone of this accreditation program is an ongoing quality control program based on daily measurements and observations and annual performance evaluation by medical physicists.

9. Liquid helium and liquid nitrogen have vaporization temperatures of 4 K and 77 K,

respectively. During a quench, the gases are released and can occlude the available oxygen. The system must be vented to the outside, and in the event of the quench, the patient and personnel should vacate the imaging room until the cryogenic gases are dissipated.

10. To inform the patient that there are known hazards associated with ferromagnetic objects inside the body. This is also a good time to explain that there are no lasting effects from the energy fields of MRI.

Answers to Practice Examinations

MRI EXAM I

1. c
2. a
3. d
4. e
5. a
6. b
7. e
8. b
9. a
10. b
11. a
12. b
13. b
14. a
15. a
16. a
17. c
18. a
19. a
20. e
21. b
22. c
23. c
24. d
25. a
26. d
27. d
28. a
29. b
30. c
31. d
32. c
33. b
34. c
35. d
36. b
37. c
38. d
39. e
40. b
41. b
42. b
43. a
44. e
45. d
46. e
47. c
48. e
49. a
50. c
51. d
52. c
53. d
54. b
55. c
56. c
57. b
58. a

59. c
60. d
61. e
62. b
63. d
64. c
65. e
66. a
67. c
68. c
69. e
70. a
71. e
72. a
73. a
74. c
75. e
76. c
77. e
78. b
79. d
80. e
81. a
82. a
83. c
84. a
85. a
86. b
87. d
88. c
89. b
90. e
91. b
92. a
93. b
94. b
95. c
96. a
97. c
98. d
99. d
100. d
101. a
102. c
103. c
104. b
105. c
106. a

107. a
108. a
109. a
110. a
111. b
112. d
113. d
114. e
115. c
116. e
117. e
118. b
119. c
120. b
121. e
122. d

MRI EXAM II

1. b
2. d
3. d
4. d
5. d
6. e
7. b
8. e
9. d
10. a
11. b
12. d
13. c
14. d
15. b
16. e
17. d
18. d
19. e
20. a
21. d
22. d
23. d
24. e
25. d
26. e
27. e
28. d
29. b

30. e
31. d
32. d
33. a
34. a
35. a
36. b
37. d
38. a
39. a
40. e
41. d
42. e
43. a
44. c
45. b
46. b
47. b
48. a
49. a
50. c
51. b
52. c
53. e
54. e
55. c
56. c
57. b
58. a
59. d
60. c
61. a
62. a
63. e
64. c
65. a
66. c
67. c
68. c
69. b
70. d
71. b
72. b
73. e
74. e
75. a
76. e
77. d

78. e
79. a
80. c
81. d
82. d
83. c
84. a
85. b
86. d
87. d
88. a
89. b
90. b
91. d
92. a
93. c
94. a
95. d
96. a
97. a
98. e
99. d
100. c
101. b
102. a
103. d
104. d
105. b
106. a
107. b
108. c
109. b
110. c
111. d
112. a
113. c
114. c
115. b
116. d
117. e
118. d
119. c
120. c
121. b
122. b

Glossary of Magnetic Resonance Imaging Terms*

α **excitation pulse** flip angle less than 90° caused by an RF pulse.

90° radiofrequency pulse see pulse, 90°.

absolute zero temperature at which material has no thermal energy and metals lose electrical resistance (0 K, −273°C, −460°F).

acceleration a change in the velocity of blood per unit time (dv/dt); can cause signal loss during MR angiography (MRA).

acquisition process of detecting and storing MR signals.

acquisition matrix the number of data points acquired in the phase- and frequency-encoded directions during 2DFT imaging (e.g., 192 × 256, 512 × 512).

acquisition time the time required for acquisition of the MR signals; distinct from reconstruction time.

acquisitions (ACQ) number of signals averaged to improve SNR; measuring and storing imaging signals; *see* number of excitations (NEX).

active shielding reduction of the fringe magnetic field through the use of secondary magnetic coils to produce a reverse magnetic field, which cancels the static magnetic field outside of the imaging volume.

air core magnet electromagnet, either resistive or superconducting, in which the conductor windings provide the magnetic field without flux enhancement by ferromagnetic materials.

aliasing artifact created by inadequate sampling of data; usually occurs when the FOV is smaller than the subject; anatomy outside the FOV is folded into the image; also called *wraparound artifact*.

analog-to-digital converter (ADC) part of the computer system that converts ordinary (analog) voltages, such as the detected MR signal, into digital numerical form.

angiography images of blood vessels; MR angiography (MRA).

angular frequency (ω) frequency of oscillation, rotation or precession, and it is commonly designated by the Greek letter ω.

angular momentum vector quantity given by the product of the momentum of a particle and its position; a rotating body tends to maintain the same axis of rotation; when a torque is applied to a rotating body, the resulting change in angular momentum results in precession; the possible values are integers or half integers: 0, 1/2, 1, 3/2, 2, 5/2, ...

---

*Some terms in this glossary have been adapted from publications by the American College of Radiology, General Electric Medical Systems, Philips Medical Systems, and Siemens Medical Systems.

annotation graphic description on the image of technique factors used, patient data, etc.

antenna device to send or receive electromagnetic radiation in the RF region of the spectrum.

array coil radiofrequency antenna composed of multiple separate elements that can be energized individually or simultaneously; useful for large area imaging, for example, total spine.

array processor optional component of computer system specially designed to speed up numerical calculations.

artifact false features of an image caused by patient instability or equipment deficiencies.

asymmetrical echo an SE or GRE with maximum intensity, which occurs when TE is not centered in the sampling window; sometimes called *fractional* or *partial echo*.

atomic number Z is the number of protons per atom.

autotuning automatic method for frequency selection and impedance matching of RF coils under different loading conditions.

axial see transverse.

B_0 conventional symbol for the main magnetic field in an MR imaging system; measured in tesla (T).

bandwidth the amount of data that can be transmitted across a communication channel over a given period of time; the range of RF frequencies in a pulse or to which an MR receiver is tuned.

bipolar gradient magnetic field gradient reversed polarity, for example, B_R in GRE imaging.

Bloch equations the equations of motion for the macroscopic net magnetization vector; they include the effects of precession about the static magnetic field and the T1 and T2 relaxation times.

Bohr magneton unit of magnetic moment; 9.3×10^{-24} J/T.

boil-off cryogens relaxing to the gaseous from the liquid state and discharging from the imaging system.

Boltzmann distribution system of particles in equilibrium that exchange energy in collisions; at room temperature, the difference in number of spins aligned with and against B_0 is about one in a million; the small excess of nuclei in the lower-energy state is the basis of the net magnetization (M) and the resonance phenomenon.

Boltzmann's constant $k = 1.4 \times 10^{-23}$ J/K.

broadband network a general term for a computer network capable of high bandwidth transmission rate.

B_X, B_Y, B_Z symbols for gradient magnetic fields produced by gradient coils. Also symbolized as B_{SS}, B_ϕ, B_R.

Carr-Purcell-Meiboom-Gill (CPMG) sequence modification of Carr-Purcell RF pulse sequence with 90° phase shift in the rotating frame of reference between the 90° pulse and the subsequent 180° pulses to reduce accumulating effects of imperfections in the 180° pulses.

Carr-Purcell (CP) sequence the sequence of a 90° RF pulse followed by repeated 180° RF pulses to produce a train of SEs.

channel the connection between two parties that mediates their communication, such as a telephone or e-mail.

chemical shift change in the Larmor frequency of a given nucleus when bound in different sites in a molecule, owing to the magnetic shielding effects of the electron orbitals.

chemical shift artifact bright band at fat-muscle interface because of slight difference in Larmor frequency (3.5 ppm) of those two tissues; occurs along the frequency-encoded axis.

coherence a constant phase relationship between rotating or oscillating waves or objects; loss of phase coherence of proton spins results in a reduction in the transverse magnetization and a decrease in the MR signal.

coil single or multiple loops of wire designed either to produce a magnetic field from current flowing through the wire or to detect a changing magnetic field by voltage induced in the wire.

contrast   relative difference of image brightness in adjacent tissues.

contrast resolution   ability of an imaging system to distinguish adjacent soft tissues from one another; this is the principal advantage of MRI.

contrast-to-noise ratio (CNR)   ratio of signal intensity of adjacent tissues (contrast) to intensity fluctuation in both (noise).

critical temperature T_c is the Curie temperature for ferromagnets.

crossed-coil   pair of coils arranged with their magnetic fields at right angles to each other to minimize their mutual electromagnetic interaction.

cryogen   atmospheric gases, such as nitrogen and helium, that have been cooled sufficiently to condense into a liquid.

cryostat   apparatus for maintaining a constant low temperature; requires vacuum chambers to help with thermal isolation.

dB/dt   rate of change of the magnetic field with time; because changing magnetic fields can induce electrical fields, this is one area of potential concern for safety limits.

decoupling   (a) method of RF irradiation to reduce spin-spin coupling of different molecules; (b) electrical method of reducing interaction of one RF coil with another.

demodulator   another term for *detector*, by analogy to broadcast radio receivers.

dephasing   loss of phase coherence within an ensemble of spins.

detector   portion of the receiver that demodulates the MR signal and converts it to a lower-frequency signal; detectors also give phase information about the MR signal.

diamagnetic   type of substance that slightly decreases a magnetic field when placed within it.

DICOM Digital Imaging and Communications in Medicine   an electronic information standard.

diffusion   process by which molecules or other particles intermingle and migrate because of the random thermal motion.

digital-to-analog converter (DAC)   part of the computer system that converts digital numbers into ordinary analog voltages or currents.

digitization   process of converting a continuous signal (analog) into a series of numbers (digital).

dipole   two poles; north and south magnetic fields.

display matrix   the number of pixels in each row and column of a digital image (e.g., 192 × 256, 512 × 512).

dynamic image   a sequence of images displayed in rapid succession so that they are perceived as continuous motion.

dynamic range   number of possible discrete values for each pixel; shades of gray for each pixel (e.g., 2^{10} = 10 bits = 1024 gray levels).

echo   signal reappearing some time after the excitation pulse as a result of the effective reversal of the dephasing of the spins.

echo planar imaging (EPI)   technique in which a complete planar image is obtained from one selective excitation pulse; the spin echo is observed while periodically switching the phase-encoding gradient in the presence of a static frequency-encoding gradient magnetic field.

echo time (TE)   see TE (echo time).

eddy currents   spurious electric currents induced in a conductor by a changing magnetic field or by motion of the conductor through a magnetic field.

electric charge   the electron charge is 1.6×10^{-19} C.

electric field (E)   the change in E produced by an electrically polarized object; expressed in V/m.

electromagnetic induction   generating an electric current with a time-varying magnetic field; generating a magnetic field with a moving electric charge; see induction.

electron spin resonance science of the response of electrons to RF and magnetic fields; similar to NMR.

encode to place a representative message onto a carrier (e.g., spatial information carried by the frequency of the MR signal).

energy the ability to do work; expressed in Joules (J).

equilibrium the state of tissue that is fully magnetized by a static magnetic field, symbolized as M_0.

excitation putting energy into the spin system by way of an RF pulse; raising protons to a higher energy level in the presence of a magnetic field.

exclusion area part of the imaging suite and surrounding areas from which people must be restricted because of possible magnetic field hazards.

Faraday shield electrical conductor placed between the MR imaging system and the environment to attenuate ambient RF radiation.

fast Fourier transform (FFT) efficient computational method of performing a Fourier transform.

ferromagnetic material substance, such as iron, that has a large positive magnetic susceptibility; it is easily magnetized.

FFE (fast field echo) a term for a family of gradient echo methods characterized by the absence of 180° RF pulses; the excitation pulses have a low and adjustable flip angle and the repetition times are short; equivalent terms: GRASS (Gradient Recalled Acquisition of Steady State), FAST (Fourier-Acquired Steady State Techniques), and FISP (Fast Imaging with Steady State Precession).

FID *see* free induction decay.

field echo *see* gradient echo.

field of view (FOV) anatomy contained within the volume imaged; determined by the product of acquisition matrix and pixel size; usually expressed in centimeters.

filling factor measure of the geometric relationship of the RF coil and the body; it affects the efficiency of irradiating the body and detecting MR signals, thereby affecting the signal-to-noise ratio. Achieving a high filling factor requires fitting the coil closely to the body.

filter an electronic circuit that passes only selective frequencies.

filtered back projection mathematical technique used in reconstruction from projections to create images from a set of multiple projection profiles.

flip angle amount of rotation of the net magnetization vector produced by an RF pulse, with respect to the direction of the static magnetic field.

flip angle sweep in turbo field echo, the image is acquired while the magnetization is approaching the steady state; the sequence starts with a low flip angle, which is gradually increased during the image, to avoid "ghost" artifacts resulting from gradient echo amplitude oscillations.

flow a measure of the volume of moving blood per unit time (cm^3/s).

flow compensation use of bipolar gradient magnetic fields to reduce flow artifacts by reestablishing phase coherence; first-order gradient moment nulling.

flow-related enhancement the increase in signal intensity of flowing blood compared with stationary tissue when fully magnetized spins replace saturated spins between RF pulses.

Fourier transform (FT) mathematical procedure to separate the frequency and phase components of a time-varying or spatially varying signal from the amplitudes as a function of time; the Fourier transform is used to generate the spectrum from the FID and is essential to most imaging techniques.

FOV (field of view) the area of the anatomical region displayed in the image.

free induction decay (FID) the signal emitted immediately after an excitation pulse; the decay is caused by progressive dephasing of the spins; the decay time constant is T2*.

frequency (f) number of repetitions of a periodic process per unit time; for RF electromagnetic radiation applied to MRI; the range is from approximately 10 MHz to 200 MHz.

frequency-encoding use of a gradient magnetic field to produce a range of frequencies along the MR signal to provide information on spatial position.

fringe magnetic field stray magnetic field that exists outside the MR imaging system; the area around any magnet having a magnetic field higher than the magnetic field of earth, which is typically between 50 and 100 μT.

gating reduction of cardiac motion artifacts by triggering signal acquisition to electrocardiogram.

gauss (G) unit of magnetic field intensity in the older CGS system; the currently preferred (SI) unit is the tesla (T); 1 T = 10,000 G.

gauss meter instrument that measures magnetic field intensity.

Gibbs artifact *see* truncation artifact.

Golay coil the coil used to create a gradient magnetic field, perpendicular to the main magnetic field.

gradient amount and direction of the rate of change in space of some quantity, such as magnetic field strength.

gradient coils (G_X, G_Y, G_Z) current-carrying coils designed to produce a desired gradient magnetic field; proper design of the size and configuration of the coils is necessary to produce a controlled and uniform gradient magnetic field.

gradient echo (GRE) MR signal produced with a bipolar read gradient.

gradient magnetic field magnetic field that changes in intensity in a given direction; a typical value is 10 to 40 mT/m.

gradient pulse briefly applied gradient magnetic field.

gradient refocused echo (GRE) see gradient echo.

gram molecular weight the mass in grams of one mole (6×10^{23} particles) of a substance.

G_X, G_Y, G_Z conventional symbols for gradient magnetic coils; used with subscripts to denote spatial direction along which the produced magnetic field changes.

gyromagnetic ratio (γ) ratio of the magnetic moment to the angular momentum of a particle; this is a constant for a given nucleus (MHz/T).

half Fourier imaging *see* partial Fourier imaging.

hardware electrical and mechanical components of a computer.

Helmholtz coil pair of current-carrying coils used to create a uniform magnetic field in the space between them.

hertz (Hz) standard (SI) unit of frequency; equal to the old unit cycles per second.

homogeneity uniformity in intensity of the static magnetic field, B_0.

image acquisition time the time required to receive all of the MR signals necessary to produce an MR image; the additional image reconstruction time is also important to determine how quickly the image can be viewed.

image reconstruction process of changing MR signals into an image (e.g., 2DFT, 3DFT).

imaginary signal out-of-phase component from a quadrature RF detector.

inductance measure of the magnetic coupling between two current-carrying coils reflecting their spatial relationship; one of the principal determinants of the resonance frequency of an RF circuit.

induction process of transferring energy from one frame of reference to another without touching; see electromagnetic induction.

inhomogeneity lack of magnetic field uniformity; the fractional deviation of the local magnetic field from the average value of the field; expressed as parts per million (ppm).

intranet a computer network that is based on World Wide Web and Internet technologies, in which the scope is limited to an organization.

inversion nonequilibrium state in which the net magnetization vector is oriented opposite to the static magnetic field.

inversion recovery (IR)   pulse sequence for MRI wherein the net magnetization is inverted and relaxes to equilibrium with the emission of an MR signal after a 90° RF pulse; a method similar to spin echo but each excitation is preceded by an inversion pulse at a time TI.

inversion time (TI)   time between the 180° RF inversion pulse and the subsequent 90° RF pulse to bring net magnetization onto the XY plane.

iron core magnet   usually a resistive electromagnet in which the conductor is wound on an iron core to increase the magnetic field.

J-coupling   interaction between two or more proton spins on the same molecule through abnormalities in the electron shells.

Kelvin   the SI unit of temperature.

k-space   mathematical space in which the Fourier transform of the image is represented; *see* spatial frequency domain.

k value   this is the mathematical coding value for the signal; the coding has the same number of dimensions (2 or 3) as the image data after reconstruction; for the reconstruction of a 2D image, a 2D set of signals with equally spaced k_X and k_Y values is needed; for the reconstruction of a 3D data set, a second preparation gradient is used to provide the needed k_Z values.

laminar flow   blood flowing in layers; maximum blood flows in the center of a vessel and slowest near the vessel wall.

LAN (local area network)   a computer network limited to servicing computers in a small locality; *see* intranet.

Larmor equation $f = \gamma B$ states that the frequency of precession of the nuclear magnetic moment is proportional to the magnetic field intensity.

Larmor frequency (f)   the frequency at which magnetic resonance can be excited; given by the Larmor equation; for hydrogen nuclei, the Larmor frequency is 42 MHz/T.

lattice   magnetic environment with which nuclei exchange energy in longitudinal relaxation; the molecule that contains the proton spins.

lodestone   a natural magnet; magnetite.

longitudinal magnetization (M_Z)   component of the net magnetization vector along the static magnetic field.

longitudinal relaxation   the relaxation of longitudinal magnetization to the equilibrium value after excitation; requires exchange of energy between the nuclear spins and the lattice.

longitudinal relaxation time   see T1.

M   symbol for net magnetization vector.

M_0   equilibrium value of the net magnetization vector directed along the static magnetic field.

magnetic dipole   north and south magnetic poles separated by a finite distance.

magnetic field gradient   *see* gradient magnetic field.

magnetic flux density   usually referred to simply as the *static magnetic field*, B_0; expressed in tesla (T) or the older unit gauss (G); 1 T = 10,000 G.

magnetic fringe field   *see* fringe magnetic field.

magnetic induction (B)   also called *magnetic flux density* and *magnetic field intensity*; it is the net magnetic effect from an externally applied magnetic field and the resulting magnetization; measured in tesla (T).

magnetic moment   measure of the magnetic properties of an object or particle (the proton) that causes it to align with the static magnetic field.

magnetic permeability   tendency of a substance to concentrate the imaginary lines of the magnetic field; $\mu_0 = 4\pi \times 10^{-7}$ H/m is the permeability of free space; $\mu_r = \mu/\mu_0$ is the relative permeability.

magnetic resonance   absorption or emission of RF by a nucleus in a B_0 field following RF excitation at the Larmor frequency.

magnetic resonance angiography (MRA)   imaging blood vessels with MRI.

magnetic resonance contrast agent   pharmaceutical that changes the relaxation times of tissues.

magnetic resonance imaging (MRI)   creation of images of patients by use of the

NMR phenomenon; image brightness of tissue usually depends on the SD and the relaxation times.

magnetic susceptibility measure of the ability of a substance to become magnetized.

magnetization transfer selective saturation of a particular spin within a multispin system; suppression of signal from a particular type of spin; useful for fat suppression.

mass density expressed in kilograms per cubic meter.

maximum intensity projection (MIP) computer technique of image reconstruction from a volume data matrix; selection of the pixel with the highest signal intensity along a ray onto a 2D image.

Maxwell coil a special kind of coil that is commonly used to create gradient magnetic fields along the direction of the static magnetic field.

megahertz (MHz) unit of frequency; equal to 1 million Hz.

misregistration artifact caused by motion or aliasing, resulting in positioning an MR signal in the wrong pixel.

multiplanar imaging the imaging of many 2D sections of anatomy simultaneously.

M_{XY} transverse magnetization.

M_Z longitudinal magnetization.

net magnetization vector (M) vector representing the magnitude and direction of the net magnetic moment of a sample in a given region; considered the integrated effect of all the individual proton magnetic moments.

noise undesirable contribution to an MR signal that reduces contrast resolution.

NSA (number of signals averaged) the number of times that an identical MR signal is collected for use in the same image; a large NSA improves signal-to-noise ratio and suppresses motion artifacts.

nuclear magnetic resonance (NMR) absorption or emission of electromagnetic energy by nuclei in a static magnetic field, after excitation by a stable RF magnetic field; the peak resonance frequency is proportional to the magnetic field and it is given by the Larmor equation.

nuclear spin property of certain nuclei; produces angular momentum and magnetic moment.

nuclear spin quantum number *see* spin quantum number.

number of excitations (NEX) number of signal acquisitions averaged to improve SNR; *see* acquisitions (ACQ), NSA.

Nyquist frequency a frequency equal to one half of the sampling rate; frequency of a signal beyond which aliasing occurs.

PACS (Picture Archiving and Communications System) a system that archives digital images and is often used to describe the viewing, printing, and annotating of the images.

paramagnetic type of substance with a small but positive magnetic susceptibility; the addition of a small amount of paramagnetic substance may greatly reduce the relaxation times of a tissue; used as contrast agents in MRI.

partial Fourier imaging image reconstructed from an MR data set that fills less than all of k-space; results in faster imaging but with reduced SNR.

partial saturation (PS) excitation technique applying repeated 90° RF pulses at times on the order of or shorter than T1; partial saturation is also commonly referred to as *saturation recovery;* the latter term should properly be reserved for the particular case of partial saturation when 90° RF pulses are far enough apart in time that the relaxation of nuclear spins to equilibrium is complete.

passive shielding use of iron around the magnet or in the walls to reduce the fringe magnetic field.

permanent magnet material, such as iron, in which the magnetic field originates with constant intensity.

permeability see magnetic permeability.

phantom artificial object of known dimensions and properties used to assay the performance of an MR imaging system.

phase in a periodic function, such as rotational or harmonic motion, the position relative to a particular part of the cycle; a position of a spin in the periodic cycle.

phase coherence multiple spins all in the same position of a periodic cycle; the origin of MR signals.

phase-encoding use of a gradient magnetic field to alter spin phase before MR signal detection for spatial localization.

pixel acronym for a picture element; the smallest discrete part of a digital image display.

planar imaging the imaging technique in which image of a plane (slice, section) is acquired from signals received from a spin echo; data are collected simultaneously from throughout the slice.

Planck's constant $h = 6.6 \times 10^{-34}$ J s.

plug flow uniform blood flow; flow profile in which flow in the center of a vessel is the same as that along the walls.

polarity assigning one of two values; for example, north or south, + or −, 0 or 1, positive or negative.

precession gyration of the axis of a spinning body so as to trace out a cone, caused by the application of a torque tending to change the direction of the rotation axis.

preparation gradient magnetic field gradient magnetic field that spatially encodes by phase in 2DFT and 3DFT imaging.

prepulse pulse applied in TFE and T1-TFE to obtain inversion or saturation before the start of imaging.

presaturation the saturation of spins outside of the imaging volume; useful in MRA.

probe part of an MR imaging system for RF emission and signal detection; the RF coils.

projection reconstruction see reconstruction from projections.

proton density (PD) density of resonating proton spins in a given region; one of the principal determinants of the strength of the MR signal from that region; hydrogen concentration.

pseudo a false image or process.

pulse length (width) time duration of an RF pulse (ms); for an RF pulse near the Larmor frequency, the longer the pulse length, the greater the flip angle of the net magnetization vector.

pulse programmer part of the computer system that controls the timing, duration, and amplitude of the RF and gradient pulses.

pulse sequence set of RF and/or gradient magnetic field pulses and time spacings between them; used to excite spins and spatially encode the received signal.

pulse, 180° radiofrequency pulse designed to rotate the net magnetization vector 180° from the static magnetic field; if the spins are initially aligned with the static magnetic field, this pulse produces inversion; if the spins are initially in the XY plane, an SE results.

pulse, 90° radiofrequency pulse designed to rotate the net magnetization vector 90° from the static magnetic field; if the spins are initially aligned with the static magnetic field, this pulse produces transverse magnetization and an FID.

quadrature detector phase-sensitive detector or demodulator that detects the components of the MR signal in phase with a reference oscillation and 90° out of phase with the reference oscillator.

quality factor (Q) applies to any electrical circuit component; most often the coil Q is limiting; inversely related to the fraction of energy in an oscillating system lost in one oscillation cycle; the Q of a coil depends on whether it is unloaded (no patient) or loaded (patient).

quantum the smallest indivisible unit of energy; a photon.

quantum mechanics physics of extremely small objects, which is based on the concept that all physical quantities can exist only as discrete units.

quench loss of superconductivity of the B_0 coil that may occur unexpectedly; as the magnet becomes resistive, heat is released, which can result in rapid evaporation of liquid helium in the cryostat; possible hazard that must be vented.

radiofrequency (RF) electromagnetic radiation lower in energy than infrared; the RF used in MRI is in the form of a burst of RF energy (pulse) in the 10- to 200-MHz range.

radiofrequency coil used for transmitting RF pulses and/or receiving MR signals.

radiofrequency pulse brief burst of RF electromagnetic energy delivered to patient by RF transmitter; if the RF frequency is at the Larmor frequency, the result is rotation of the net magnetization vector and phase coherence of the proton spins.

radiofrequency shield *see* Faraday shield.

read gradient magnetic field (B_R) a gradient magnetic field energized while the MR signal is detected; the frequency-encoding gradient magnetic field.

real image that component of an MR image reconstructed from the part of the signal that is in phase with a reference signal, as opposed to the imaginary component.

receiver portion of the MR imaging system that detects and amplifies RF signals picked up by the receiving coil; includes a preamplifier, an amplifier, and a demodulator.

receiver bandwidth the range of frequencies detected; 32 kHz is a typical value for MR imaging systems.

receiver coil the coil of the RF receiver; detects the MR signal; sometimes used for RF transmission and excitation of spins.

reconstruction from projections magnetic resonance imaging technique in which a set of projection profiles of the body is obtained by observing MR signals in the presence of a suitable corresponding set of rotated gradient magnetic fields.

refocus the relaxation of spins to phase coherence by application of an RF pulse or gradient magnetic field.

region of interest (ROI) specified area of a digital image chosen for analysis.

relaxation rate reciprocal of relaxation time (e.g., R1 = 1/T1, R2 = 1/T2).

relaxation time after excitation, the proton spins tend to relax to their equilibrium position, in accordance with these time constants; T1 is the spin-lattice (longitudinal) relaxation time; T2 is the spin-spin (transverse) relaxation time.

repetition time (TR) the period between the beginning of a pulse sequence and the beginning of the succeeding and identical pulse sequence.

rephasing gradient the gradient magnetic field applied briefly after a selective excitation pulse, in the opposite direction from the gradient magnetic field used for the selective excitation; the result of the gradient reversal is a rephasing of the spins, forming GRE.

resistive magnet a magnet in which magnetic field originates from current flowing through an ordinary electrical conductor.

resolution *see* spatial resolution and contrast resolution.

resonance vibration in an electrical or mechanical system caused by a relatively small periodic stimulus with a frequency at or close to a natural frequency of the system.

REST (regional saturation technique) the technique for saturation of the proton spins in all regions of the body that are not imaged; REST slabs can be parallel to the imaged section or at any angle; equivalent term: PRESAT (presaturation).

rotating frame of reference frame of reference with corresponding coordinate systems that rotate around the axis of the static magnetic field (B_0) at a frequency equal to that of the applied RF.

saddle coil radiofrequency coil design; commonly used when the static magnetic field is coaxial with the axis of the coil along the long axis of the body.

saturation nonequilibrium state in MRI in which equal numbers of spins are aligned against and with the static magnetic field so that there is no net magnetization.

saturation recovery (SR) particular type of partial saturation pulse sequence in which the preceding pulses leave the spins in a state of saturation so that recovery to equilibrium is complete by the time of the next pulse.

SE (spin echo imaging) the classic method for acquisition in MR imaging systems; a spin echo is formed at a given time TE after each excitation pulse and data are sampled around this echo; later spin echoes can be formed and sampled as well.

security zone part of the MR imaging suite where ferromagnetic objects are intercepted so they do not enter the imaging room; usually incorporates a metal detector.

selective excitation controlling the frequency spectrum of an irradiating RF pulse while imposing a gradient magnetic field on nuclear spins, such that only a desired region has a suitable resonant frequency to be excited; commonly used to select a plane for excitation and imaging; restriction of excitation to a volume or section.

self shielding reduction of fringe magnetic field by incorporating iron around the magnet (passive shield) or reverse polarity magnetic fields (active shield).

semiconductor material, such as silicon and germanium, that controls electron flow as a gate by application of a small voltage.

sensitive plane the technique of selecting a plane for imaging by using an oscillating gradient magnetic field and filtering out the corresponding time dependent part of the MR signal.

sensitive point the technique of selecting a point for imaging by applying three orthogonal oscillating gradient magnetic fields so that the local magnetic field is time dependent everywhere, except at the desired point, and then filtering out the corresponding time-dependent portion of the NMR signal.

sensitive volume region of the patient from which the MR signal is predominantly acquired because of strong magnetic field inhomogeneity elsewhere; the effect can be enhanced by use of a shaped RF field that is strongest in the sensitive volume.

sensitivity ability to detect weak MR signal; ability to image a diseased or abnormal state.

sequential line imaging magnetic resonance imaging techniques in which the image is built up from successive lines through the object.

sequential plane imaging magnetic resonance imaging techniques in which the image is built from successive planes in the object.

shielded gradient coils reverse polarity secondary gradient coils to reduce the fringe magnetic field inside the cryostat; also help reduce eddy currents.

shim coils the coils carrying a relatively small current that are used to provide auxiliary magnetic fields to compensate for inhomogeneities in the static magnetic field, B_0; used to improve B_0 field homogeneity.

shimming correction of inhomogeneity of the static magnetic field, B_0, of an MR imaging system owing to imperfections in the magnet or to the presence of external ferromagnetic objects.

signal averaging method of improving SNR by averaging several FIDs, SEs, or GREs.

signal-to-noise ratio (SNR) used to describe the relative contributions to a detected signal of the true signal and random superimposed noise; the SNR can be improved by averaging several MR signals, by sampling larger volumes or by increasing the strength of the B_0 magnetic field.

SI unit universally accepted Systeme Internationale d'unites as defined by The General Conference on Weights and Measures.

software set of instructions or programs that controls the activities of the computer.

solenoid coil coil of wire wound in the form of a long cylinder; when a current is passed through the coil, a magnetic field is produced along the axis of the coil.

SPAMM (spatial modulation of magnetization) a saturation technique that is applied in a periodic pattern perpendicular to the imaged slice and is visible in the slice as a chessboard pattern; equivalent term: tagging.

spatial relating to space; a specific location in space.

spatial frequency domain a dimension of the Fourier transform space (like k-space) having units of inverse distance.

spatial resolution ability of an imaging process to distinguish small adjacent high-contrast structures in the object.

specific absorption rate (SAR) radiofrequency energy deposited in the patient; magnetic resonance imaging exposure quantity; measured in watts per kilogram.

spectrum array of the intensity of the components of the MR signal according to frequency.

speed of light 3×10^8 m/s.

spin intrinsic angular momentum of an elementary particle or system of particles; a nucleus that is responsible for the magnetic moment; property of nuclei with either an odd number of protons or neutrons or both.

spin density (SD) *see* proton density.

spin echo (SE) reappearance of an MR signal after the FID has disappeared; the result of the effective reversal of the dephasing of the nuclear spins.

spin echo imaging any one of many MRI techniques in which the SE MR signal rather than the FID is used.

spin-lattice relaxation time (T1) longitudinal relaxation time; the characteristic time constant for spins to align themselves with the external static magnetic field.

spin quantum number property of all nuclei related to the largest measurable component of the nuclear angular momentum; the possible values are integers or half integers; 0, 1/2, 1, 3/2, 2, 5/2, ...

spin-spin coupling *see* J-coupling.

spin-spin relaxation time (T2) spin-spin or transverse relaxation time; the characteristic time constant for loss of phase coherence among spins oriented at an angle to the main magnetic field owing to interactions between the spins; T2 never exceeds T1.

spin-warp imaging form of Fourier transform imaging in which phase-encoding gradient magnetic field pulses are applied for a constant duration but with varying amplitude; different from the original methods with pulses of constant amplitude but varying duration.

spoiler pulse a gradient magnetic field applied to eliminate residual signal by dephasing spins.

steady state free precession (SSFP) method of MRI excitation in which strings of RF pulses are applied rapidly and repeatedly with interpulse intervals short compared with both T1 and T2.

STIR (short tau inversion recovery) the term *tau* in the expression stands for the inversion time, TI; the value is relatively short, resulting in an image contrast that is useful for some special applications.

superconducting magnet magnet in which magnetic field originates from current flowing through a superconductor, which has no electrical resistance at very low temperature; such a magnet must be enclosed in a cryostat.

superconductor substance in which electrical resistance essentially disappears at temperatures near absolute zero; the superconductor used in MR imaging systems is niobium-titanium.

surface coil simple, flat RF receiver coil placed over a region of interest; it has an approximate imaging volume equal to the coil circumference and one radius deep from the coil center; designed to improve SNR for a small FOV.

susceptibility *see* magnetic susceptibility.

T1 longitudinal relaxation time; quantity that describes the rate of regrowth of the longitudinal magnetization to the equilibrium value after a disturbance such as that caused by an RF pulse; for most tissues, T1 has a value of a few hundred milliseconds.

T1-FFE FE with enhancement of T1 contrast; equivalent terms: FLASH (Fast Low Angle Shot) and SPGR (SPoiled GRass).

T1-TFE TFE with enhancement of T1 contrast; equivalent terms: Turbo FLASH, Rapid

SPGR (Rapid Spoiled GRass) or for 3D imaging, 3D MP RAGE (3D Magnetization-Prepared Rapid Gradient Echo).

T2 transverse relaxation time; quantity that determines loss of transverse magnetization after generation by an RF pulse, assuming that the external magnet field is homogenous; T2 is always less than T1; in tissue, T2 ranges between 10 and 50 ms; in body liquids, T2 can be several hundred milliseconds.

T2* time constant for loss of phase coherence among spins oriented perpendicular to the static magnetic field, B_0; principally due to magnetic field inhomogeneities and spin-spin relaxation; T2* is always much shorter than T2.

T2-FFE FE with enhancement of T2 contrast; equivalent terms: CE-FAST (Contrast-Enhanced FAST), PSIF (Mirrored FISP), and SSFP (Steady State Free Precession).

T2-TFE TFE with enhancement of T2 contrast.

tailored pulse a shaped RF pulse in which the magnitude is varied with time in a predetermined manner; affects the frequency components of an RF pulse in a manner determined by the Fourier transform of the pulse.

TE (echo time) time interval between the middle of the excitation pulse and the middle of the echo signal that is observed.

tesla (T) preferred (SI) unit of magnetic flux density or magnetic field intensity:

$$1 \text{ T} = 10,000 \text{ G} = \frac{1 \text{ N}}{\text{A–m}}.$$

TFE (Turbo Field Echo) FFE with very short TR and TE and special provisions for optimizing contrast and signal-to-noise ratio; these provisions optionally include "flip angle sweep" and "prepulses."

thermal equilibrium state in which all parts of a system are at the same effective temperature; when the relative alignment of the spins with the magnetic field is determined solely by the thermal energy of the system.

three-dimensional Fourier transform imaging (3DFT) signal acquisition/reconstruction method in which a volume of tissue is sampled; thin-slice 2D images with high SNR result.

TI (inversion time) time between the middle of the inversion pulse and the middle of the subsequent excitation pulse.

TI inversion time the time after middle of inverting RF pulse to middle of 90° pulse to detect amount of transverse magnetization.

time of flight (TOF) magnetic resonance angiography imaging technique that relies primarily on flow-related enhancement to distinguish moving from stationary spins.

time reversal the technique of producing an SE by subjecting excited spins to a gradient magnetic field and then reversing the direction of the gradient magnetic field.

torque a force that causes or tends to cause a body to rotate; it is a vector quantity given by the product of the force and the position vector where the force is applied.

TR (repetition time) *see* repetition time.

transaxial *see* transverse.

transmitter part of the MR imaging system that produces RF current and delivers it to the transmitting coil.

transverse perpendicular to the external magnetic field (B_0); perpendicular to the long axis of the body.

transverse magnetization (M_{XY}) component of the net magnetization vector at right angles to the static magnetic field.

transverse relaxation time *see* T2.

truncation artifact ripples that appear near a tissue discontinuity, which results from image reconstruction from only a portion of the Fourier transform.

TSE (turbo spin echo) this is a spin echo technique for fast imaging based on the use of multiple spin echoes per excitation; each echo has a different preparation gradient encoding and all echoes are used for one image; equivalent terms: MEMS (Multi Echo Multi Shot), RARE (Rapid Acquisition by Repeated Echo).

tuning the process of adjusting the resonant frequency of the RF circuit to the Larmor frequency.

tunnel   an opening into the MR imaging system for the patient; it is sometimes called the *patient aperture.*

turbo factor   in TSE imaging, the number of profiles per excitation, which is equal to the number of spin echoes generated after each excitation.

turbulence   blood flow with a random velocity profile; results in spin dephasing and signal loss.

unsaturated spins   spins at equilibrium magnetization; spins that have not been exposed to an RF pulse within several T1s.

vector   quantity having both magnitude and direction, frequently represented by an arrow in which length is proportional to the magnitude and an arrowhead to indicate direction.

velocity   measure of blood flow (cm/s).

viscosity   resistance of blood to flow because of friction of blood elements.

volume imaging   magnetic resonance signals are collected simultaneously from a large volume of the patient; 3DFT imaging.

voxel   volume element; the element of three-dimensional space corresponding to a pixel for a given slice thickness.

zero filling   substitution of zeros for unmeasured MR data points; useful for fast imaging.

zeugmatography   term for MRI coined from Greek roots suggesting the role of the gradient magnetic field in joining the RF to a desired local spatial region through nuclear magnetic resonance.

Index

A

A. *See* Ampere.
AAPM. *See* American Association of Physicists in Medicine.
Abdomen, surgical clips and sutures in, 428
ABSIR. *See* Absolute inversion recovery.
Absolute inversion recovery (ABSIR), 266
Absorptiometry, 98
AC. *See* Alternating current.
ACMP. *See* American College of Medical Physics.
Acq, signal averaging and, 218
ACR. *See* American College of Radiology.
Action potentials, visual images and, 226
Active shielding, 163, 163t
   superconducting electromagnet and, 133, 135
Adenosine diphosphate (ADP), 107
Adenosine monophosphate (AMP), 107
Adenosine triphosphate (ATP), 107
Adipose tissue. *See* Fat.
Adjusting screws, permanent magnets and, 126
ADP. *See* Adenosine diphosphate.
Alias, 95
Aliasing, 84
   artifacts, 84, 94-95, 95f, 379, 385-386
   computed tomography and, 180, 182f
   digital imaging and, 180, 182f
   Fourier transform and, 84, 94-95
   sampling and, 180
   two-dimensional Fourier transform and, 189
Alnico magnet, 125
Alpha pulse, 54, 61
   echo planar imaging and, 312
   gradient echo imaging and, 288, 289, 291, 299
Alternating current (AC), 24, 25f

Aluminum, resistive electromagnets and, 130
AM radio, 6, 39
American Association of Physicists in Medicine (AAPM), 159, 421
American College of Medical Physics (ACMP), 159
American College of Radiology (ACR), 159, 421, 422, 426, 427
American National Standards Institute (ANSI), 402, 403f
American Registry of Radiologic Technologists (ARRT), 413
Ampere (A), 24
Ancillary equipment, MRI and, 411-412, 412b
Angiography
   computed tomography, 258
   contrast agents and, 372
   coronary artery, 360-361
   digital subtraction, 330
   magnetic resonance, 258, 275, 285, 372
   phase contrast magnetic resonance, 327, 328-329
   time of flight, 301
   time of flight magnetic resonance, 320, 327, 328
   x-ray contrast, 330
   x-ray coronary, 349
Angular momentum, 11
ANSI. *See* American National Standards Institute.
APC. *See* Apparent diffusion coefficient.
Apparent diffusion coefficient (APC) image, 346, 347f
ARRT. *See* American Registry of Radiologic Technologists.
Artifacts, 131
   aliasing, 84, 94-95, 95f, 379, 385-386
   attenuation, 349
   bleeding, 390
   blood flow, 389
   chemical shift, 106, 280, 315, 377-378
   ghost, 388
   magnetic and RF field distortion, 375-379

Figures denoted by *f;* tables denoted by *t;* boxes denoted by *b.*